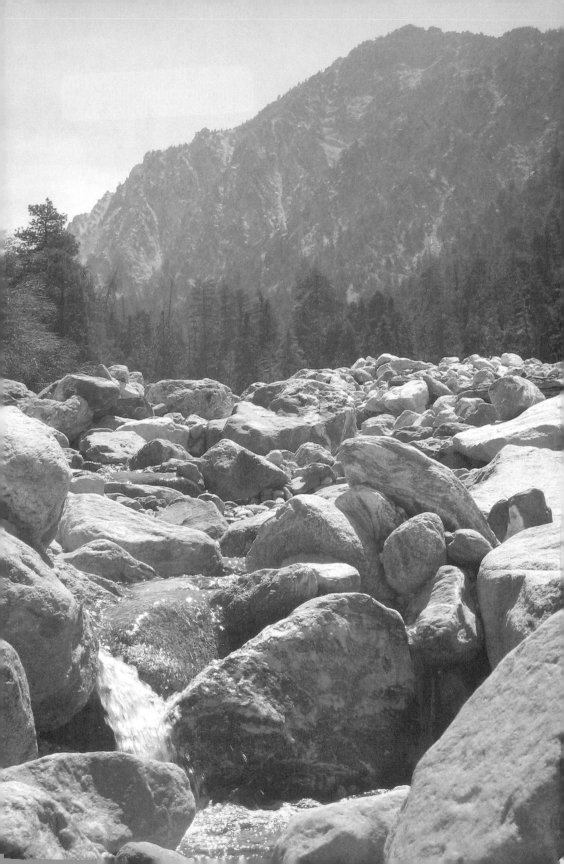

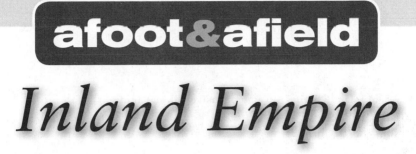

afoot & afield

Inland Empire

A comprehensive hiking guide

David & Jennifer Money Harris

 WILDERNESS PRESS . . . *on the trail since 1967*

BERKELEY, CA

To Abraham and Samuel

Afoot & Afield Inland Empire: A Comprehensive Hiking Guide

1st EDITION 2009
  2nd printing October 2009

Copyright © 2009 by David and Jennifer Money Harris

Front cover photos copyright © 2009 by David Money Harris
Interior photos, except where noted: David Money Harris
Maps: David Money Harris
Cover design: Larry B. Van Dyke
Book design and layout: Larry B. Van Dyke
Book editor: Roslyn Bullas

ISBN 978-0-89997-462-0

Manufactured in United States of America

Published by: **Wilderness Press**
               1345 8th Street
               Berkeley, CA 94710
               (800) 443-7227; FAX (510) 558-1696
               info@wildernesspress.com
               www.wildernesspress.com

Visit our website for a complete listing of our books and for ordering information.

Cover photos (clockwise from top): Headstone Rock (Joshua Tree National Park);
                          Big Bear Lake; Desert Divide (Trip 10.7)
Frontispiece: Galena Peak above Mill Creek (Trip 5.3)

SAFETY NOTICE: Although Wilderness Press and the author have made every attempt to ensure that the information in this book is accurate at press time, they are not responsible for any loss, damage, injury, or inconvenience that may occur to anyone while using this book. You are responsible for your own safety and health while in the wilderness. The fact that a trail is described in this book does not mean that it will be safe for you. Be aware that trail conditions can change from day to day. Always check local conditions and know your own limitations.

Acknowledgments

We are grateful to many people for their help with this project.

Hiking is safer and more enjoyable with companions. We would like to particularly thank the following friends and family for their company on the trail: Tony Condon, Sian Davies-Vollum, Brian Elliot, Emil Feisler, Rick Graham, Daniel Harris, Mark Headricks, Alex Honnold, Alfred Kwok, Aaron Money, Melissa Money, Cidney Scanlon, Joe Sheehy, and Elizabeth Thomas. We also have enjoyed the company of several hiking clubs, including Delta H, On the Loose, the Sierra Club, and the Coachella Valley Hiking Club.

We thank our able editor, Roslyn Bullas, for first envisioning this book, for putting her confidence in us to write it, and for encouragement along the way. Larry Van Dyke is responsible for the exceptional design and layout of the book.

Many reviewers have helped improve this book. They include: Sharon Barfknecht, Christina Burns, Tony Condon, Caroline Conway, Buford Crites, Don Davidson, Brad Eells, Jim Foote, Frazer Haney, Sally Harris, Tim Hough, Bradley Mastin, David Miller, Bart O'Brien, Bob Romano, Audrey Scranton, Joe Sheehy, Ginny Short, Kevin Smith, Wayne Steinmetz, Paula Taylor, Rocky Toyama, Pam Tripp, and Betty Zeller.

The remaining errors are our own.

Wild lands are a precious resource. Each of the trips in this book owes its existence to the vision and effort of many people, from grass-roots volunteers to conservation organizations to civil servants to far-sighted political leaders, who have protected the land and constructed and maintained the trails that we now enjoy.

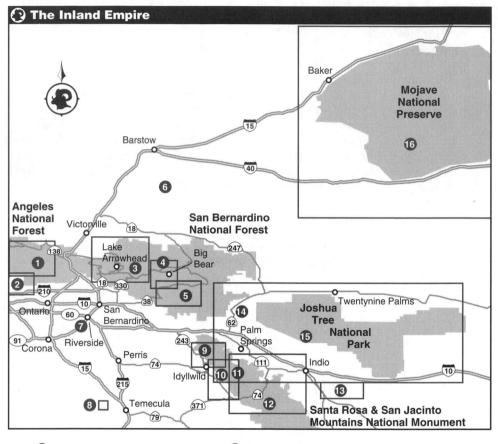

The Inland Empire

1. Mount Baldy Area
2. San Dimas-Claremont Hills
3. Western San Bernardinos
4. Big Bear Lake Area
5. San Gorgonio Wilderness
6. High Desert
7. Urban Parks
8. Santa Rosa Ecological Reserve
9. San Jacinto National Monument
10. Desert Divide
11. Palm Springs & Indian Canyons
12. Santa Rosa National Monument
13. Mecca Hills Wilderness
14. Desert and Mountain Preserves
15. Joshua Tree National Park
16. Mojave National Preserve

Contents

Preface

This book covers over 200 hikes around the Inland Empire. While the region is too large to include every trail worth hiking, the authors personally enjoyed each of the selected trips.

This book has been a nearly three-year project. One of the pleasures of writing a guidebook is exploring trails that we might not otherwise have visited. We continue to be amazed by the wonderful places that we discover. We scouted a few trips that were left out of the book because of excessive brush, access problems, or lack of distinguishing features, but the vast majority of our days on the trail have been tremendously enjoyable. Learning about the plants, animals, and geology and watching the seasons change in the deserts and mountains have added new dimensions to our hiking pleasure.

Another joy of this work has been hiking with our son Abraham, who was born near the start of the project. One of us, David, once had little interest in easy hikes where the drive exceeded the hiking time. But now, spending a morning helping Abraham climb rocks, jump off logs and smell the wildflowers is as much fun as taking on the most challenging mountains. We hope that these experiences nurture in him a life-long love of wild places. And we hope that we've selected a diverse collection of trips so that readers of all ages and experience levels can find their own perfect hikes.

These trips are constantly changing. Roads and trails get rerouted. Wildfire scours the mountains, and chaparral grows over seldom-visited tracks. Property owners deny access to trails, and far-sighted leaders open up new areas. Authors have even been known to make mistakes, writing "left" when they mean "right." When the facts on the ground seem inconsistent with the trip descriptions, use your best judgment and err on the side of safety.

We have established a companion web site, www.afootafieldie.com, to offer live updates to the book. You can check for recent changes, find some bonus hikes, download GPS data, and post your own updates. The authors would greatly appreciate hearing about changes that affect trips in this book

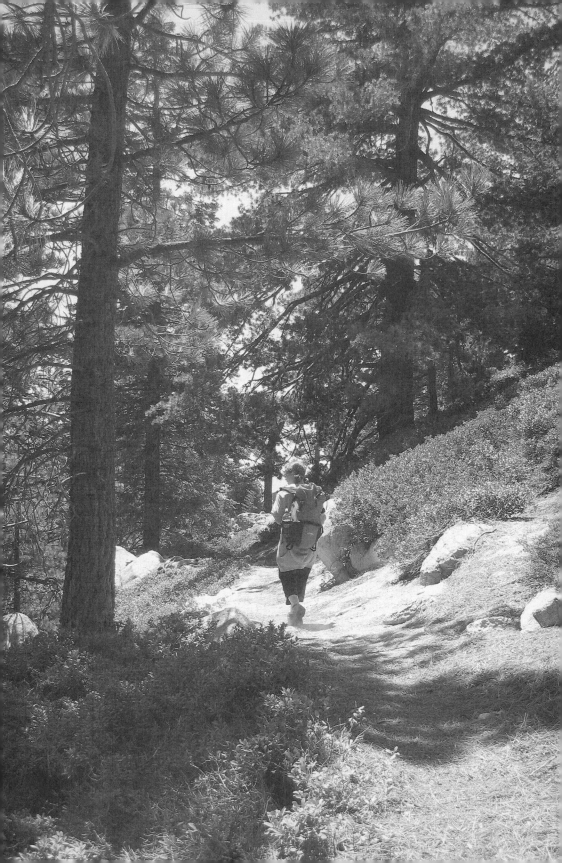

Introducing the
Inland Empire

The origin of the term *Inland Empire* is shrouded in the mists of history, but one theory says it was coined by real estate developers to lure buyers to this purported paradise. The boundaries of the Inland Empire are even murkier. One definition, adopted in this guide, is that the Inland Empire spans Riverside and San Bernardino counties and eastern Los Angeles County including Claremont, San Dimas, Pomona, and La Verne. Though these borders are inexact, few would dispute that the Inland Empire is a hiker's paradise.

The Inland Empire is home to California's best and most diverse hiking south of the Sierra Nevada. It includes Southern California's three tallest mountains, Mojave National Preserve, the Santa Rosa and San Jacinto Mountains National Monument, and the world-famous Joshua Tree National Park. There are hundreds of lesser known, but tremendously enjoyable, hikes to be found just about anywhere you live or visit in this area. It is remarkable that these hikes, many of them in the peaceful tranquility of the mountains or desert, are located in the fastest-growing region of California, within a short drive of more than 15 million residents.

Prior to the arrival of European invaders, the Inland Empire was lightly populated by Native Americans who were keenly adept at living in the unforgiving deserts and mountains. The Spanish arrived in the late 16th Century, established a few missions and ranches, and named the major geographical features, but considered the region poorly suited for colonization. A hardy band of Mormon settlers were the first white Americans to arrive in numbers, coming by wagon over Cajon Pass in 1851. They established an outpost near present day San Bernardino, but soon returned to Salt Lake City. The development of railroads and irrigation drastically changed the Southern Californian landscape. The citrus industry took root in the 1870s, and soon industrious farmers (one of the author's great-grandparents included) flocked to the area to seek their fortune growing oranges and shipping them back to the East Coast.

California joined the United States in 1850 in the wake of the Gold Rush, and the government moved promptly to survey the new state. In November of 1852, Colonel Henry Washington and a team of surveyors made the arduous ascent of San Bernardino Peak, where they established the initial point from which all of Southern California was measured. Curious hikers can take in the expansive views where his survey monument still stands on the shoulder of the peak. Baseline Avenue loosely follows his survey line from Highland to San Dimas.

Colonel Washington's Monument on San Bernardino Peak

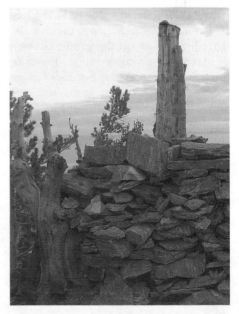

When explorers and miners first set foot in the San Bernardino Mountains, they found a vast forest of great pines, firs, and cedars. The lumber potential was not overlooked and, starting in 1852, wagon roads were painstakingly carved up the foothills and the huge trees were felled to build the burgeoning cities of Los Angeles and San Bernardino. The loggers worked with great diligence and by the end of the 19th Century, most of the forest had been chopped to the ground. By this point, the interests of the cities began to conflict with the interests of the lumber companies: residents and ranchers were dependent on the mountain streams for their water, and the mountain watersheds, denuded of timber, were becoming polluted and drying up. Intensive lobbying led to the Forest Reserve Act of 1891, which gave the President authority to protect forests on public lands. In the next two years, Benjamin Harrison established Forest Reserves in the San Gabriel, San Bernardino, and Santa Ana Mountains. At first, protections were lax, but in 1905, the reserves were reorganized under the leadership of Gifford Pinchot. He renamed them National Forests and laid the foundation of today's Forest Service.

More recent stories of the Inland Empire are chronicled in each chapter of this book. A recurring theme is the tension between development and conservation. The same threads continue to play out today as we balance the benefits of access with the threat of loving our wilderness to death. Tread lightly so that our grandchildren can enjoy the same special places that we do today.

Geography and Weather

The greater Los Angeles Basin is cut off from the vast Mojave and Colorado Deserts by three tall mountain ranges: the San Gabriels, San Bernardinos, and San Jacintos. The San Jacintos form the northern end of the Peninsular Ranges that stretch all the way to the tip of Baja California. The San Gabriels and San Bernardinos are part of the Transverse Ranges, an anomalous mountain group running east and west rather than the prevailing southeast to northwest direction. These complex mountains were pushed up by the San Andreas Fault at the interface between the Pacific and North American plates. The topography of Southern California strongly influences the weather patterns that hikers will encounter.

The Los Angeles Basin exhibits a classic Mediterranean climate, with rainy winters and dry summers. In the summer, a high-pressure system over the eastern Pacific dominates the weather patterns, ensuring warm, dry weather. The high-pressure system also creates an inversion layer over the cooler ocean, forming a marine layer of low clouds known as "June gloom." Moreover, this inversion layer traps the pollution produced by Southern California's factories and freeways, resulting in notorious smog. While aggressive air quality management has led to a gradual improvement over the past three decades, there are still days when the air in the basin is unhealthy for vigorous activity. On these days, climbing above 5000 feet brings dramatically improved air quality and views. The Inland Empire experiences hot summers, routinely over 100°F. In the winter, the high-pressure system shifts and Southern California is exposed to intermittent Pacific storms that carry the bulk of the year's rain. Occasional cold fronts can bring subfreezing temperatures, which were the bane of the citrus farmers.

The San Bernardinos and San Jacintos present a formidable barrier to moisture moving in from the Pacific, so the lands to the east and north receive far less rainfall. For example, Riverside averages 10 inches of rain a year. The exposed western slopes of the San Bernardino Mountains receive 40 inches or more of rain and snow, while Palm Springs, in the rain shadow, averages only 6 inches annually. Beyond these mountains lie the legendary deserts of the

American Southwest, which stretch all the way to the Rocky Mountains.

The deserts are divided into two major regions. The Sonoran Desert is the lower and hotter, extending south and east from Joshua Tree National Park to Mexico and central Arizona. The portion of the Sonoran Desert in California is called the Colorado Desert; it receives the occasional Pacific storm, which can lead to outstanding wildflowers in the spring. Nevertheless, when Ontario is cloudy on a dreary February morning, you can likely drive to Palm Springs and find clear blue skies and temperatures perfect for hiking. The Mojave Desert is higher and cooler, extending from Joshua Tree northward toward the Great Basin. Winter snowfall is not uncommon at the higher elevations. However, hiking any of the deserts on a summer afternoon is an activity only for the perversely masochistic.

Not surprisingly, the interfaces between these climate zones experience unusual weather. In particular, hot dry winds exceeding 70 mph blow through the Cajon and Banning passes several times a year. These winds are caused when a high-pressure region develops over the Great Basin, forcing warm air down through the narrow passes and out to the ocean. They are called Santa Ana winds and occur most often in the spring and fall. They have been known to topple big rigs on Interstate 15 and fan the flames of the most devastating wildfires in Southern California. Banning Pass has some of the most consistently strong winds. The famous wind farm along Interstate 10 converts a fraction of this wind into electricity. Hiking in these strong winds tends to be unpleasant, but the wind speed drops dramatically as soon as you get away from the mouths of the passes.

Safety

Hiking is a relatively safe activity. While reliable statistics are hard to come by, fewer than one in a million Yosemite National Park visitors have a fatal hiking accident in a typical year. Comparing this with auto-mobile accident statistics (approximately one fatality per 100 million miles driven), the risk of getting killed while driving to the hike apparently exceeds the risk of dying in the outdoors. Nevertheless, hiking does have its own special risks and prudent hikers manage these risks through preparation and awareness.

Always be prepared for an emergency, even on a short hike. The bare essentials to have along include:

- water
- map and compass or GPS (and knowledge of how to navigate)
- headlamp
- matches or lighter
- extra food
- extra clothing (enough to survive an unplanned night out)

Other items that can be very helpful include:

- whistle
- sunscreen, sun glasses, hat
- toilet paper
- first aid kit
- cell phone (but there is not always coverage in the wilderness)

Some of the perils in the outdoors include weather, slippery footing, getting lost, old mine shafts, animals, plants, and unsafe drinking water. The best way to learn about safety in the outdoors is to travel with experienced and prudent hikers.

Get a weather report before you go, but always be prepared for an unexpected change in the weather. The winter and early spring are the rainy season in the Inland Empire, and snow is common at higher elevations. Hypothermia is a particular risk if your clothes become wet. Carry warm and waterproof clothes. The summer can be dangerously hot in the desert, leading to heat exhaustion and heat stroke. Temperatures can exceed 100°F as early as April and

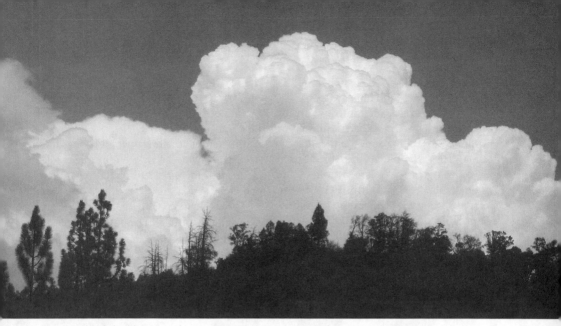

Cumulus clouds building over the San Bernardino Mountains before an August afternoon thunderstorm

as late as October. Carry a generous supply of water, even on short hikes. Summer afternoons are also the most common time for thunderstorms over the mountains; don't get caught exposed on a mountaintop in an electrical storm or in a canyon during a flash flood.

Cross-country hiking often involves walking on unstable boulders, where it is easy to slip and twist an ankle. The best way to develop cross-country travel skills is through practice on easier hikes. Many hikers find that a trekking pole (or two) helps with balance and relieves one's knees on downhill trails. Ice is a much more serious

Cramponing up a slope on a spring snow climb.

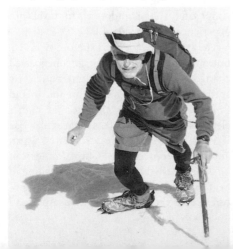

threat. Highly experienced hikers have had fatal falls on Mt. Baldy and San Gorgonio in recent years. Ice can remain in north-facing gullies long after most of the mountain appears free of snow. Under these conditions, carry an ice axe and crampons and know how to use them. If you are unfamiliar with these mountaineering tools, take a mountaineering class before trying them out on your own.

Always let somebody know where you are going and when you expect to return. If you do get lost, the best advice is to stay in one spot. If search and rescue teams know where to look for you, they are almost certain to find you. Make yourself easy to spot by wearing bright clothes (for these reasons, a red jacket is obviously preferable to a green one). With sufficient water and clothing, an unplanned night out is inconvenient but not catastrophic. A fire is helpful in an emergency for warmth and visibility, but thoroughly clear the area first. (In 2003, a lost hunter set a fire in the Cleveland National Forest to signal rescuers. It got out of control, fanned by Santa Ana winds. The Cedar fire ended up burning more than a quarter-million acres and 2000 homes and killed 15 people.) Hiking alone is statistically more dangerous than hiking with a group. The cautions about letting somebody know where you are going are even more important when hiking solo. If a hiker is overdue, call local law enforcement to initiate a search.

On the other hand, being lost is partly a matter of perspective. Henry David Thoreau wrote, "If a person lost would conclude that after all he is not lost, he is not beside himself, but standing in his own old shoes on the very spot where he is, and that for the time being he will live there; but the places that have known him, they are lost,—how much anxiety and danger would vanish." With proper navigation equipment and careful attention to one's surroundings, an experienced hiker may not always be certain exactly where he or she is, but should certainly be able to get to a known destination.

Many trips in this book lead to old mines or through areas of historical or active mining. Resist the temptation to enter these mines; hikers have died while exploring some of the mines near trails in this book. Besides the obvious risks of structural collapse and falling down shafts, there are other hazards including hantavirus from rodents, poison gas, and even radiation. Keep an especially close eye on children near mines.

Rattlesnakes, scorpions, bees, ticks, bears, and mountain lions are occasionally encountered in the wilds. Rattlesnakes want to stay away from you at least as much as you want to stay away from them. 75% of snake bites happen to men between the ages of 19 and 30 years, and most of these bites occur when the victim is drunk and/or playing with the snake. Avoid putting your feet or hands anywhere that you can't see. If you have to cross dense grass or brush, make plenty of noise to warn away any snakes. In the unlikely event of a snake bite, seek medical attention as rapidly as possible.

Scorpions sting with their barbed tails. The only dangerous scorpions in California live near the Colorado River; stings of scorpions encountered on hikes in this book are no more poisonous than bee stings. If you leave your boots outside while camping, turn them over and shake them first in the morning in case a critter has crawled in overnight.

Africanized bees, popularly known as killer bees, have migrated into California after escaping from a botched agricultural experiment in Brazil in the 1950s. Some have established hives in Joshua Tree National Park. They are aggressive and tend to attack in large numbers when disturbed.

Adit (horizontal mine shaft) on Silver Peak near Holcomb Valley

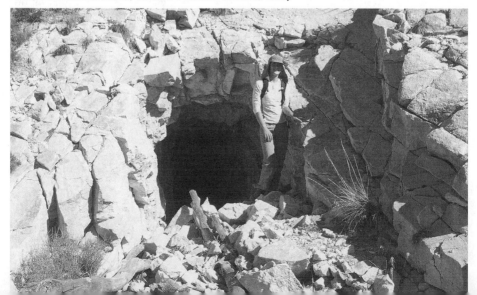

The best way to avoid trouble is to not disturb bees. If you are pursued by a swarm, run away as fast as possible and seek shelter. Medical attention may be necessary if you receive a large number of stings.

Ticks are found in the brush in California. They range in size from poppy seeds to sesame seeds. Ticks drop onto hikers and like to crawl to a protected spot before attaching themselves and sucking blood. If you must walk through brush, wearing long pants and gaiters (worn over the boot and lower leg) eliminates many opportunities for ticks to reach your skin. Bug repellents, such as those containing DEET, are also effective at deterring ticks. Be sensitive to slight sensations that might be a clue that a tick is crawling on you, and check yourself in the shower after a hike to be sure you haven't picked up a tick. The greatest problem with tick bites is that deer ticks sometimes carry Lyme disease. They usually must be attached for at least 36 hours to convey the disease to a human. Symptoms of Lyme disease include rashes, fever, headache, fatigue, and joint pain. Lyme disease is treated with antibiotics and is readily cured if treated when symptoms first appear, but can lead to complications if left untreated.

Grizzly bears, once common enough to be celebrated on the California State Flag, were hunted to extinction in the state by 1922. Fortunate hikers might still see evidence of black bears: scat, footprints, or even the back end of a bear shambling into the woods. Black bears seldom cause trouble for dayhikers in Southern California, but it is prudent to store your food in a bear-proof canister while backpacking in bear habitat such as the San Gorgonio Wilderness. Canisters are available for rent at the Mill Creek Ranger Station and the Barton Flats Visitor Center. Bears are usually more afraid of people than people are of bears. Bears attacks are extremely rare. Don't get between a mother bear and her cubs. If you do see a bear on the trail, stop and let it pass.

Mountain lions, also called cougars, are North America's largest cats. They are notoriously shy and hikers should consider themselves lucky to see one in a lifetime outdoors. Mountain lion attacks were almost unheard of before 1986, but the encroachment of humans on their habitat has increased pressure on the cats and made them more aggressive. There have been about a dozen attacks in the last two decades, three of which were fatal. If you do encounter a mountain lion, shout loudly, wave your hands, throw rocks, and make a point of not looking like cat food. If attacked, fight back. Do not run or play dead. Children and petite women have been the predominant victims. Hiking in groups is always safer. Don't allow young children to run out of sight, especially in areas where mountain lions are known to live.

Hazardous plants include poison oak, cactus, and yucca. Poison oak, not a true oak, is a plant all hikers should learn to identify. It has shiny green or red leaflets in clusters of three. It grows as a vine in shady canyons and as a bush or dense thicket in direct sun. Moist, shady canyon bottoms are the most common place that you will encounter poison oak on trips in this book. Poison oak secretes an oil called urushiol that causes a highly irritating rash in more than 80% of people. The rash is occasionally serious enough to require hospitalization.

Poison oak thicket in the San Gabriel foothills. "Leaves of three, let it be."

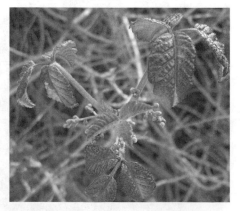

In winter, the leafless stalks still carry the oil and cause skin irritation. Even if you are lucky enough to be immune, your immunity can wear off after repeated exposure. Wearing long pants helps reduce the risk of contact. If you do come in contact with poison oak, wash with soap and water as soon as possible after exposure. Also, take care handling clothes that might have been exposed, and wash the clothes thoroughly in hot water. A rash usually develops about 24 hours after exposure and lasts up to two weeks. Antihistamines can help treat severe rashes.

Yucca and cactus have sharp tips or barbs that can inflict nasty jabs to the unwary hiker. Long pants and gaiters can help, especially when hiking cross-country through the desert, but a direct hit by a yucca will penetrate even the sturdiest of clothes. The best defense is alertness. Cactus barbs tend to lodge in your skin. Jumping cholla cactus get their name because of their propensity to latch onto anyone who comes nearby. Don't try to remove a cactus barb with your hands; you will only get it embedded in your fingers. Tweezers, pliers, or a wide-toothed comb are helpful, but a pair of rocks will do in a pinch.

Unfortunately, untreated water in Southern California should generally be considered unsafe to drink. Thoroughly boil it first, or use a pump or chemical treatment kit available from outdoor equipment stores. The availability of water is also a problem; springs and creeks can dry up. Never get in a situation where you depend on finding water in a spring or creek and cannot get yourself to a reliable source if the first is dry.

Vehicle break-ins, while rare, do occur in Southern California. Don't leave valuables in your vehicle. Report incidents to law enforcement.

Courtesy

While you enjoy yourself afoot and afield, follow simple courtesies so that others will enjoy themselves too, and so that the wilderness will be there for future generations to discover.

The general rule is to leave no trace. It is common sense not to litter or vandalize our wild places, and it is even better style to pick up litter when you come across it. Don't cut switchbacks; this causes erosion. Deposit human waste in a cathole at least 200 feet from water. Limit campfires to already

Cute but not-so-cuddly teddy bear cholla cactus in Pinto Basin, Joshua Tree National Park. Fallen stem joints are a common desert hazard.

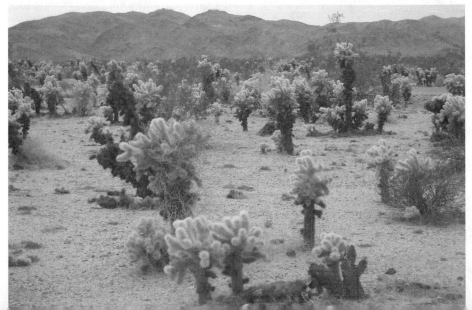

existing fire rings. It is preferable to cook on a gas stove, which does not consume wood or scar the rocks. Some wilderness areas have more specific campfire rules. Collecting rocks, pine cones, wild flowers, Native American artifacts, and so forth is forbidden in many areas. Leave these things for the next visitors to enjoy too. If you must smoke, do so seated in an area cleared of flammable materials. Serious wildfires have been caused by cigarettes. In areas where dogs are allowed, they generally must be kept on a leash. Loud and aggressive dogs should stay at home.

Each jurisdiction has its own specific regulations, and visitors are responsible for knowing them.

Camping

There are many established campgrounds in the Inland Empire. To assure yourself a site, make reservations in advance. Many of the most popular campgrounds fill up well ahead of time in high season; for example, Joshua Tree is heavily visited in the spring and fall. Camping fees have been on the rise and are approaching $20 in some locations.

The best deal in the National Forests is the "yellow-post" campsites. These dispersed, unimproved sites are mostly sprinkled along dirt roads in the San Gabriel, San Bernardino, and San Jacinto Mountains and are marked with numbered yellow posts. They are free and you rarely have to deal with noisy neighbors. You can't reserve these sites, but it is rare for all the sites in an area to be occupied. Keep your eyes out as you explore the back roads, or call the local ranger station for more information. Some of the yellow-post site locations include: the areas northwest of Lytle Creek off Forest Road 3N06, the Keller Peak Road near Running Springs, the ridge south above Big Bear off Forest Road 2N10, the Coon Creek Jumpoff area northeast of San Gorgonio on Forest Road 1N02, and the Fuller Ridge Road (4S01) on San Jacinto above Black Mountain Campground.

Backpackers can camp at established sites along many trails. Each area has different regulations regarding backcountry camping.

Using this Book

This book is organized into 16 chapters, each covering a different region of the Inland Empire. It is not intended to be read cover-to-cover. Instead, browse for trips that look interesting, or turn to a specific chapter when you are looking for hikes in an area that you plan to visit.

TRIP SUMMARIES

Each trip begins with a summary of key information to help you choose the right one.

DISTANCE

The total distance of the trip is given. For out-and-back trips, both directions are included. Some trips have alternative paths that change the distance. Your mileage may vary.

Distances measured with an odometer or GPS are generally reported to the nearest tenth of a mile. Beware that two different GPS units will read slightly different mileages, even when carried by the same person at the same time. Total trip distance is generally rounded to the nearest mile for longer trips.

HIKING TIME

An estimate of the hiking time is given. It is important to note that this is just the time spent walking; it does not include breaks, lunch, or time to smell the flowers. The time is only an average; trail runners will clearly be faster, and many hikers prefer a more leisurely saunter. If you are carrying a heavy backpack, the times may double. The very strenuous trips in this book assume that you are exceptionally fit and will be walking faster than on the more moderate trips.

ELEVATION GAIN

Elevation gain accounts for the entire elevation a hiker must climb. For example, if a trail starts at 500 feet and climbs to a 2500-foot summit but has a 400-foot dip in the middle, the elevation gain for the round trip is 2800 feet because the hiker must climb out of the dip in both directions. You can reduce the elevation gain for some one-way trips by hiking in the downhill rather than uphill direction.

DIFFICULTY

The difficulty depends on the terrain as well as the distance and elevation. There are four general categories, each roughly twice as difficult as the previous.

Easy: suitable for families with young hikers

Moderate: suitable for anyone of ordinary fitness

Strenuous: suitable for strong and highly motivated hikers

Extremely strenuous: profoundly long and difficult, harder than a marathon

Extremely strenuous trips are not recommended unless you are already intimately familiar with an area and highly skilled at navigation, are in excellent condition, and are equipped to spend an unplanned night in the wilderness. The extremely strenuous trip descriptions tend to be less detailed.

Some trips in this book involve what rock climbers call *third-class climbing*: scrambling up rocks using one's hands and feet. The hand and foot holds are large and fairly obvious, but a fall could cause serious injury or death. Such climbing is not advisable for hikers who are uncomfortable with heights or unsure of their balance. If the group includes a competent rock climber and some inexperienced hikers, the climber might belay the novices on a rope.

Fourth- and fifth-class climbing involves smaller holds and more severe consequences for a fall, so even experienced climbers will likely want a rope. None of the trips in this book require fourth- or fifth-class climbing, but occasionally interesting rock climbs near the trips are mentioned.

TRAIL USE

All trips are open to hikers. It is noted if the trip is also well suited for dogs, horses, mountain bikes, families with children, or backpacking.

BEST TIMES

The best times listed are generally those where the trailhead can be reached and the trail is not excessively hot or covered in snow. However, if you have proper equipment and experience, many of these trips are great fun in the snow on skis or snowshoes.

AGENCY

The office of the agency that manages the area is listed. Contact information for the agencies appears in Appendix B.

PERMITS

Many wilderness areas require permits for entry. Details are listed here. Some popular areas have quotas that fill up long in advance on summer weekends, so plan ahead.

A recent development is that many parts of the Angeles and San Bernardino National Forests require parked cars to display a National Forest Adventure Pass. These passes cost $5 for a day or $30 for a year. You may also use an Interagency Annual Pass (which covers admission to national parks and most other federal lands). These passes charging the public for access to public land are quite controversial. The Forest Service argues that they are needed to make up for budget shortfalls and help fund parking, outhouses, and trash pickup. Critics are concerned about lumber companies receiving government subsidies to build roads on public land while hikers are charged to park on these roads. Critics are also concerned about the significant portion of the pass proceeds being spent on enforcement rather than on user benefits.

Forest Adventure passes can be purchased at ranger stations and many outdoor stores. Purchasing a day pass is rather inconvenient if you are starting before nearby stores open. At the time of this writing, if you cannot obtain a pass in advance and receive a Notice of Noncompliance on your vehicle, you can pay the day-use fee after the fact with no other penalties.

Forest Adventure Passes and Wilderness Permits sometimes confuse visitors. They are two separate items. The Forest Adventure Passes cost money and are required to park your car. The Wilderness Permits are free, subject to quota limits, and are required to enter wilderness areas.

Any person who is 16 years of age or older must possess and wear a California sport fishing license while fishing. Licenses are good for one calendar year and presently cost $38.85 for California residents. They can be purchased from the State Department of Fish and Game or from authorized agents.

MAPS

Locator maps for the trails appear in each chapter. These maps may be sufficient for easy trips and are also helpful for newer trails and cross-country routes that do not appear on published maps. However, for many trips, there is no substitute for a good topographic map and the knowledge of how to use it. Most of the maps described below can be purchased from local outdoor equipment stores, ranger stations, and rei.com, as well as directly from the publishers.

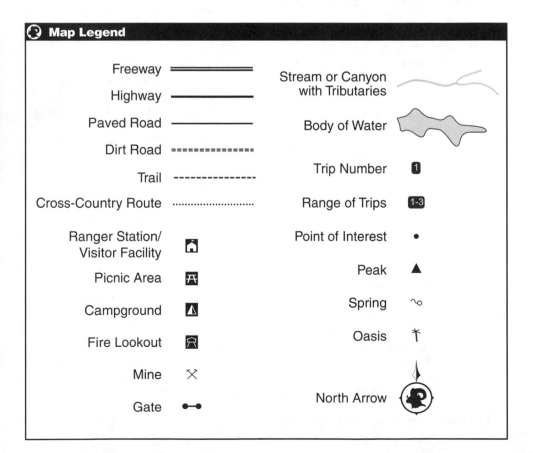

Map Legend

Freeway	═══	Stream or Canyon with Tributaries		
Highway	────			
Paved Road	────	Body of Water		
Dirt Road	▪▪▪▪▪			
Trail	-----	Trip Number	**1**	
Cross-Country Route	·········	Range of Trips	**1-3**	
Ranger Station/ Visitor Facility	🏠	Point of Interest	•	
Picnic Area	⛱	Peak	▲	
Campground	⛺	Spring	∿	
Fire Lookout	🛖	Oasis	🌴	
Mine	✕			
Gate	●—●	North Arrow	↑	

For trips in this book maps are categorized as optional, recommended, or required. If you already know an area well, you may be able to do without a recommended map. However, required maps are essential for successful navigation.

Tom Harrison Maps publishes the best maps for many popular regions in California. The maps highlight the critical features, are waterproof, and are significantly less expensive than buying the equivalent set of USGS quad maps. The maps can be purchased at www.tomharrisonmaps.com. His relevant maps in the Inland Empire include:

- Angeles High Country
- San Gorgonio Wilderness
- San Jacinto Wilderness
- Mojave National Preserve

The *Santa Rosa and San Jacinto Mountains National Monument* map, published in 2008, is by far the best map for hikes in this area. This large waterproof map shows trails that are not depicted anywhere else, and covers a vast amount of territory. It can be purchased through the monument visitor center at www.desertmountains.org.

National Geographic publishes a Trails Illustrated-series map of Joshua Tree National Park. The Trails Illustrated map shows many trails (including several that are described in this book) that do not appear on the Tom Harrison map. The Trails Illustrated *Mojave National Preserve* map is also very good. Trails Illustrated maps can be purchased from www.natgeomaps.com.

The entry fee to the Indian Canyons south of Palm Springs includes a helpful trail guide. A larger trail map with contour lines is available at the Trading Post at the Hermits Bench trailhead, but this map is unnecessary unless you plan to hike some of the more obscure trails.

In other regions, the United States Geological Survey 7.5′ series of topographic maps are the next best choice. Each map covers approximately 7 x 9 miles and has contours on 40 foot or 80 foot intervals. The USGS maps are sold at some hiking stores or can be ordered from store.usgs.gov. USGS maps are also available in electronic format. National Geographic TOPO!, for example, allows you to print your own custom maps (www.topo.com).

The *San Bernardino National Forest Atlas* contains 42 USGS 7.5′ maps shrunk to fit on 8.5 x 11″ pages covering the entire San Bernardino National Forest, including the Mt. Baldy area, the western San Bernardino Mountains, the Big Bear area, the San Gorgonio Wilderness, and the San Jacinto area. The atlas is the most cost-effective way to obtain maps covering the trails in this national forest. It can be purchased from www.nationalforeststore.com.

Finding some of the trailheads can be challenging, especially on the maze of ever changing dirt roads. AAA maps provide good general coverage of the area and are free to members. The *San Bernardino Mountains Guide* map covers the western San Bernardinos, Big Bear, and San Gorgonio areas. The *San Diego Region* map covers Palm Springs, the Santa Rosa Mountains, and the Mecca Hills. The *San Bernardino County* map covers the vast county at a coarse level of detail, and includes Mojave National Preserve.

The *San Bernardino Mountains Recreation* topo map from Fine Edge Productions has especially good coverage of the dirt roads in the San Bernardino Mountains. The Forest Service's *San Bernardino National Forest* map covers the roads through the entire National Forest.

DRIVING DIRECTIONS

Many of these trips are reached by dirt roads. These roads are classified as excellent, good, fair, or 4WD. Normal passenger vehicles should have no trouble with excellent and good roads. Driven slowly and carefully, they can often navigate fair dirt roads too, but high clearance makes driving on such roads easier. 4WD roads have large rocks, serious ruts, or sandy sections that make 4WD vehicles advisable, but an experienced driver in a 2WD pickup truck can likely handle these roads too.

Forest Service roads and trails are identified by a four-character code such as 7W02 that appears on some maps and signposts. These codes are given in parentheses after the road or trail name to help identify the route.

Mountain and desert roads are constantly changing. Roads get washed out and covered with debris. New roads are constructed and old ones are rerouted. Use your discretion.

Hiking with a GPS

Global Positioning Satellite (GPS) receivers are revolutionizing hiking. While navigation skills, a map and compass, and experience will always be critical, a GPS can make finding the trailhead or following the trail significantly easier. Properly used, a GPS also adds a level of safety by helping one find the way home even through darkness, fog, or snow. The locator maps include GPS waypoints for trailheads, destinations, and critical points along the hikes. Entering coordinates and receiving turn-by-turn driving directions to an unfamiliar trailhead is especially convenient. However, all of the hikes in the book can be done without a GPS.

GPS tracks and waypoints for many of the trips in this book can be downloaded from www.afootafieldie.com. Tracks and waypoints can be downloaded into many GPS receivers, and also displayed on a map using software such as Google Earth, MapSource, and TOPO! Use the WGS 84 datum.

GPS coordinates include altitude, latitude, and longitude. Latitude and longitude are given in degrees and minutes. For purposes of estimating distances on a map, 1 minute is approximately 1 mile.[1]

A GPS often has errors of up to 50 feet horizontally and even more vertically. Do not worry if your position varies slightly from a coordinate in this book. Also, GPS units have poor or nonexistent reception under trees and in canyons, have limited battery life, and occasionally lockup in normal use. Be certain that you can navigate on your own if your GPS fails. Carry spare batteries. Some of the newer receivers have sophisticated electronics that can keep their lock in canyons where older units fail to see the satellites; this is definitely worthwhile for serious GPS users. At the time of this writing, the Garmin GPSmap 60CSx is the gold standard for hiking GPS units, but it will undoubtedly be surpassed by even better models soon.

Plant Identification

One of the rewards of spending time on the trail is learning to recognize the local trees, wildflowers, chaparral, and cacti. This section includes a brief guide to some of the most common plants you will see in the Inland Empire wilderness. A flower guide is useless if not in color, and there are plenty of good flower books on sale at local ranger stations and outdoors stores, so this section intentionally omits wildflowers.

California has one of the world's most diverse assortments of plants, with approximately 8000 species, nearly half of which are found only within the state. The state can be loosely divided into plant communities. Philip Munz, a former professor at Pomona College and director of the Rancho Santa Ana Botanical Garden in the 1960s, proposed a system of plant communities and many refinements have been made since then.

---

1. A minute of latitude is technically 1 nautical mile, or 1.15 ordinary (statute) miles. A minute of longitude varies with your distance from the equator, but is almost exactly 1 statute mile in the Inland Empire.

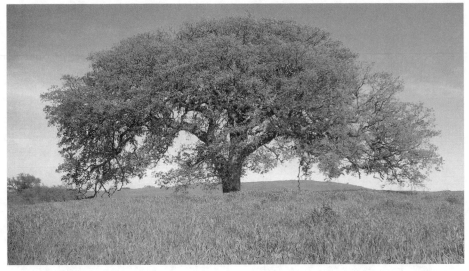

Oak grassland at Santa Rosa Plateau

Moving from west to east and up the mountains, hikers first encounter the coastal sage scrub zone containing sagebrush and other subshrubs. Many of the urban parks in the Inland Empire are within this zone. As one climbs, the vegetation transitions to chaparral, the elfin forest of tough and wiry brush that presents an almost impenetrable barrier to cross-country travel. Despite its obvious problems for hikers, chaparral possesses a contagious beauty that infects most of those subjected to prolonged exposure. The upper slopes of the mountains are covered in splendid conifer forests with their stately Jeffrey and Coulter pines, white firs, and incense cedars, all of which need cooler temperatures and more reliable rainfall. The highest reaches of San Jacinto, San Gorgonio, and Mt. Baldy host the narrow subalpine forest zone of limber and lodgepole pines. These hardy trees become gnarled

and stunted, then vanish entirely at treeline just below the summit. Descending onto the dry eastern slopes, the hiker is likely to pass through the delightful pinyon-juniper woodlands or Joshua tree woodlands before reaching the desert scrub. Scattered along the journey are occasional patches of riparian woodlands, mountain meadows, and palm oases, worthy destinations for many trips in this book.

Thankfully, for the hiker learning plant names, a few species dominate each of these plant communities. With a few exceptions for space reasons, this section contains most of the frequently encountered conifers, cacti, yuccas, and desert trees. There are far too many species of shrubs to list here, so only a handful of especially common and distinctive ones are called out.

A number of excellent books on California plants are listed in Appendix D.

CONIFERS

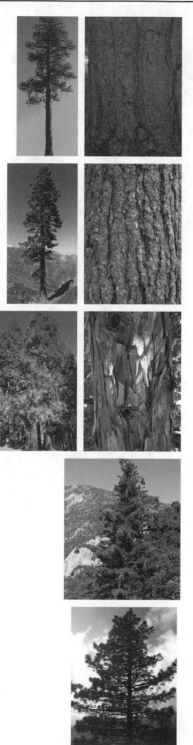

Jeffrey Pine
Pinus jeffreyi

The most common evergreen tree along trails in the SoCal mountains. Usually found from 6000–9800′. 5–9″ needles in bundles of 3. Shapely 4–10″ cones. Deeply fissured reddish-brown bark smelling of vanilla or pineapple. Similar in appearance to Ponderosa pine, which are found up to 8000′, lack the distinctive odor, and have smaller 2.5–4″ cones with outward-pointing barbs.

White Fir
Abies concolor

Another ubiquitous evergreen tree in the SoCal mountains. Found from 3000–10,000′. Readily identified by the 1–2″ solitary needles lined along the branches, with white bands on one side. Grayish-brown bark. When ripe, the cones fall apart on the tree and are rarely seen on the ground.

Incense Cedar
Calocedrus decurrens

Graceful and fragrant evergreen tree with bright green scales rather than needles. Grows to 120–200′ tall. Fire-resistant red-brown bark is flaky to fiberous and does not splinter. Found to 7000′. Member of the cypress family.

Sugar Pine
Pinus lambertiana

2–4″ needles in groups of 5 at the end of thin branches. New wood is white and flexible, while older bark is reddish. Branches tend to droop near the ends. Found to 9800′. Long (12–18″), skinny pine cones, the longest of any pine species. Sugar pines also grow to be the tallest of any pine, over 200′, although such monumental trees are becoming scarce.

Coulter Pine
Pinus coulteri

Famous for enormous "widowmaker" pinecones up to 5 pounds. Found from 600–7500′. Tree grows to 30–80′ tall, with horizontal to upcurving branches. 6–12″ needles in groups of 3. Most easily distinguished from Jeffrey pines by the huge cones found at the base. Mostly scattered in mixed forests; plentiful around Big Bear Lake and on the Spitler Peak trail.

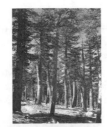

Lodgepole / Tamarack Pine
Pinus contorta

1.5–3″ needles in pairs. Thin and flaky smooth bark. Common on the San Bernardino Divide at 10,000′ above the other pines. See Trip 4.9 for the world's largest lodgepole pine.

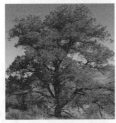

Pinyon Pine
Single-leafed pinyon (Pinus monophylla)
Parry pinyon (Pinus quadrifolia)

Common in the transition zone between desert and mountain from 3500′–9500′, often mixed with juniper. 2–3″ cones. 2″ curving needles alone or in pairs. Pine nuts are a staple of the Native American diet.

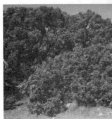 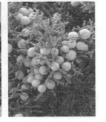

Juniper
Juniperus californica

Distinctive blue berries and tiny scale-like leaf. Numerous species varying from bushes to trees. Californica is the most common bush-like juniper, often mixed with pinyon pine in the transition zone between desert and mountain.

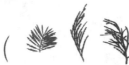

Coulter Pine, similar to Jeffrey and Ponderosa Pine

Sugar Pine **Pinion Pine** **White Fir** **Incense Cedar** **Juniper**

0″   2″   4″   8″

Cones, Needles and Scales

The easiest way to distinguish among most common conifers is by the shape, number, and size of needles or scales or by examing the fallen cones.

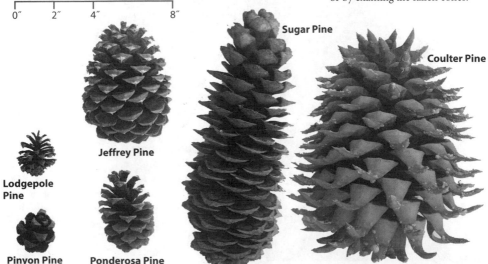

Lodgepole Pine

Jeffrey Pine

Pinyon Pine

Ponderosa Pine

Sugar Pine

Coulter Pine

CACTUS AND OCOTILLO

Teddy Bear Cholla Cactus
Cylindropuntia bigelovii

Cuddly-looking but vicious. Green tops, with brownish lower old growth. Reproduces through dropped joints, which can catch on your clothes. Sometimes called "Jumping Cholla" for its tendency to latch onto passersby. 100'–3500'. Common in Palm Canyon, lower Santa Rosa Mountains, Pinto Basin of Joshua Tree NP. Pronounced "choya."

Silver Cholla Cactus
Cylindropuntia echinocarpa

Bushy, with short trunk and fat branches bristling with silver (or gold) spines. Widespread from 200'–6000'. Common in Joshua Tree NP.

Pencil Cholla Cactus (Diamond Cactus)
Cylindropuntia ramosissima

Branches slightly thicker than a pencil, with long spines. 1000'–4200'. Common in Joshua Tree NP.

Engelmann's Hedgehog (Calico Cactus)
Echinocerus engelmannii

Numerous fat and tall green to brown stems. Found in clumps throughout the desert below 7000', especially in Joshua Tree National Park. Distinguished from Mojave Mound cactus by the less-dense stems and the flat, rather than rounded central spines. Bright pink flowers.

Mojave Mound Cactus (Claret Cup Cactus)
Echinocerus triglochidiatus

Low, dense cactus with dozens to hundreds of green globular stems. Scattered through pinyon-juniper woodlands, especially in rocky habitat around Joshua Tree NP. Bright red flowers.

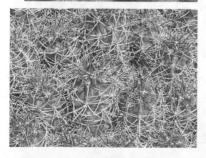

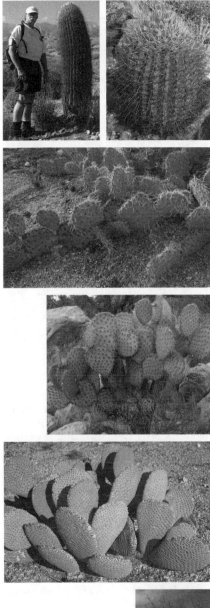

California Barrel Cactus
Ferocactus cylindraceus

Cylindrical cactus. Found from sea level to 5200´. Contrary to popular myth, the vile fluid stored inside the barrel is of no help to thirsty travelers. Common in Santa Rosa Mountains and Mojave National Preserve.

Prickly Pear Cactus
Opuntia phaeacantha

Large circular green pads with long spines. Common throughout the high desert. Many species, some of which are difficult to distinguish. Two of the distinctive ones are the tree-like Pancake Prickly Pear with a well-defined trunk and the Old Man Prickly Pear with shaggy spines.

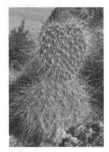

Pancake Prickly Pear
Opuntia chlorotica
(left)

Old Man Prickly Pear
Opuntia polyacantha
(right)

Beavertail Cactus
Opuntia basilaris

Prickly pear with no long spines, only tiny barbed dot-like glochids. Brilliant magenta flowers in April and May. Fruits were eaten by Cahuilla Indians. Found from sea level–9000´. Common throughout Joshua Tree, the Santa Rosa Mountains, and dry slopes of higher mountains.

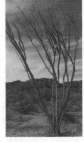

Ocotillo (Coachwhip)
Fouquieria splendens

Not a cactus, but rather a plant with many slender canes armed with inch-long thorns. Grows as tall as a house. Usually naked, but sprouts small leaves and red flowers in the spring after a good rain (multiple times per year). Prefers hot low desert; common above La Quinta Cove, in the Anza Borrego Desert, and in the Mecca Hills.

YUCCA AND AGAVE

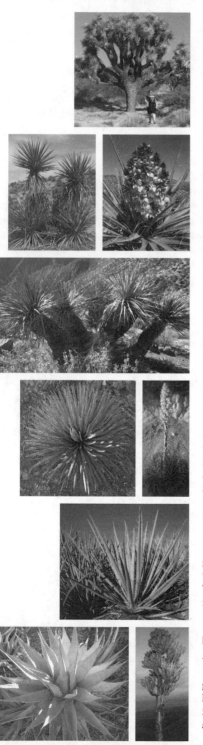

Joshua Tree
Yucca brevifolia

King of the yuccas, with many arms and rough bark. Short, stiff blades. The characteristic tree of the Mojave Desert, common in Joshua Tree National Park and elsewhere from 3000′–6000′. Blooms in March and is pollinated by the yucca moth.

Mojave Yucca
Yucca schidigera

Readily distinguished from most other yuccas by the coarse hairs on the edges of the stiff blades. Common in Joshua Tree National Park and throughout the Mojave desert to 7000′.

Giant Nolina
Nolina parryi

Fat rough bare trunks, often topped with dead curley-cues below the crown of blades. Distinguished from Mojave Yucca by lack of hairs on the blades. Young nolinas without trunks can be mistaken for chaparral yucca, but have flexible blades.

Chaparral Yucca (Our Lord's Candle)
Hesperoucca whipplei

Short rigid armor-piercing blades are hazardous to hikers even through thick clothes. Common throughout the desert and chaparral, especially around Mount Baldy. In our region, most bloom once, then die, though some produce "pups" that live on and can form dense colonies.

Banana Yucca (Blue Yucca)
Yucca baccata

Bluish-green stiff blades growing from the ground. Coarse hairs on the blades, but clearly distinguished from Mojave yucca by the lack of a trunk. Tend to grow in clumps of several plants. Common in Mojave NP, but not elsewhere in this book's trips.

Desert Agave (Century Plant)
Agave deserti

Succulent gray leaves with teeth along the margins and a stiff terminal spine. Common in Coachella Valley and lower Santa Rosa Mtns. Ranges from 500′– over 4000′. Sends up a single 8–20′ flower stalk after 5–50 years of life. Pronounced "Ah-gah-vey."

DESERT TREES

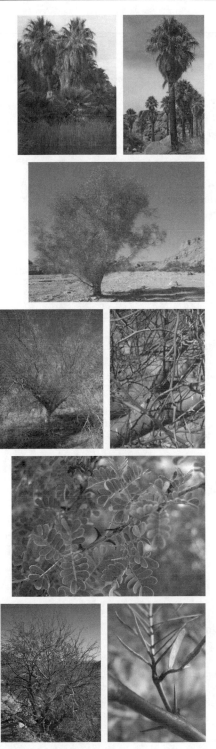

California Fan Palm
Washingtonia filifera

The monarch of the desert oasis and the only native palm in the western United States. Grows to 70′. Dead fronds bend down and form a brown skirt around the trunk. The skirt burns in wildfires, but the rest of the tree usually survives, leaving a black trunk. Common in Palm Canyon and other oases in the Santa Rosas and Joshua Tree NP.

Smoke Tree
Psorothamnus spinosus

Wispy foliage resembling a cloud of smoke. Commonly found in dry washes in the Santa Rosa Mountains and Joshua Tree NP.

Blue Palo Verde
Parkinsonia florida (a.k.a. *Cercidium floridum*)

Despite its name, a trunk and branches of bright green wood that performs photosynthesis. Another thirsty desert dweller, common in dry washes in the Santa Rosa Mountains and Mecca Hills. 12–30′ tall. Yellow blossoms in late spring. "Palo Verde" is Spanish for "greenstick."

Cat's Claw Acacia
Acacia greggii

A perennial hiker's nuisance, with curved thorns that tear at clothing and exposed flesh. It is prudent to go around rather than through cat's claw. Also called Devil's claw or "wait-a-minute" tree. Common in desert washes. Protein-rich beans are an important part of the Native American diet. Common in Joshua Tree and much of the desert.

Honey Mesquite
Prosopis glandulosa

Leaves somewhat similar to acacia, but easily differentiated by the pairs of straight thorns. Also produces protein-rich beans that are important to Native Americans.

DESERT BUSHES

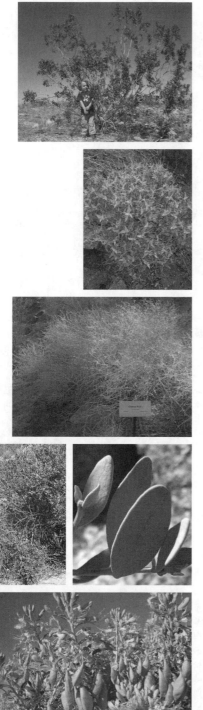

Creosote Bush
Larrea tridentata

The dominant shrub of California deserts. Tiny waxy leaves have a distinctive odor, especially after rain. Yellow flowers in the spring, followed by fuzzy white seed balls. Lives to over 10,000 years, with new parts growing in a ring as the old branches at the center die.

Brittlebush
Encelia farinosa

Dry white leaves turn bright green after the first winter rains. Interspersed with longer stalks, which grow bright yellow flowers and light up the desert in the winter and spring. Very common in the Santa Rosa Mountains and in many other hot dry parts of Southern California to 3000′.

Cheesebush
Hymenoclea salsola

Sprawling bush with greener foliage on top and yellow to tan below. Gives off a cheese-like scent when crushed.

Jojoba
Simmondsia chinensis

Succulent oval leaves about 1″ in diameter. Eaten by most desert animals for their water and protein content. Pronounced "Ho ho buh."

Bladderpod
Isomeris arborea

3′–6′ shrub found to 4000′. Spectacular yellow flowers and large green pea-like pods in winter and spring time even in dry years. Foul smell to bruised foilage. Scattered at lower elevation in Joshua Tree NP.

CHAPARRAL

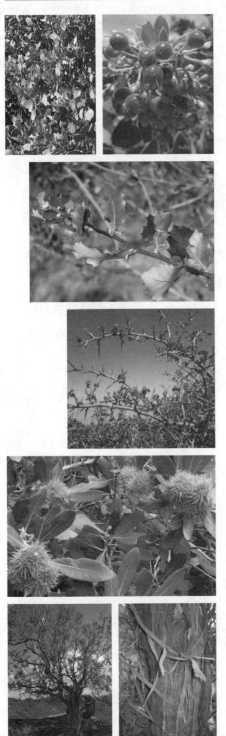

Manzanita
Arctostaphylos spp.

Attractive, yet a formidable obstacle to cross-country travel, manzanita species vary from ground-hugging bushes to tree-like stands. Smooth red bark and green elliptical leaves identical on the front and back. Produce large numbers of small round fruit Manzanita is Spanish for "little apple."

Scrub Oak
Quercus spp.

Bushy oaks, generally less than 12' tall, with a dense pattern of branches that is nearly impenetrable for the hiker. Spiny-edged gray to green leaves remain on the tree year round. Several species, *Quercus berbidifolia* being most widely distributed. "Chaparral" is Spanish for "a place of scrub oaks."

Mountain Whitethorn
Ceanothus cordulatus

Low-growing flat-topped deciduous thorn bush in the Buckthorn family. White blooms from May–July. Penetrable, but at some cost to the hiker. Often simply called "buckthorn" by hikers. Common above 6000' on San Gorgonio, San Jacinto, and the Desert Divide.

Chinquapln
Chrysolepis sempervirens

Evergreen shrub with oblong leaves and distinctive spiny nuts. Part of a mountain chaparral comunity, where it comingles with manzanita and mountain whitethorn to form nearly impenetrable stands. Also grows alone at higher elevations. Common on south-facing slopes in the San Jacintos.

Ribbonwood/Red Shanks
Adenostoma sparsifolium

A striking tall shrub, up 12–20', readily recognizable by the peeling red ribbon-like bark. Common near the town of Ribbonwood on Highway 74 and on the Desert Divide, but not naturally found at similar altitudes in the San Jacinto or San Bernardino mountains.

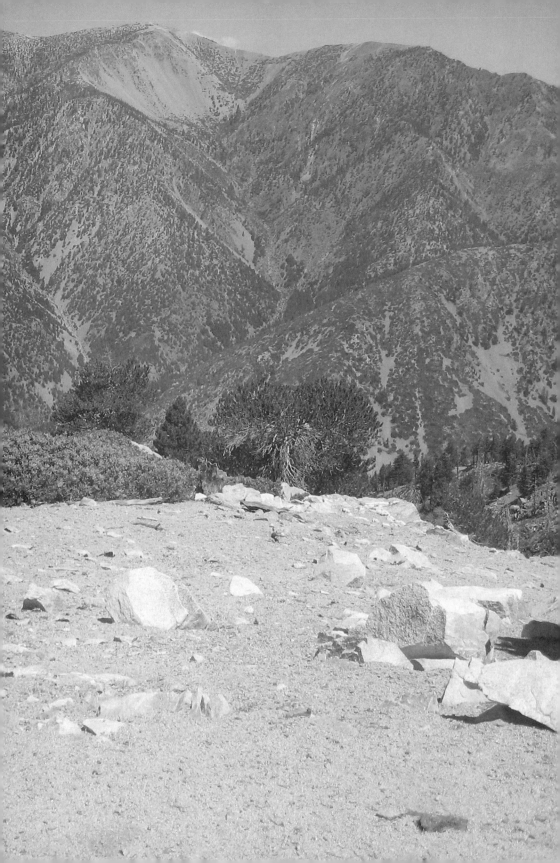

chapter 1

Mt. Baldy Area

Mt. Baldy, also known as Mt. San Antonio, is one of the four towering saints standing watch over the Inland Empire. At 10,064 feet, it stands well above any other summit in the San Gabriel Mountains, and is taller than the Zugspitze, Germany's highest peak. The bare, snow-capped top is readily recognizable from great distances in Southern California and constantly reassures tens of millions of suburban residents that wilderness is within sight. In 1923, Charles Francis Saunders wrote of Baldy in *Southern Sierras of California*, "If you have anything of the Californian in you, you mark it for the objective of an outing sometime." The summit has been a Southern California hiker's favorite for more than eight decades now.

Numerous lower peaks surrounding Mt. Baldy also offer superb hiking opportunities. The 44,000-acre Sheep Mountain Wilderness to the west is the largest roadless area in the San Gabriel Mountains. The 12,000-acre Cucamonga Wilderness to the southeast protects many of the best hiking opportunities in Southern California. Between the two wilderness areas is the quiet mountain resort of Mt. Baldy Village and a small ski area that offers excellent runs immediately after good winter storms.

Sheep Mountain Wilderness is named for the desert bighorn sheep (*Ovis canadensis nelsoni*) that once roamed these mountains in large herds. Their numbers plummeted from about 750 in 1982 to about 90 in 1995, most likely because of predation by mountain lions, but they have slowly recovered and number almost 300 due to conserva-

tion efforts. Sightings are not uncommon near the Mt. Baldy Bowl and in the more remote parts of the wilderness.

A wilderness permit is required to enter Cucamonga Wilderness, and can be obtained, at no charge, in person or by mail from the Mt. Baldy Visitor Center or Cajon Ranger Station. Most hikers enter this area via the Icehouse Canyon Trail. Campfires are not allowed at any backcountry campsites; bring a camp stove. A fire permit is required for the use of a stove. Dogs are permitted on a leash no longer than 6 feet. Leave vicious or noisy dogs at home.

A wilderness permit is required for entry into Sheep Mountain Wilderness from the East Fork Trailhead only. The only trip this affects is Iron Mtn. A permit can be obtained, at no charge, in person or by mail from the San Gabriel River Ranger District office (see Appendix B); mailed requests must arrive at least two weeks in advance.

Nelson Bighorn Sheep

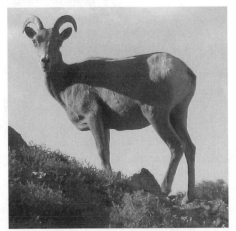

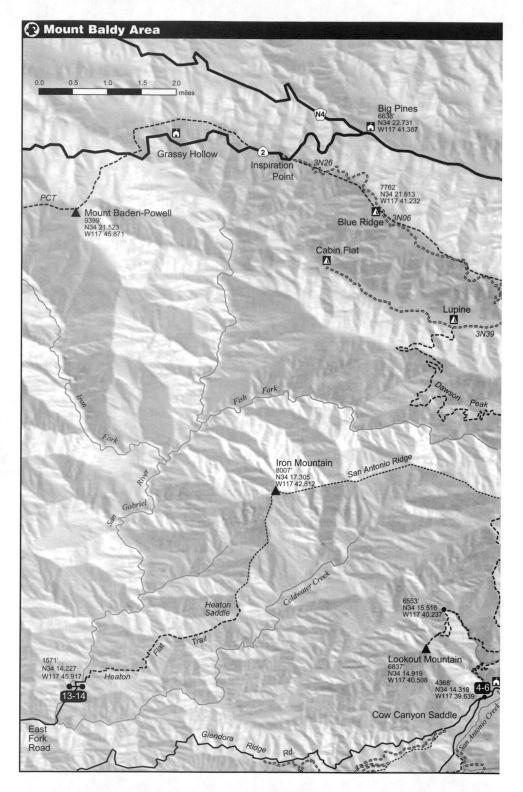

Mount Baldy Area

0.0   0.5   1.0   1.5   2.0
miles

N4

Big Pines
6638'
N34 22.731
W117 41.387

Grassy Hollow

Inspiration
Point

2

3N26

7762'
N34 21.613
W117 41.232

PCT

Mount Baden-Powell
9399'
N34 21.523
W117 45.871

Blue Ridge

3N06

Cabin Flat

Lupine

3N39

Dawson Peak

Iron

Fish   Fork

Fork

Iron Mountain
8007'
N34 17.305
W117 42.812

San Antonio Ridge

River

San   Gabriel

Coldwater Creek

6553'
N34 15.516
W117 40.237

Heaton
Saddle

1571'
N34 14.227
W117 45.917

Flat   Trail

Lookout Mountain
6837'
N34 14.919
W117 40.508

4368'
N34 14.318
W117 39.639

4-6

13-14

Heaton

Cow Canyon Saddle

East
Fork
Road

Glendora   Ridge   Rd.

San Antonio Creek

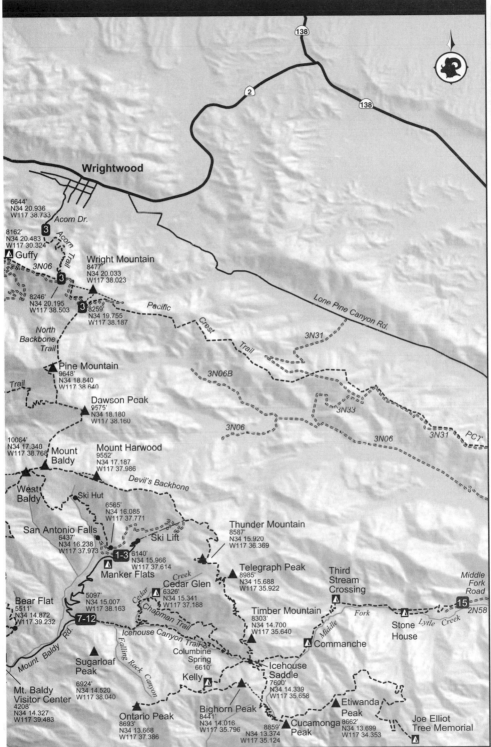

Directions to Mt. Baldy Village

Many trips in this chapter start from Mt. Baldy Rd. near the village of Mt. Baldy. The road can be reached from either the 210 or 10 freeways by taking the Mountain Ave. exit in Upland and driving north. The top of Mountain Ave. turns right, then back left (west), passes San Antonio Dam, then leads north to the Lower San Antonio Fire Station, across San Antonio Creek and back south and west to a T-junction with Mt. Baldy Rd. Turn right and drive 5 miles up to Mt. Baldy Village. The Mt. Baldy Visitor Center is on the left (west) side of the road just past Mt. Baldy Lodge.

Alternatively, if you are coming from west of Claremont, exit the 210 Freeway at Baseline. Go west 0.1 mile, then turn north on Padua. At the top of Padua, turn right on Mt. Baldy Rd. and follow it 7.5 miles up to Mt. Baldy Village.

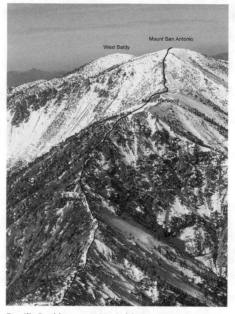

Devil's Backbone on Mt. Baldy in winter

trip 1.1 Mt. Baldy Loop

Distance	12 miles (loop)
Hiking Time	6 hours
Elevation Gain	3900'
Difficulty	Strenuous
Trail Use	Dogs
Best Times	June–October
Agency	Angeles National Forest (Mt. Baldy Visitor Center)
Recommended Map	Tom Harrison *Angeles High Country* or *Mount San Antonio* 7.5' (trail not entirely shown)

see map on p. 24

DIRECTIONS (See directions to Mt. Baldy Village above) From the ranger station in Mt. Baldy Village, continue up the Mt. Baldy Rd. for 4.2 miles to Manker Flats. Park on the side or middle of the divided road near San Antonio Falls Rd.

Mt. Baldy is one of the most popular hikes in Southern California. Its summit is high and offers breathtaking views, yet the route is straightforward for a hiker of average ability. There are many routes on the mountain, but this one is especially enjoyable because it makes a loop up past the Baldy Bowl and down along the stunning Devil's Backbone to the ski area at the Baldy Notch. From here, one can follow a dirt service road back to Manker Flats.

Alternatively, it is possible to do the loop in reverse and ride the chair lift up, saving 1300 feet and 3.5 miles of climbing. The lift begins 0.4 mile above Manker Flats at the top of Mt. Baldy Rd. At the time of this writing, the chair lift is open on weekends and holidays 8 A.M.–5 P.M., and costs $15 round-trip or $10 one-way. Call Mt. Baldy

Ski Area at (909) 981-3344 for more information.

From Manker Flats, walk west through a gate and up a service road. In 0.5 mile, the road makes a hairpin turn, and you have an excellent view of San Antonio Falls (see Trip 1.2). In another 0.3 mile, look for a trail switchbacking up the slope to the left. It is easy to miss; if you get to a point directly overlooking Manker Flats, you have gone too far.

This unmarked path is known as the Baldy Bowl Trail or Ski Hut Trail. Follow the trail 2 miles through an open forest of Jeffrey and lodgepole pines up to a Sierra Club ski hut, built by volunteers in 1937, located off the right side of the trail. This marks the halfway point in distance and elevation gain. Just beyond, cross the head of San Antonio Creek beneath the scree-filled Baldy Bowl. This area is a backcountry skier's paradise in the winter and early spring. On a rare quiet day, it is also a good place to look for bighorn sheep.

The trail continues around the southwest edge of Baldy Bowl, crossing a field of talus and switchbacking up to the ridge. Shady spots along this part of the trail remain icy long after most of the mountain has melted out. Expert mountaineers have had serious and fatal slips on this seemingly innocuous stretch of trail. The trail then follows the ridge north, climbing above treeline, and reaching the summit 2 miles beyond the ski hut.

After taking in the magnificent scenery, descend east along the Devil's Backbone Trail. This 3-mile trail passes along the south side of Mt. Harwood, and then follows a knife-edge ridge down to the ski area at Baldy Notch. Again, be especially careful because a slip down one of the steep chutes may be your last.

From the lodge at Baldy Notch, follow the service road descending to the southwest. In 3 miles, reach the original junction with the Baldy Bowl Trail, and in 1 more mile arrive back at Manker Flats.

Author hiking on the Devil's Backbone

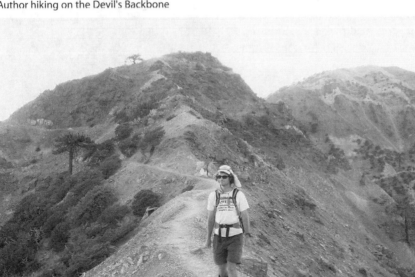

trip 1.2 San Antonio Falls

Distance	1.2 miles (out-and-back)
Hiking Time	1 hour
Elevation Gain	200'
Difficulty	Easy
Trail Use	Dogs, good for children
Best Times	April–November
Agency	Angeles National Forest (Mt. Baldy Visitor Center)
Optional Map	Tom Harrison *Angeles High Country* or *Mount San Antonio* 7.5'

see map on p. 24

DIRECTIONS (See directions to Mt. Baldy Village p. 26) From the ranger station in Mt. Baldy Village, continue up the Mt. Baldy Rd. for 4.2 miles to Manker Flats. Park on the side or middle of the divided road near San Antonio Falls Rd.

San Antonio Creek begins as a snow-fed trickle high up on the east face of Mt. Baldy. It gains strength as it descends the canyon, then cascades down a series of steep drops. The final and most impressive three-level drop is called San Antonio Falls. This short hike leads to a viewpoint near the falls. Go on a warm spring day, when the creek is in full flow and the chaparral is in bloom.

From Manker Flats, walk west through a gate and up a service road past some cabins. In 0.5 mile, the road makes a hairpin turn. This is the best viewpoint for San Antonio Falls.

If you want a closer view, it is possible to follow a narrow and tenuous dirt trail 150 yards to the base of the falls. Rock climbers sometimes practice alongside the falls.

VARIATION

It is possible to follow San Antonio Creek up the falls all the way to the Sierra Club ski hut, but this involves some fourth-class climbing and a rope is advisable. Stay left of the first waterfall, then right of the next ones. The walking then eases until you reach another waterfall just below the ski hut. Climb loose rock on the left side or bushwack up the steep slope farther left.

San Antonio Falls

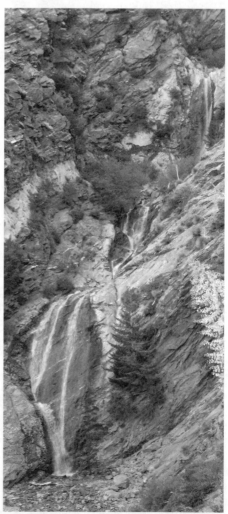

Mt. Baldy Area

trip 1.3 North Backbone Traverse

Distance	12 miles (one-way)
Hiking Time	7 hours
Elevation Gain	5100'
Difficulty	Strenuous
Trail Use	Dogs
Best Times	June–October
Agency	Angeles National Forest (Mt. Baldy Visitor Center)
Recommended Map	Tom Harrison *Angeles High Country* or *Mount San Antonio* 7.5'

see map on p. 24

DIRECTIONS This trip requires a lengthy car shuttle. From Interstate 15 south of the Cajon Pass, drive northwest on Highway 138 for 8.8 miles, and then west on Highway 2 for 5.3 miles to Wrightwood. Turn left on Spruce, then immediately right on Apple, then immediately left again on Acorn Dr. Follow Acorn for 0.6 mile to where it becomes a private road, and park off the pavement. Drive the other car back down to Interstate 15, and then south to the 210 Freeway and up to Mt. Baldy Village (see directions to Mt. Baldy Village on p. 26). Then continue 4.2 miles up Mt. Baldy Rd. to Manker Flats.

This trip traverses the San Gabriel Mountains from south to north, climbing over Mt. Baldy and following its rugged north backbone over Dawson Peak and Pine Mtn. down to Wrightwood. It features grand views from the rarely visited north face of Baldy down into the remote Fish Fork of the San Gabriel River. The long drive is justified by the fantastic scenery and seclusion of Sheep Mountain Wilderness. With an early start, you can reach Wrightwood in time for lunch with a friend who picks you up. Beware: these north slopes hold snow and ice in the spring long after the south face snow has completely melted.

Follow the Baldy Bowl Trail 5 miles to the summit of Mt. Baldy (see Trip 1.1).

Descend the steep North Backbone Trail on the north side to a saddle of 8800 feet, then follow the trail that climbs steeply up to Dawson Peak, 1.5 miles from Baldy. Descend the far ridge for 0.5 mile past a junction with the Dawson Peak Trail, which drops westward into Fish Fork Canyon. Continue north on the Backbone Trail over Pine Mtn.; a 100-foot detour is necessary to reach the true summit. Then drop back down to a saddle and up to an unmarked trailhead on Forest Road 3N06.

ALTERNATIVE FINISH

It is possible to end the hike here. Park your car at the trailhead, which is reached from Inspiration Point on Highway 2 by driving 7.2 miles east on the fair dirt Blue

Mt. Baldy's North Backbone

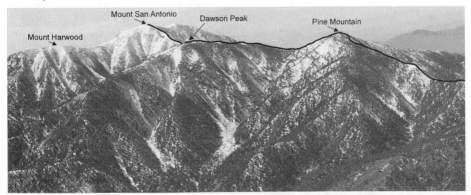

Ridge Rd. (labeled 3N26 at the start, but soon becoming 3N06) to the point above the prominent saddle between Pine and Wright Mountains. The driving time may exceed the time you save hiking, but the views of the North Backbone, Iron Mtn., the San Antonio Ridge, and the San Gabriel River Canyon are breathtaking.

VARIATION

Peak baggers may choose to make a short excursion to the summit of Wright Mtn. Cross the road and continue, very steeply for the first few yards, straight up the toe of the ridge. Soon, cross the Pacific Crest Trail (PCT) and look for traces of an old jeep trail. In 0.1 mile, the slope levels out under the Jeffrey pines and white firs. In another 0.2 mile, the jeep trail dips and climbs back up to reach a T-junction on top of the ridge. Turn left and walk 100 yards to a yellow triangular sign. Look for a faint climber's trail on the right leading north 100 feet to the indistinct summit, which is marked with a large cairn. Then continue west on the jeep trail to rejoin the PCT. This option adds 200 feet of climbing and negligible distance.

Find the PCT on the north side of the road and follow it west as it contours around Wright Mtn. In 0.8 mile, turn north onto the Acorn Trail and follow it 2.1 miles down to the top of Acorn Dr. Continue 0.2 mile to a gate, then another 0.4 mile down the paved private road to your vehicle.

trip 1.4 Bear Flat

Distance	3.2 miles (out-and-back)
Hiking Time	2 hours
Elevation Gain	1200'
Difficulty	Moderate
Trail Use	Dogs, suitable for backpacking
Best Times	All Year
Agency	Angeles National Forest (Mt. Baldy Visitor Center)
Recommended Map	Tom Harrison *Angeles High Country* or *Mount Baldy* 7.5'

see map on p. 24

DIRECTIONS (See directions to Mt. Baldy Village p. 26) From Mt. Baldy Rd. in Mt. Baldy Village, directly across from Mt. Baldy Lodge, turn onto Bear Canyon Dr. It is the first road on the west-side just south of the Mt. Baldy Visitor Center. The beginning of the road passes through the parking lot of Mt. Baldy Village Church. Drive 0.2 mile west through the parking lot and up the road beyond, and park in a small dirt lot on the right side just below a gate. Take care not to block private driveways. If the lot is full, there is additional parking at the Mt. Baldy Visitor Center.

Bear Flat is actually a sloping valley at the head of Bear Canyon and is only flat in comparison to the rugged slopes of Mt. Baldy. The short but steep trail leads along Bear Creek and past numerous cabins, through forest and chaparral. It is enjoyable either for a quick workout; or for a leisurely tour of the oaks, bigcone Douglas-firs, cedars, and spring wildflowers. Lucky and patient observers might catch sight of bighorn sheep roaming the mountainside nearby. Ambitious hikers may continue from the flat to Lookout Mtn. (see Trip 1.6), or all the way to the summit of Mt. Baldy (see Trip 1.5).

Walk up the road along Bear Creek past the gate and numerous cabins. When the road ends in 0.3 mile, just beyond a large water tank, cross the creek on wooden planks and continue up the Bear Canyon Trail (7W12) beyond. In 0.2 mile is an unmarked junction. Turn sharply right to stay on the main trail.

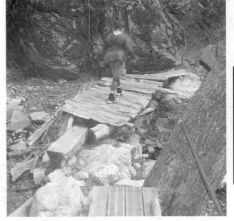
Bridge over Bear Creek

see map on p. 24

VARIATION

An interesting alternative is to continue straight up the canyon on the Bear Canyon Loop Trail (7W12A). This trail passes more cabins and crosses a truly ramshackle bridge, then climbs very steep steps cut into the rocky hillside. When you reach the next to last cabin in the canyon, cross Bear Creek on some logs; you may have to look hard for the crossing. The trail then climbs out of the creek bed, and joins with the main Bear Canyon Trail.

The Bear Canyon Trail and Bear Canyon Loop Trail rejoin at a signed junction on the hillside in 0.2 mile. Beyond this second junction, the Bear Canyon Trail switchbacks across the sun-baked slope, then reenters the shady canyon. In 0.9 mile, it passes a small clearing beneath an oak tree, not far from the east fork of Bear Creek, shortly before it arrives at the signed Bear Flat. The clearing is large enough for a tent, but campfires are not allowed. Near the top of the flat, there are several more clearings in which to enjoy a picnic and take in the views.

Bear Flat is an ecological anomaly. The stream issues from a spring a few hundred yards upstream from the trail, and rarely dries up. Ferns grow profusely in an area exposed to the sun. Geologists offer an explanation: the water table is unusually high here because of the San Antonio Fault.

In May 2008, the Bighorn Fire charred 500 acres of chaparral from the edge of Bear Flat up to the ridge. This is a great place to watch the cycle of regrowth. The cute Bear Flat sign at edge of the meadow miraculously survived the blaze.

trip 1.5 Bear Ridge

Distance	12 miles (out-and-back)
Hiking Time	7 hours
Elevation Gain	5800'
Difficulty	Strenuous
Trail Use	Dogs
Best Times	June–October
Agency	Angeles National Forest (Mt. Baldy Visitor Center)
Recommended Map	Tom Harrison *Angeles High Country* or *Mount Baldy* and *Mount San Antonio* 7.5'

DIRECTIONS (See directions to Mt. Baldy Village p. 26) From Mt. Baldy Rd. in Mt. Baldy Village, directly across from Mt. Baldy Lodge, turn onto Bear Canyon Dr. It is the first road on the west-side just south of the Mt. Baldy Visitor Center. The beginning of the road is the parking lot of the Mt. Baldy Village Church. Drive 0.2 mile west through the parking lot and up the road beyond, and park in a small dirt lot on the right side just below a gate. Take care not to block private driveways. If the lot is full, there is additional parking at the Mt. Baldy Visitor Center.

The great south ridge of Mt. Baldy rises directly from Mt. Baldy Village to the summit, and climbs nearly 6000 feet in 3.5 horizontal miles. The trail offers the greatest sustained elevation gain of any in the San Gabriel Mountains. This is a tough

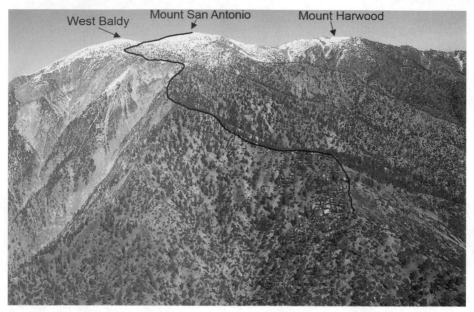

West Baldy   Mount San Antonio   Mount Harwood

Bear Ridge from the south

climb, but the views are fantastic and you avoid the usual Baldy crowds until reaching the summit.

Walk up the road past the gate and numerous cabins. When the road ends in 0.3 mile, cross Bear Creek on wooden planks and continue up the Bear Canyon Trail (7W12) beyond. In another 0.2 mile, come to an unmarked junction. The main trail turns sharply right. Follow the switchbacks across the sun-baked slope, then reenter the shady canyon and cross Bear Creek, in another mile arrive at the Bear Flat sign.

The 2008 Bighorn Fire burned from Bear Flat up to the ridge. The trail switchbacks up through the burn area onto Bear Ridge, then climbs relentlessly for 4.7 miles. This is a good place to watch for elusive desert bighorn sheep. The trail passes close by West Baldy before reaching the true summit. Return the way you came.

ALTERNATIVE FINISH

If you left a vehicle at Manker Flats, descend the Devil's Backbone or Baldy Bowl Trails (see Trip 1.1). These options are highly recommended because they are spectacular, you avoid retracing your steps, and you save your knees from the brutal descent.

Bear Ridge   *photo by Wayne Steinmetz*

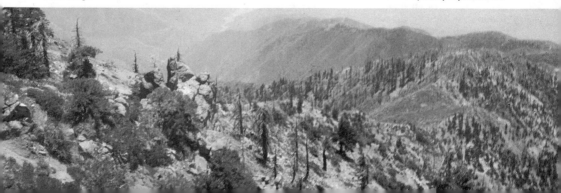

trip 1.6 Lookout Mtn.

Distance	9 miles (out-and-back)
Hiking Time	6 hours
Elevation Gain	2400'
Difficulty	Strenuous
Trail Use	Dogs
Best Times	March–November
Agency	Angeles National Forest (Mt. Baldy Visitor Center)
Required Map	Tom Harrison *Angeles High Country* or *Mount Baldy* and *Mount San Antonio* 7.5'

see map on p. 24

DIRECTIONS (See directions to Mt. Baldy Village, p. 26) From Mt. Baldy Rd. in Mt Baldy Village, directly across from Mt. Baldy Lodge, turn onto Bear Canyon Dr. It is the first road on the west-side just south of the Mt. Baldy Visitor Center. The beginning of the road is the parking lot of the Mt. Baldy Village Church. Drive 0.2 mile west through the parking lot and up the road beyond, and park in a small dirt lot on the right side just below a gate. Take care not to block private driveways. If the lot is full, there is additional parking at the Mt. Baldy Visitor Center.

Lookout Mtn., a seemingly minor bump on the south ridge of Mt. Baldy, plays an important role in the history of science. In 1915, a fire lookout was constructed on the summit to take advantage of the commanding views. In 1926, Albert Michelson conducted a groundbreaking experiment here to measure the speed of light. He placed a prism on Mt. Wilson and a large mirror on Lookout Mtn. The United States Geodetic Survey team surveyed the distance between the two peaks with unprecedented accuracy. By bouncing a beam of light from the prism off the mirror and carefully measuring the round trip travel time, he determined that the speed of light is nearly 300,000 kilometers per second or about 670 million miles per hour. In 1927, a windstorm destroyed the fire lookout and now all that remains are some concrete pilings.

This trip follows a trail to the rarely visited summit of Lookout Mtn. The trail has suffered from years of disuse and parts of it are blocked by downed trees and washouts. The trail is not depicted on maps. However, the serious brush has been chopped back and the path can still be followed without undue difficulties. As you hike through the rugged terrain, imagine the struggles that Michelson and the lookout builders must have overcome. Bighorn sheep frequent this area, so do not camp here; just enjoy it as a day hike.

Follow the Bear Canyon Trail (7W12) 1.6 miles up to Bear Flat (see Trip 1.4). This area burned in the Bighorn Fire of 2008. Just above the Bear Flat sign, look to the left for a path chopped through the bushes. This old trail curves around the hillside into the West Fork of Bear Canyon, passing through oaks, yuccas, and cedars. The going can be slow because of the fire damage and obstacles on the trail. Beware of missing the switchbacks and wandering off the trail. Near the head of the canyon, the

Succulent Dudleya along West fork of Bear Canyon

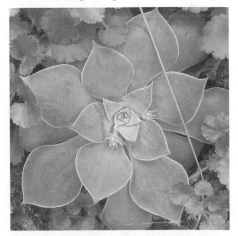

trail turns sharply left and crosses the creek (usually dry), then climbs into a grassy clearing where it vanishes, a long 1.5 miles from Bear Flat. From here, hike 0.3 mile up the pinecone-laden floor of the canyon to a saddle at the top at about 6553 feet. There are dramatic views down the other side into Cattle Canyon and the Big Horn Ridge beyond, where former tungsten mining operations are still visible.

From the saddle, a ridge leads south. Hike south 0.1 mile up a bump for a view of the route ahead. There are two more bumps beyond. The next is labeled 6930′ on the Mount San Antonio USGS map. The farther and lower one is Lookout Mtn., located 1 mile away at the south end of the ridge. You may be able to make out faint traces of trail along the way. Descend to a notch, then start climbing toward Peak 6930′.

Look for a trail across the open slope on the northeast side of the hill. The trail becomes a corridor hacked through the buckthorn on the southeast side. If you miss the trail, you can also go directly over the top of Peak 6930′ and down to the saddle on the south side. Beyond, the trail continues threading through low manzanita bushes to the summit of Lookout Mtn.

On a clear day, you can enjoy views in all directions. Nearby are Ontario, Timber, Telegraph, Thunder, Baldy, and Iron Mountains. To the west are Mt. Wilson and the rest of the San Gabriels.

Lookout Mtn. can also be accessed via a short and steep trail/firebreak from Cow Canyon Saddle (see Trip 2.8). Stop at the Mt. Baldy Ranch RV Park and pay a $2 fee to park and hike across their land.

trip 1.7 Icehouse Canyon

Distance	7 miles (out-and-back)
Hiking Time	4 hours
Elevation Gain	2600′
Difficulty	Strenuous
Trail Use	Dogs
Best Times	May–November
Agency	Angeles National Forest (Mt. Baldy Visitor Center)
Recommended Map	Tom Harrison *Angeles High Country* or *Mount Baldy* and *Cucamonga Peak* 7.5′
Permit	Cucamonga Wilderness Permit Required

see map on p. 24

DIRECTIONS (See directions to Mt. Baldy Village p. 26) From the ranger station in Mt. Baldy Village, continue up the Mt. Baldy Rd. for 1.5 miles. Turn right into Icehouse Canyon, then park at the trailhead on the left.

Icehouse Canyon is the most accessible hike in the beautiful Cucamonga Wilderness. The canyon was formed by earthquake fault activity. It is part of a larger system of east-west running canyons that stretches along the southern San Gabriel Mountains out to the west fork of the San Gabriel River. The shady recesses remain cool well into the summer and the canyon gets its name from purveyors of ice that supplied

Southern California residents in the 1850s or 60s. This trip climbs through a forest of incense cedars to the saddle at the head of the canyon. A five-way junction on the saddle tempts the ambitious hiker with numerous ways to continue exploring (see Trips 1.8–1.10 and 1.14).

Hike east along the popular Icehouse Canyon Trail past numerous cabins along the north side of the creek. Icehouse Canyon had its heyday during the great age of hiking and mountain resorts in the 1920s and 1930s. The devastating floods of 1938 wiped out many cabins. Fires and avalanches have also taken their toll.

In 0.5 mile, pass the mouth of the first tributary canyon carved between steep cliffs on the right (south). This is Falling Rock Canyon, and is a possible descent route from Ontario or Sugarloaf Peaks (see Trips 1.9 and 1.12). In another 0.5 mile, pass an intersection with the Chapman Trail to the left (see Trip 1.8).

As you ascend, the canyon bottom becomes dry. Pass the wilderness boundary, and then watch for Columbine Spring on the downhill side of the trail, 2.4 miles from the start. The spring is located immediately before a series of switchback and is often surrounded by a patch of columbine in the summer. In 0.5 mile of serious climbing, pass the second junction with the Chapman Trail, and then saunter up the last 0.6 mile to Icehouse Saddle.

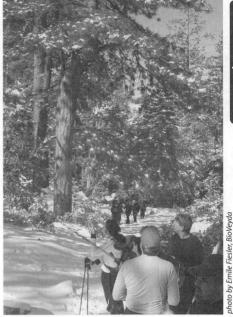

photo by Emile Fiesler, BioVeyda

Winter wonderland in Icehouse Canyon

trip 1.8 Cedar Glen

Distance	4.5 miles (out-and-back), or 7.5 miles (loop)
Hiking Time	2.5–4 hours
Elevation Gain	1200' or 2100'
Difficulty	Moderate
Trail Use	Dogs, suitable for backpacking
Best Times	May–November
Agency	Angeles National Forest (Mt. Baldy Visitor Center)
Recommended Map	Tom Harrison *Angeles High Country* or *Mount Baldy, Cucamonga Peak*, and *Telegraph Peak* 7.5'
Permit	Cucamonga Wilderness Permit Required

see map on p. 24

DIRECTIONS (See directions to Mt. Baldy Village p. 26) From the ranger station in Mt. Baldy Village, continue up the Mt. Baldy Rd. for 1.5 miles. Turn right into Icehouse Canyon, then park at the trailhead on the left.

Cedar Glen Trail Camp is perched on a bench overlooking Icehouse Canyon. This beautiful trip up to the glen follows the shady Icehouse Canyon Trail to the Chapman Trail, and then climbs the wall of the canyon, alongside Cedar Creek, passing chaparral and wildflowers. Cedar Glen has one of the most diverse conifer groves in Southern California, with most of the local species growing together. This trip can be done as a short out-and-back jaunt, or better yet, as a loop continuing on to rejoin Icehouse Canyon and returning via the canyon floor. It is also an enjoyable destination

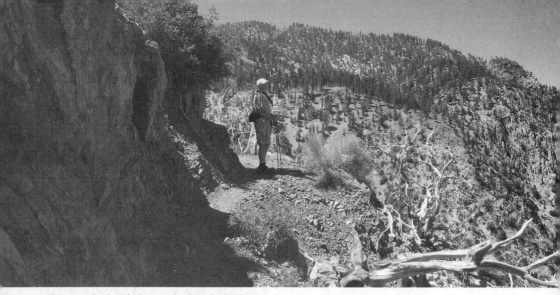
Chapman Trail with Ontario Peak in the background

for a short backpacking trip. The climb to Cedar Glen is steep and shadeless. If you are going in the summer, start in the morning before it gets too hot.

From the popular Icehouse Canyon Trailhead, hike east up the canyon past cabins. The dirt road soon narrows to a trail and continues along the north bank of the rushing creek beneath oaks, incense cedars, and broad-leaf trees. In the summer, expect to pass a field of fragile red and yellow flowered columbines growing along the trail.

In 1.0 mile, reach a trail junction with the Chapman Trail; at the time of this writing, the sign was damaged. Turn sharply left and follow the Chapman Trail up the north slope of the canyon along Cedar Creek. This slope is exposed to the searing sun and is covered with yuccas, buckthorns, manzanitas, and other chaparral adapted to the harsh conditions. Watch for rattlesnakes, especially in the summer. The trail crosses to the west side of Cedar Creek, then crosses back east again in a lush field of vines and wildflowers. This is the best place to get water if you are camping. Follow one more switchback and arrive at Cedar Glen, 1.3 miles up from Icehouse Canyon.

The small grove on the bench includes Jeffrey, ponderosa, and sugar pines, bigcone Douglas-firs, white firs, and, of course, incense cedars. It is a great place to study the trees and learn to identify the different species. Incense cedars have distinctive scale-like leaves instead of needles. White firs and bigcone Douglas-firs have short needles, which grow individually rather than in bundles. White fir cones are rarely seen at the base of the tree; the barrel-shaped cones grow near the top of the tree and decompose on the branch rather than falling. Bigcone Douglas-fir, also called bigcone spruce, is neither a fir nor a spruce. Its cones grow up to 7 inches long. Pines have longer needles growing in bundles. Sugar pines have bundles of five needles, about 4 inches long, and are easily recognized by their long, skinny cones; sugar pine cones are the world's longest, usually exceeding 12 inches. Jeffrey and ponderosa have long needles in bundles of three and are much more difficult to distinguish. The size of the cones is your best clue: Jeffrey pine cones grow up to 10 inches, while ponderosa pine cones are 3–5 inches long.

Return the way you came.

ALTERNATIVE FINISH

You can make a wonderful loop by continuing 2.2 miles up the Chapman Trail to where it rejoins the Icehouse Canyon Trail. This stretch offers fantastic views of the north wall of Ontario Peak across the canyon, and out to Sunset Peak and Bear Ridge to the west. Reach the Icehouse Canyon

Trail at a switchback beneath some sugar pines. It is possible to head uphill for 0.6 mile to Icehouse Saddle, and then on to any of several terrific peaks (see Trips 1.9–1.11). But for now, turn right and follow the switchbacks downhill for 0.6 mile. At the base of the last switchback is Columbine Spring, whose clear, cold waters gush forth beneath the trail in a patch of columbine and red monkeyflowers. Continue down the trail past the wilderness boundary into a talus field, and soon reach the stone foundations of old cabins. Icehouse Creek begins flowing strongly again. In 1.3 miles from Columbine Spring, reach the lower junction with the Chapman Trail, then hike the final mile down to the trailhead.

trip 1.9 Ontario Peak

Distance	12 miles (out-and-back)
Hiking Time	7 hours
Elevation Gain	3600'
Difficulty	Strenuous
Trail Use	Dogs, suitable for backpacking
Best Times	June–October
Agency	Angeles National Forest (Mt. Baldy Visitor Center)
Recommended Map	Tom Harrison *Angeles High Country* or *Mount Baldy* and *Cucamonga Peak* 7.5'
Permit	Cucamonga Wilderness Permit Required

see map on p. 24

DIRECTIONS (See directions to Mt. Baldy Village p. 26) From the ranger station in Mt. Baldy Village, continue up the Mt. Baldy Rd. for 1.5 miles. Turn right into Icehouse Canyon, then park at the trailhead on the left.

O ntario and Cucamonga Peaks form an imposing wall overlooking the western end of the Inland Empire. They rise more than a vertical mile from the endless subdivisions at the 2000-foot base to the summits at almost 9000 feet. Ontario Peak is one of the classic climbs of Southern California. It is named for the town of Ontario, which in turn was named by the founding Chaffey brothers for their home province of Ontario, Canada. The easiest way to the summit is to ascend the Icehouse Canyon Trail, then turn southwest and hike up past Kelly Camp along the long ridge to the summit. The north side of the ridge can be deceptively icy in early summer and after the first storms of the fall.

Follow the Icehouse Canyon Trail 3.5 miles to the signed five-way junction at Icehouse Saddle (see Trip 1.7). Turn sharply right and take the Ontario Peak Trail 0.9

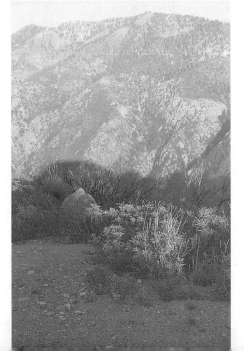
Ontario Peak from Sunset Peak

mile to Kelly Camp. John Kelly began prospecting here in 1905 and Henry Delker turned the site into a backcountry resort in 1922. It is now a simple trail camp and an excellent place to stay if you are backpacking. In the early summer, you may find water trickling from a small spring by the camp. It is always prudent to treat water before drinking.

Beyond Kelly Camp, continue 0.4 mile to the ridge, where there are breathtaking views down into Cucamonga Canyon and out over the Inland Empire. Continue west along the undulating ridge. This area is in a burn zone, and travel is hampered by the occasional need to scramble over large fallen timber. Most of the annoying deadfalls across the trail have been removed by enterprising Boy Scouts. In a seemingly endless 1.2 miles, reach the 8693-foot summit, which is readily recognizable by a granite spire.

ALTERNATIVE FINISH

Most parties descend the way they came. It is also possible to take cross-country routes down Falling Rock Canyon or Shortcut Ridge, but these routes are only recommended for experienced cross-country travelers. Yet another option is to follow the ridge east over Bighorn Peak, then down and up to Cucamonga Peak (see Trips 1.9 and 1.11).

Falling Rock Canyon is accessed from the broad bowl beneath the trail 0.3 mile east of Ontario Peak. Pick a way down to the north through the fallen timber. The canyon steepens and passes a small saddle next to Sugarloaf Peak. It then veers right and descends through talus fields before reaching the bottom of Icehouse Canyon 0.5 mile east of the trailhead. This route saves substantial distance but not much time because of the difficult terrain. Be careful not to be lured down the wrong canyon because some of the canyons have cliff bands of decomposing rock.

Shortcut Ridge descends from Kelly Camp and reaches Icehouse Canyon near the wilderness boundary.

VARIATIONS

Truly adventurous mountaineers can reach Ontario Peak from the southwest ridge starting near Stoddard Flat or from any of several ridges rising from Cucamonga Canyon. These cross-country routes were burned clear of chaparral in the vast Grand Prix Fire of October 2003, but are becoming less enjoyable as the vegetation returns. They require a good map and excellent navigation skills.

trip 1.10 Cucamonga Peak

Distance	12 miles (out-and-back)
Hiking Time	7 hours
Elevation Gain	3800′
Difficulty	Strenuous
Trail Use	Dogs
Best Times	June–October
Agency	Angeles National Forest (Mt. Baldy Visitor Center)
Recommended Map	Tom Harrison *Angeles High Country* or *Mount Baldy* and *Cucamonga Peak* 7.5′
Permit	Cucamonga Wilderness Permit Required

see map on p. 24

DIRECTIONS (See directions to Mt. Baldy Village p. 26) From the ranger station in Mt. Baldy Village, continue up the Mt. Baldy Rd. for 1.5 miles. Turn right into Icehouse Canyon, then park at the trailhead on the left.

Ontario and Cucamonga Peaks form an imposing wall overlooking the western end of the Inland Empire. They rise more than a vertical mile from the endless subdivisions at the 2000-foot base to the summits at almost 9000 feet. Cucamonga Peak is another of the classic climbs of Southern California. It is named for the Cucamonga Rancho, established in the valley below in 1839 by Tiburcio Tapia. The ranch, in turn, got its name from the Tongva/Shoshonean word *kukill-mongo*, whose meaning is uncertain. The easiest way to the summit is to hike to Icehouse Saddle, then follow a good trail to the summit. The north-facing leg beyond Icehouse Saddle traverses a steep slope and holds unconsolidated snow late into the spring, rendering it nearly impassable long after the snow has melted away on the surrounding mountains.

Ontario-Cucamonga Ridge from above Baldy Bowl

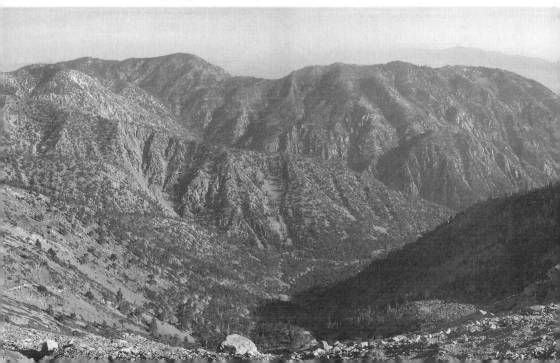

Follow the Icehouse Canyon Trail 3.5 miles to the signed five-way junction at Icehouse Saddle (see Trip 1.7). Cross the saddle and follow the trail southeast for 0.9 mile as it contours around the steep east slope of Bighorn Peak. It reaches another saddle separating the rugged drainages of Cucamonga Canyon and Lytle Creek, then switchbacks steeply up through a forest of lodgepole pines and white firs to Cucamonga Peak. Reach the 8859-foot peak in 1.4 strenuous miles. The last 0.2 mile of trail on the flattish top can be faint and confusing, but aim for the highest point with unobstructed views south over the Inland Empire.

VARIATIONS

Highly motivated mountaineers can also reach Cucamonga Peak from either of two great ridges rising up on the sides of Deer Canyon. These cross-country routes were burned clear of chaparral in the vast Grand Prix fire of October 2003, but the routes are becoming less enjoyable as the vegetation regains its hold on the ridges. They require a good map and excellent navigation skills.

trip 1.11 The Three T's

Distance	13 miles (one-way with short shuttle)
Hiking Time	8 hours
Elevation Gain	5000'
Difficulty	Moderate
Trail Use	Dogs
Best Times	June–October
Agency	Angeles National Forest (Mt. Baldy Visitor Center)
Recommended Map	Tom Harrison *Angeles High Country* or *Mount Baldy*, *Cucamonga Peak*, and *Telegraph Peak* 7.5'
Permit	Cucamonga Wilderness Permit Required

see map on p. 24

DIRECTIONS This trip requires a short car or bicycle shuttle. (See directions to Mt. Baldy Village p. 26) From the ranger station in Mt. Baldy Village, continue up the Mt. Baldy Rd. for 4.2 miles to Manker Flats, where you leave one vehicle. Drive or pedal 2.7 miles down the hairpin turns and turn left into Icehouse Canyon, then park at the trailhead on the left.

Timber, Telegraph, and Thunder Mountains form the undulating northeast wall of San Antonio Canyon. This superb romp over the three T's begins up Icehouse Canyon and descends through the ski resort at Baldy Notch. For an easier hike with only 9.5 miles of distance and 2100 feet of elevation gain, take the ski lift from the top of Mt. Baldy Rd. up to the notch and do the trip in reverse.

Follow the Icehouse Canyon Trail 3.5 miles to the signed five-way junction at Icehouse Saddle (see Trip 1.7). Turn left and climb north 0.7 mile toward Timber Mtn. The trail curves around the west side, so you will have to make a 0.2 mile detour to reach the true summit. Follow the trail 2.0 miles down to a saddle and up to Telegraph Peak. Again, make a short detour on a use trail to the northeast to reach the summit, which is the highest point of the trip. Return to the trail and drop steeply to a third saddle, and then climb back up to the final summit, reaching Thunder Mtn. in 1.2 miles. From here, the Gold Ridge ski road leads 1.5 miles back down to Mt. Baldy Notch.

From the notch, hike down the service road 3.2 miles to Manker Flats. Alternatively, the ski lift runs on weekends and is a tempting way to save the wear and tear on your knees.

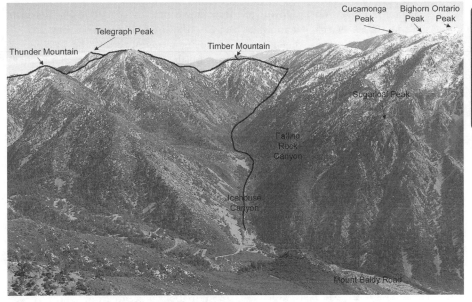

Aerial view of the Ontario-Cucamonga ridge and the Three T's

trip 1.12 Nine Baldy Area Peaks

Distance	28 miles (one-way, with a short shuttle)
Hiking Time	15 hours
Elevation Gain	10,600′
Difficulty	Very strenuous
Trail Use	Suitable for backpacking
Best Times	June–October
Agency	Angeles National Forest (Mt. Baldy Visitor Center)
Recommended Map	Tom Harrison *Angeles High Country* or *Mount Baldy, Mount San Antonio, Cucamonga Peak*, and *Telegraph Peak* 7.5′
Permit	Cucamonga Wilderness Permit Required

see map on p. 24

DIRECTIONS This trip requires a short car or bicycle shuttle. (See directions to Mt. Baldy Village p. 26) From the ranger station in Mt. Baldy Village, continue up the Mt. Baldy Rd. for 4.2 miles to Manker Flats, where you leave one vehicle. Drive or bike 2.7 miles down the hairpin turns and turn left into Icehouse Canyon, then park at the trailhead on the left.

This is the mother of all hikes in Southern California. It tours nine major summits around San Antonio Canyon: Ontario, Bighorn, Cucamonga, Timber, Telegraph, Thunder, Harwood, Baldy, and West Baldy. There is substantial elevation gain and loss between most of the peaks, making this the toughest of the multi-mountain challenges in this book. Standing on top of Ontario Peak at dawn, mighty Mt. Baldy beckons to you from across the deep canyon separating the peaks. Standing atop Baldy at dusk, you will look back at the dramatic ridges of Ontario. This is a great trip to do when there is a full moon because the extra light may be helpful. Bring a headlamp, a generous supply of water, and boundless enthusiasm.

Hike 3.5 miles up Icehouse Canyon to Icehouse Saddle. Turn sharply left and hike up past Kelly Camp to the ridge, then follow the trail along the ridge to Ontario Peak. Return along the ridge; when the main trail begins descending to Kelly Camp, stay on the ridge and follow a use trail east to Bighorn Peak. Make a cross-country descent of the southeast ridge of Bighorn Peak to a saddle, where you join the Cucamonga Peak Trail and switchback up to the summit. Then return via the trail to Icehouse Saddle.

At this point, you have climbed 5700 feet and toured three magnificent peaks. If time or energy is waning, follow the Icehouse Canyon Trail back to your vehicle. Otherwise, continue north up to the three T's (see Trip 1.10) and on to the Mt. Baldy Notch.

If you reach the top of the notch before 5 P.M., you may be able to get water or snacks at the Top-of-the-Notch Restaurant. This is also your next escape route. You can either hike down the service road to Manker Flats or take the chair lift if it is running.

Again, if energy permits, begin climbing west up the Devil's Backbone. Before making the final push up Baldy, take a short detour from the trail to the summit of Mt. Harwood. Then top out on Mt. Baldy before taking an easy 0.5-mile jaunt to West Baldy. Return to Baldy and descend via the Baldy Bowl Trail to Manker Flats.

VARIATIONS

If you are in supremely good condition and know the trails of this region well, consider adding even more peaks. Climb Ontario by way of Falling Rock Canyon to scale Sugarloaf Peak. Follow the Cucamonga Peak Trail a mile east to the 8662-foot Etiwanda Peak (not named on most maps). Descend from Baldy by way of Pine and Dawson Peaks, or, even more boldly, down the grueling San Antonio Ridge to Iron Mtn.

trip 1.13 Iron Mtn.

Distance	13 miles (out-and-back)
Hiking Time	8 hours
Elevation Gain	6200'
Difficulty	Strenuous
Trail Use	Dogs
Best Times	October–November, April–May
Agency	Angeles National Forest (Mt. Baldy Visitor Center)
Required Map	Tom Harrison *Angeles High Country* or *Glendora, Mount Baldy,* and *Mount San Antonio* 7.5'
Permit	Sheep Mountain Wilderness Permit Required

see map on p. 24

DIRECTIONS From the 210 Freeway in Azusa, exit north on Azusa Ave. (Highway 39) and take it up into San Gabriel Canyon. In 11.9 miles, turn right (east) on East Fork Rd. At a hairpin turn in 5.3 miles, stay straight (east) on a minor road that crosses a bridge and ends in 0.9 mile at a parking lot and closed gate.

Big Bad Iron Mtn. stands west of Mt. Baldy, towering over the headwaters of the San Gabriel River. It is the toughest single peak hike in the San Gabriel Mountains, and the second hardest (after Rabbit Peak) in this book. The hike begins near the river at 2000 feet and climbs to the 8007-foot summit. The first half is on good trail to Heaton Saddle, but the second half follows a steep climber's path up the interminable south ridge of Iron Mtn. The mountain is defended by sharp yuccas, so wear sturdy pants and gaiters. Most people will want at least 4 quarts of water on a cool day; don't even think about this shadeless climb on a hot day. This is also a popular conditioning hike and gets regular use by a number of sturdy mountaineers. The route is south-facing and lower than many others in the region, so it can often be done in the winter months if snowfall has been light.

Hike north past the gate along the dirt road to Heaton Flat Campground. Near the outhouse, turn right and follow the Heaton Flat Trail 3.9 miles to Heaton Saddle. The maintained trail ends here, but a surprisingly good climber's path leads up the south ridge for 2 intense miles with 3500 feet of elevation gain. The route is distinct and straightforward to follow, even on a foggy day.

Return the way you came. Or, if you have plenty of time and are feeling extremely strong, follow the great San Antonio Ridge east to Mt. Baldy (see Trip 1.14).

---

trip 1.14 **San Antonio Ridge**

Distance	16 miles (one-way)
Hiking Time	14 hours
Elevation Gain	10,200'
Difficulty	Very strenuous
Best Times	October–November
Agency	Angeles National Forest (Mt. Baldy Visitor Center)
Required Map	Tom Harrison *Angeles High Country* or *Glendora, Mount Baldy,* and *Mount San Antonio* 7.5'
Permit	Sheep Mountain Wilderness Permit Required (for entry from East Fork only)

see map on p. 24

DIRECTIONS This trip requires a long car shuttle. Follow the directions on p. 26 to Mount Baldy Village, then continue up Mt. Baldy Rd. 4.2 miles and leave a vehicle at the Manker Flats Trailhead. Return to the 210 Freeway and drive west to Azusa. Exit north on Azusa Ave. (Highway 39) and take it up into San Gabriel Canyon. In 11.9 miles, turn right (east) on East Fork Rd. At a hairpin turn in 5.3 miles, stay straight (east) on a minor road that crosses a bridge and ends in 0.9 mile at a parking lot and closed gate.

The great San Antonio Ridge connects Iron Mtn. to Mt. Baldy. This is a monster hike: strenuous, with interesting rock scrambling, completely devoid of water, and absolutely spectacular. It should be done when temperatures in the canyons have cooled but while Baldy is still free of ice. This is most common in late fall, but sometimes conditions are still good in early winter during a light snow year. It is good to know the Baldy area well so you can find the descent trail in the dark. Headlamps are usually necessary and some parties have spent an unplanned night (or two!) on the ridge. Most climbers will want at least 6 quarts of water on a cool day. The trip is easier if you do it in reverse, but still involves more than 5000 feet of climbing. It is theoretically possible to backpack this trip and camp on Iron Mountain, the San Antonio Ridge, or Mt. Baldy, but there is no water on the route and you may need to carry 10 quarts or more.

Follow the Heaton Flat Trail and south ridge to Iron Mtn. (see Trip 1.13). Look east along the San Antonio Ridge and pick out Mt. Baldy, only 4 miles away and 2000 feet higher. Despite appearances, getting there is at least as hard as the climb of Iron Mtn. that you have just completed. Unless it is still early in the day and you are bubbling with energy, this is the last good place to turn around.

Pick a path down the dramatic trailless ridge to the east through rocks and brush. Cross the aptly-named Gunsight Notch, which involves exposed third-class moves on poor quality rock. There is little benefit

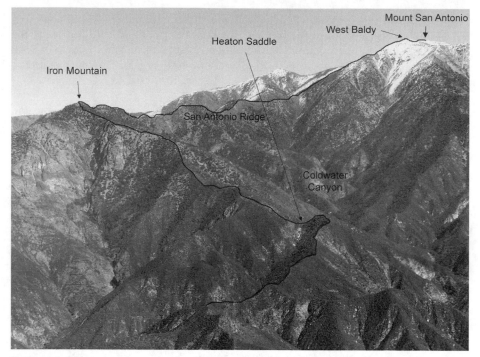

San Antonio Ridge

in bringing a rope because it would be hard to establish a trustworthy anchor. Eventually reach the low point on the ridge, 1 mile from Iron Mtn. Follow the undulating ridge 1.5 miles over two bumps to the eastern saddle before the steep rise to Mt. Baldy. There are a few manzanita patches along the way, but you can stay on bighorn sheep trails to avoid the worst of the chaparral.

Then make the final 2200-foot climb up the west ridge of Baldy, going over West Baldy to the true summit of Mt. Baldy.

Descend via the Baldy Bowl Trail to Manker Flats. Remember that this trail is prone to ice on the switchbacks above the ski hut; take special care as this area is especially treacherous in the dark.

trip 1.15 Icehouse Saddle from Lytle Creek

Distance	12 miles (out-and-back, with a possible overnight camp)
Hiking Time	6 hours
Elevation Gain	3600'
Difficulty	Strenuous
Trail Use	Dogs, suitable for backpacking
Best Times	June–October
Agency	San Bernardino National Forest (Cajon/Lytle Creek Ranger Station)
Recommended Map	Tom Harrison *Angeles High Country* or *Telegraph Peak* and *Cucamonga Peak* 7.5'
Permit	Cucamonga Wilderness Permit Required

see map on p. 24

DIRECTIONS From Interstate 15 between the 210 and 215 freeways, exit north on Sierra Ave., which becomes Lytle Creek Rd. Proceed 5.2 miles to the ranger station, where you can pick up your wilderness permit. Continue 1.7 miles, then turn left on Middle Fork Rd., which soon becomes the fair dirt Forest Road 2N58. In 2.9 miles, reach the trailhead parking at the end of the road beside an outhouse, at 3955 feet.

This trip takes the back way up to Icehouse Saddle. It follows the middle fork of Lytle Creek past three pleasant trail camps before making the steep climb to the saddle. A herd of bighorn sheep roam the crumbling canyon walls. Chickadees sing from the trees and wildflowers decorate the trail. You are much more likely to find solitude on this side of Icehouse Saddle, though the trail camps are favored by Boy Scout troops.

Boy Scout backpacking on the Lytle Creek Trail   *photo by Wayne Steinmetz*

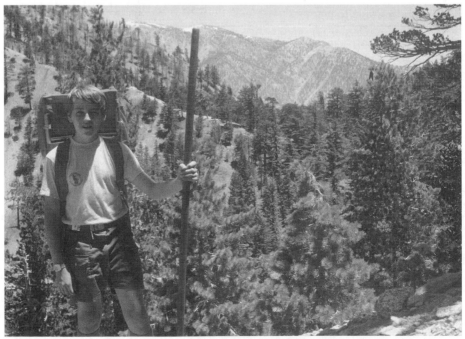

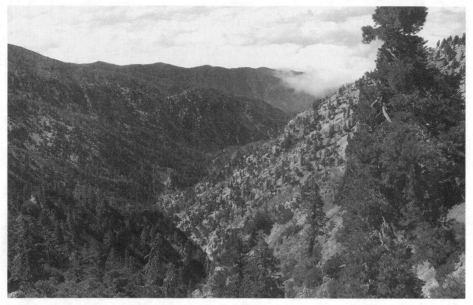

Looking down Icehouse Canyon from Icehouse Saddle

The trail leads west, climbing onto the slope north of the creek, passing yuccas and scrub oak. This part of the canyon burned in the catastrophic Grand Prix fire of 2003. The chaparral is growing back on the north side of the creek, but the toothpick forest on the south side will take decades to recover. After climbing some switchbacks, round a corner and reach an unmarked junction in 0.6 mile. The old trail to the left descends to Stone House Trail Camp at 4403 feet. In another 0.8 mile, reach a second junction with the old trail leading back to Stone House. By now, you have passed the end of the burn area and entered a forest of live oak and bigcone Douglas-fir.

In 1.1 miles, turn left and cross the Middle Fork to reach Third Crossing Trail Camp at 5194 feet. (This would have been your third creek crossing if you had taken the old trail.) The section near the creek crossing is somewhat indistinct; look for a rock-lined trail resuming at the campsite.

The trail now switchbacks up onto a ridge and joins a southern tributary of the Middle Fork above a spectacular section of narrows. (Some canyoneers enjoy making a technical descent of this gorge.) It crosses some scree and talus slopes with poor tread and reaches Commanche Trail Camp in 1.5 miles, at 6132 feet. The camp is beautifully situated beneath oaks, firs, incense cedars, and ponderosa pines. The choice and spelling of camp name is curious as the Comanche Indians lived east of the Rockies.

The last part of the trail is the toughest, climbing 1.7 miles to Icehouse Saddle. Along the way, you can enjoy the dramatic views of the rugged canyons as they abruptly drop to the San Andreas Fault. Return the way you came, or follow any of the other four trails radiating from Icehouse Saddle (see Trips 1.7–1.11).

VARIATION

The three trail camps along the way are great backpacking destinations.

chapter 2

San Dimas–La Verne–Claremont–Upland Foothills

Residents of communities around San Dimas, La Verne, Claremont, and Upland enjoy remarkable hiking, biking, running, bird watching, and equestrian opportunities at the base of the foothills on the north edge of their towns. In particular, Marshall Canyon Regional Park and Claremont Hills Wilderness Park are extremely popular and are worthy of the occasional visit from hikers who live farther away.

As suburban sprawl has taken over the open space at the base of the foothills, Los Angeles County set aside 678 acres in the oak-filled Marshall and Live Oak canyons for a regional park. Now, a maze of shady trails tempts hikers, equestrians, and mountain bikers to lose themselves in the canyons. In 1997, the city of Claremont established a wilderness park on the north edge of town with a system of fire roads through the chaparral-clad hills offering visitors excellent hiking opportunities and panoramic views. These parks form the heart of a planned 5-mile corridor of protected open space and natural habitat.

This chapter describes several hikes within these parks and on nearby foothills. If you have a little more time, consider combining several of the hikes for a longer workout exploring more of the trails.

Live Oaks in Marshall Canyon

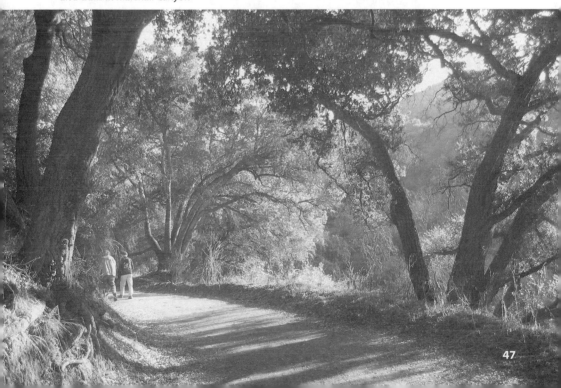

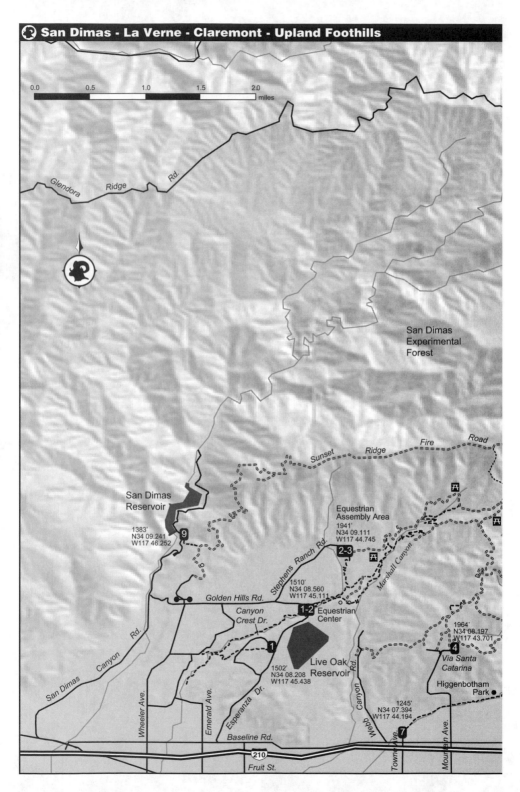

San Dimas - La Verne - Claremont - Upland Foothills

0.0   0.5   1.0   1.5   2.0
miles

Glendora Ridge Rd.

San Dimas
Experimental
Forest

Sunset Ridge Fire Road

San Dimas
Reservoir

1383'
N34 09.241
W117 46.252

9

Equestrian
Assembly Area
1941'
N34 09.111
W117 44.745

2-3

Stephens Ranch Rd.

Marshall Canyon

1510'
N34 08.560
W117 45.111

Golden Hills Rd.

Canyon
Crest Dr.

1-2 Equestrian
Center

1964'
N34 08.197
W117 43.701

San Dimas Canyon Rd.

1

1502'
N34 08.208
W117 45.438

Live Oak
Reservoir

4

Via Santa
Catarina

Higginbotham
Park

Emerald Ave.

Esperanza Dr.

Wheeler Ave.

Webb Canyon Rd.

1245'
N34 07.394
W117 44.194

7

Townsend Ave.

Mountain Ave.

Baseline Rd.

210

Fruit St.

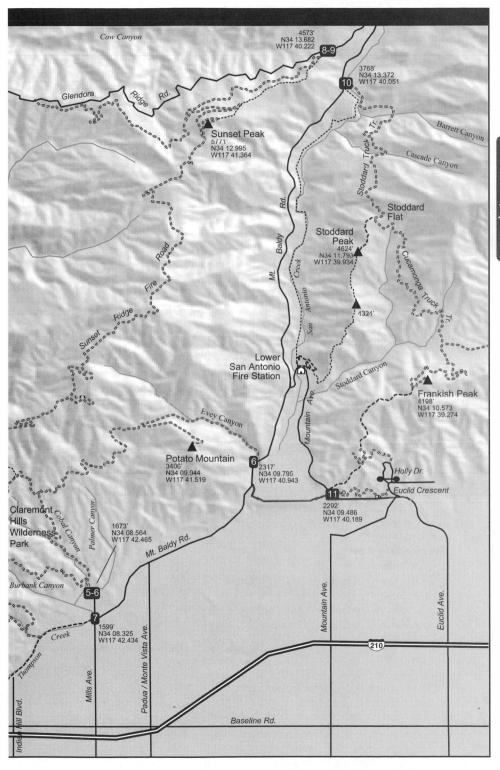

Cow Canyon

4573'
N34 13.682
W117 40.222

8-9

3768'
N34 13.372
W117 40.051

10

Glendora

Ridge Rd.

Barrett Canyon

Stoddard Truck Tr.

Cascade Canyon

Sunset Peak
5771'
N34 12.995
W117 41.364

Stoddard
Flat

Stoddard
Peak
4624'
N34 11.793
W117 39.934

Fire Road

Cucamonga Truck Tr.

Mt. Baldy Rd.

San Antonio Creek

Sunset Ridge

4324'

Lower
San Antonio
Fire Station

Stoddard Canyon

Frankish Peak
4198'
N34 10.573
W117 39.274

Evey Canyon

Mountain Ave.

Potato Mountain
3406'
N34 09.944
W117 41.519

6

2317'
N34 09.795
W117 40.943

Holly Dr.

Euclid Crescent

11

2292'
N34 09.486
W117 40.189

Claremont
Hills
Wilderness
Park

Cobal Canyon

Palmer Canyon

1673'
N34 08.564
W117 42.465

Mt. Baldy Rd.

Burbank Canyon

5-6

7

1599'
N34 08.325
W117 42.434

Mills Ave.

Padua / Monte Vista Ave.

Mountain Ave.

Euclid Ave.

Thompson Creek

Indian Hill Blvd.

210

Baseline Rd.

trip 2.1 Lower Marshall Canyon

Distance	2.3 miles (semi-loop)
Hiking Time	1.5 hours
Elevation Gain	300'
Difficulty	Easy
Trail Use	Dogs, equestrians, cyclists, good for children
Best Times	All year, but hot in summer
Agency	LA County Dept. of Parks and Recreation
Optional Map	none

see map on p. 48

DIRECTIONS From Interstate 210 in La Verne, exit north on Fruit Ave. Drive 0.1 mile, then turn left on Baseline Rd. After 0.3 mile, turn right on Esperanza Dr. Follow Esperanza for 1.2 miles, and then turn left on Canyon Crest Dr. and park near the intersection.

Marshall Creek flows past endless subdivisions alongside the Sierra La Verne golf course. One might be surprised to discover a trail along the creek shaded under the oaks that whisks you away and gives you the feeling of being in the wilderness. Runners, bikers, and hikers all enjoy this short but beautiful loop hike.

The signed Marshall Canyon Equestrian and Hiking Trail starts on the south side of Canyon Crest Dr. Follow the trail east under the power lines between rows of houses. In 0.3 mile, cross Canyon Crest again and climb a hill for views of the golf course and Sunset Ridge beyond the chaparral.

In another 0.2 mile reach a junction with another trail coming down from a housing development. Stay right and drop into the oak-lined canyon. When you reach the bottom in 0.2 mile, turn right, and then immediately right again to follow the path upstream for a mile alongside Marshall Creek. The trail crosses the creek at several points and travels alongside the golf course, but for the most part you enjoy the feeling of seclusion. When you reach the tunnel under Esperanza, climb up to the sidewalk. Turn right and walk 0.6 mile southwest alongside Esperanza to return to the starting point.

trip 2.2 Middle Marshall Canyon

Distance	2 miles (loop)
Hiking Time	1 hour
Elevation Gain	300'
Difficulty	Easy
Trail Use	Dogs, equestrians, cyclists, good for children
Best Times	All year, but hot in summer
Agency	LA County Dept. of Parks and Recreation
Optional Map	Tom Harrison *Angeles High Country* or *Mt. Baldy* 7.5'

see map on p. 48

DIRECTIONS From Interstate 210 in La Verne, exit north on Fruit Ave. Drive 0.1 mile, then turn left on Baseline Rd. After 0.3 mile, turn right on Esperanza. Follow Esperanza for 3.0 miles, and then turn right on Stephens Ranch Rd. Proceed 1.0 mile past a golf course to the signed Equestrian Assembly Area, a large dirt parking area on the right side of the road.

Marshall Canyon Regional Park at the top of Live Oak Canyon is popular with local hikers and riders and features a creek lined with stately oaks. In the spring during good rainfall years, wildflowers are in abundant bloom. This trip explores a short loop around the middle part of the canyon. There are many possible variations and, if you have time to spare, it is fun to just roam the maze of trails and see where you come out. Poison oak is common in Marshall Canyon, so don't stray off the trail.

From the parking area take a footpath south winding steeply down the hill and passing beneath power lines. The trail crosses a small creek and runs alongside another creek. Although the Marshall Canyon Golf Course is only yards away, the dense trees in the canyon give you the feeling of complete seclusion.

In 0.5 mile, reach a T-junction. The right fork leads to the stables at the Marshall Canyon Equestrian Center, but our short loop stays left and begins climbing back up the hill. In 0.2 mile, reach a dirt road at the south end of an equestrian training area. Locate a trail that continues east and then north around the perimeter of the training area. In 0.3 mile, drop down to the east to join another trail running along Marshall

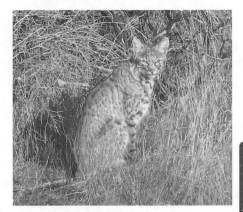

Bobcat along the Marshall Canyon Trail

Creek. Turn left again and hike 0.2 mile north along the creek through the fine oaks. At your first opportunity, stay left, then left again to work your way out of the canyon to the west through a maze-like area and emerge at the signed Fred Palmer Equestrian Camping and Training facility. From here, a dirt road leads 0.4 mile west back to where you started or, better yet, stay on the pleasant trail paralleling the road.

trip 2.3 Upper Marshall Canyon

Distance	4.5 miles (semi-loop)
Hiking Time	2 hours
Elevation Gain	750′
Difficulty	Moderate
Trail Use	Dogs, equestrians, cyclists, good for children
Best Times	All year, but hot in summer
Agency	LA County Dept. of Parks and Recreation
Optional Map	Tom Harrison *Angeles High Country* or *Mount Baldy* 7.5′

see map on p. 48

DIRECTIONS From Interstate 210 in La Verne, exit north on Fruit Ave. Drive 0.1 mile, then turn left on Baseline Rd. After 0.3 mile, turn right on Esperanza. Follow Esperanza for 3.0 miles, and then turn right on Stephens Ranch. Proceed 1.0 mile past a golf course to the signed Equestrian Assembly Area, a large dirt parking area on the right side of the road.

Much like Middle Marshall Canyon, Upper Marshall Canyon is popular with local hikers and riders. It also features a creek lined with stately oaks. In the spring, wildflowers burst into joyous bloom. This trail through the steep upper part of the canyon is a great way to get exercise while enjoying the outdoors. Poison oak is common in Marshall Canyon, so don't stray off the trail.

From the east end of the parking lot, drop down to a paved road and follow the trail along the north side of the road. Pass a yellow gate in 0.2 mile, and then come to the signed Fred Palmer Equestrian Camping and Training facility in another 0.2 mile. Turn left at the sign and follow a fire road as it winds generally northeast through shady oaks above the creek. In 0.6 mile, come to a three-way junction with two other trails leading to the right. Stay left on the fire road. You will make a loop that returns on the rightmost trail to this point. The middle trail is a shortcut that rejoins the fire road.

As you continue up the fire road, you will soon come to another trail on the right that parallels the fire road for 0.2 mile before rejoining; you may take either path. Soon after, the fire road starts climbing in earnest. Pass a picnic area nestled in the oak trees beside the creek at the head of the canyon. The fire road turns south and comes to another junction where a trail on the right shortcuts back to the three-way junction you passed earlier. But this hike continues east up the fire road 0.4 mile more until it reaches the gate to the Claremont Wilderness Park (see Trip 2.5).

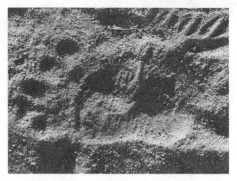

Bear print in Marshall Canyon

Turn right and follow another broad fire road southwest for 0.4 mile, pass a set of benches, and continue until you can turn right on another fire road that leads back to Marshall Canyon. Descend for 0.5 mile until you reach a trail junction; take the trail right and switchback down the hill and across the creek, returning to the three-way junction. Turn left on the fire road and retrace your steps for a mile back to the parking area.

trip 2.4 Johnson's Pasture

Distance	2.2 miles (out–and–back)
Hiking Time	1 hour
Elevation Gain	400'
Difficulty	Easy
Trail Use	Dogs, cyclists, equestrians, good for children
Best Times	All year
Agency	City of Claremont
Optional Map	Tom Harrison *Angeles High Country* or *Mount Baldy* 7.5'

see map on p. 48

see map on p. 48

DIRECTIONS From the 10 Freeway, exit north on Indian Hill in Claremont and drive north past the 210 Freeway, then turn left on Baseline. From the 210 Freeway, exit at Baseline in Claremont and drive west. Turn right on Mountain Avenue in Claremont (caution: there is another parallel Mountain Avenue in Upland only a few miles to the east). Go up the steep hill for a mile to the top, and then make a right on Via Santa Catarina. Park at the end of Via Santa Catarina, taking care not to block private driveways. It is possible that designated trailhead parking will be established by the time you take this trip.

Johnson's Pasture is a 180-acre plot of land overlooking Claremont. In 2006, city voters passed a bond measure to purchase the land, saving it from development and annexing it to the Claremont Wilderness Park. This short and gentle hike is popular with families and for strolls at sunset.

The trail, actually a dirt road, starts on the north side of the cul-de-sac on Via

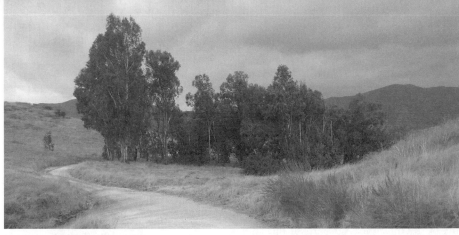
Eucalyptus grove in Johnson's Pasture

Santa Catarina. This is a quiet neighborhood; please respect the residents. The trail climbs steeply for the first few yards. In 0.1 mile, pass a side road on the right leading to power lines and down to Thompson Creek. In another 0.2 mile, pass a side road on the left leading down to the High Point condominiums. Straight ahead, arrive at a pleasant grove of eucalyptus, where another power line road leads left down into Webb Canyon. 0.2 mile later, a short side road on the left climbs up to a hill offering panoramic views of the San Gabriel Mountains, Claremont, and the Inland Empire. But the main road continues, passing yet another side road to an antenna farm on the right, arriving at a switchback junction with the Claremont Wilderness Park loop, 1.1 miles from the start (see Trip 2.5). Return the way you came, or wander off to explore some of the side roads. Note that none of the side roads return you to the trailhead.

trip 2.5 Claremont Hills Wilderness Park

Distance	5 miles (loop)
Hiking Time	2.5 hours
Elevation Gain	950'
Difficulty	Moderate
Trail Use	Dogs, cyclists, equestrians, good for children
Best Times	All year, dawn to dusk
Agency	City of Claremont
Optional Map	Tom Harrison *Angeles High Country* or *Mount Baldy* 7.5'

see
map on
p. 48

DIRECTIONS From the 10 Freeway, exit north on Monte Vista in Montclair and drive north past Foothill Blvd., then turn left on Baseline. From the 210 Freeway, exit at Baseline in Claremont and drive west. Proceed 0.7 mile, and then turn right on Mills. Go up the hill 1.4 miles to the trailhead parking on the left just before Mills turns into a private driveway. If the trailhead is overflowing, park on the street or at a large lot 0.3 mile down Mills.

The Claremont Wilderness Park, established in 1997, has become the region's most popular loop for hiking, biking, running, and strollers. On a clear winter day, it offers views of the snow-capped summits of San Jacinto, San Gorgonio, and Ontario Peaks, and out to the skyscrapers of downtown Los Angeles towering beyond countless subdivisions. On a perfect day you can even see Catalina Island. The trail is on a good fire road that is normally well-graded, but it can wash out during winter rains. The park can be unpleasantly hot on summer

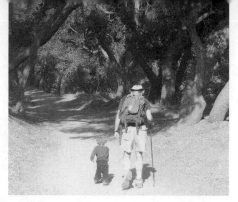

afternoons and is occasionally closed during times of extreme fire danger.

From the west end of the parking lot, follow the dirt road past the Thompson Creek Dam flood control basin and across a small creek. The path forks in 0.2 mile. You will follow the right fork up Cobal Canyon, and then loop around to return to this junction via Burbank Canyon. Hiking alongside Cobal Creek in the oak-shaded canyon is one of the most pleasant parts of this trip. After 0.8 mile, the road leaves the canyon at a switchback and climbs unrelentingly up the ridge. At a water tank in another 0.5 mile, a side road leads east toward Palmer Canyon and Potato Mtn. (see Trip 2.6), but the Wilderness Park loop veers west and in 0.5 mile reaches a saddle at the northernmost point of the park.

The loop continues along an undulating ridge to the southwest. This area burned on Halloween night in 2003 leaving a scorched, barren landscape, but the vegetation has rebounded remarkably well. In 0.1 mile, pass a gate on the right at the top of the fire road leading up from Marshall Canyon (see Trip 2.3). Soon after, hikers will pass shaded

The Claremont Wilderness Park delights young and old.

benches placed on the hill by the Rotary Club in memory of Claremont mayor Nick Preseam, who helped preserve the park. In 0.4 mile from the last gate, pass a second fire road again leading to the right down into Marshall Canyon.

In another 0.5 mile, crest the last of the hills and begin the steady descent. In 0.4 mile, reach yet another junction. Turn hard left and descend the switchback. The other path connects to Johnson's Pasture (see Trip 2.4). Drop down the chaparral-covered slopes of Burbank Canyon overlooking Thompson Creek Dam and return to the main fork where you started the loop. Turn right, cross the creek, and reach the parking lot.

trip 2.6 Potato Mtn.

Distance	4.5 miles (out-and-back)
Hiking Time	2.5 hours
Elevation Gain	1100′
Difficulty	Moderate
Trail Use	Cyclists
Best Times	October–May
Agency	Herman Garner Biological Preserve
Optional Map	Tom Harrison *Angeles High Country* or *Mount Baldy* 7.5′
Permit	Herman Garner Biological Preserve Permit Required

see map on p. 48

DIRECTIONS From the 210 Freeway, exit on Baseline Rd. and drive west to the first intersection, Padua Ave. Turn right on Padua and travel north for 1.8 miles, until reaching Mt. Baldy Rd. Turn right and go up Mt. Baldy Rd. for 2.4 miles. Park your vehicle at a gated turnout on the left side of the road.

Potato Mtn. is a seemingly unremarkable bump overlooking the city of Claremont. Though the mountain itself is nothing special, the hike up Evey Canyon is beautiful. The views from the summit on a clear day are far-reaching, and the short but steep trail is popular for exercise. The springtime is an especially good time to visit because the wildflowers are in bloom. Avoid this hike on summer afternoons, when you are certain to get baked under the unrelenting sun.

The shortest way to reach Potato Mtn. is via Evey Canyon. Evey Canyon is private property owned by Pomona College and managed as the Herman Garner Biological Preserve. A free permit, which is good for one year, is required to enter the canyon. Call the Pomona College Biology Department at (909) 607-2993 to request a permit, which you must read, sign, and send back.

The hike follows a fire road up Evey Canyon. This canyon was once among the most beautiful in the San Gabriels, with tall oaks branching over the road alongside the stream. The 2002 Williams Fire swept through the foothills and wiped out many trees, but a remarkable number survived and the canyon is gradually returning to its former glory. In 1.4 miles, the road veers left and reaches a saddle at the top of the canyon. From here, turn left and follow a spur road 0.8 mile to the summit of Potato Mtn.

ALTERNATIVE FINISH

If you have arranged a car or bicycle shuttle, you can make a fine one-way hike by returning to the saddle, and then following the fire road west for 2.1 miles to the Claremont Wilderness Park and another 1.6 mile down to the trailhead at the north end of Mills Ave.(see Trip 2.5).

trip 2.7 Thompson Creek Trail

Distance	4.5 miles (out-and-back)
Hiking Time	2 hours
Elevation Gain	300′
Difficulty	Easy
Trail Use	Dogs, cyclists, good for children
Best Times	All year
Agency	City of Claremont
Optional Map	Tom Harrison *Angeles High Country* or *Mount Baldy 7.5′*

see map on p. 48

DIRECTIONS From the 10 Freeway, exit north on Monte Vista in Montclair and drive north past Foothill Blvd., then turn left on Baseline. From the 210 Freeway, exit at Baseline in Claremont and drive west. Proceed 0.7 mile, and then turn right on Mills. Go up the hill 1.1 miles to the large parking lot on the right at the corner of Mt. Baldy Rd.

Thompson Creek is fed by the many canyons overlooking Claremont and is sadly channeled into a concrete canal to reduce the flood risk at the expense of natural habitat. Fortunately, a paved trail now follows the side of the canal through pleasant landscaping and past Higginbotham Park. This Thompson Creek Trail is popular for jogging, cycling, and strollers.

The Thompson Creek Trail starts on the west side of Mills opposite the parking area. It leads west across the plain beneath Thompson Creek Dam and soon meets the canal. In 1 mile, it passes a parking area at the north end of Indian Hill Blvd. Just 0.3 mile farther, it reaches Higginbotham Park, complete with a restroom, drinking fountain, and Wild West-themed play area. In the spring, you may see a camp on the far side of the canal where a herd of goats grazes the hillside to reduce the amount of brush before fire season.

The trail continues west, crossing Mountain Avenue, passing stables, and terminating in 0.9 mile at the north end of Towne Ave. just north of Baseline and the 210 Freeway. Return the way you came.

trip 2.8 Sunset Peak

Distance	3–7 miles (loop)
Hiking Time	2–3 hours
Elevation Gain	1300'
Difficulty	Moderate
Trail Use	Dogs
Best Times	All year
Agency	Angeles National Forest (Mt. Baldy Visitor Center)
Recommended Map	Tom Harrison *Angeles High Country* or *Mount Baldy* 7.5'

see map on p. 48

DIRECTIONS From the 210 Freeway, exit on Baseline Rd. and drive west to the first intersection, Padua Ave. Turn right on Padua and travel north for 1.8 miles, until reaching Mt. Baldy Rd. Turn right and go up Mt. Baldy Rd. for 7 miles. On the outskirts of Mt. Baldy Village, turn left onto Glendora Ridge Rd. Travel 0.8 mile up the road to Cow Canyon Saddle. Park your vehicle along the south side of the road (the lot on the north side is signed no parking). If the gate at the bottom of Glendora Ridge Rd. is closed, park outside the gate and hike the road.

Sunset Peak offers the perfect hike for stepping out of city life for an afternoon. It is not a long drive into the mountains, and the hike is relatively short, yet the trail travels through the rugged and picturesque San Gabriel Mountains. There are two options for hiking Sunset Peak. One is a steep and rough firebreak that follows the ridge 1.6 miles up to the peak. The other is a dirt service road that switchbacks 3.6 miles up the mountain. From the summit one can see miles of the San Gabriel Mountains, as well as great views of the cities below. A recommended loop is to climb the fire road, enjoy a picnic at sunset, and descend the dirt road by headlamp.

The firebreak and the road both start on the south side of the paved Glendora Ridge Rd. The firebreak starts very steeply and follows the ridge over one major crest and a couple minor bumps before passing a bend in the fire road at 1.2 miles. Continue up the ridge for another 0.4 mile to rejoin the road just before reaching the summit. The chaparral encroaches on the trail at points, so wearing long pants is a good idea.

If you choose to take the road instead, walk past the gate near the parking area. Follow the road southwest for 1.9 miles until reaching the first junction; take a sharp left at this junction. Hike another 0.6 mile and pass the firebreak trail at a hairpin turn. Hike another 0.7 mile until reaching a final junction; take a sharp left here and reach the summit in 0.4 mile.

Sunset over the San Gabriel Mountains from Sunset Peak

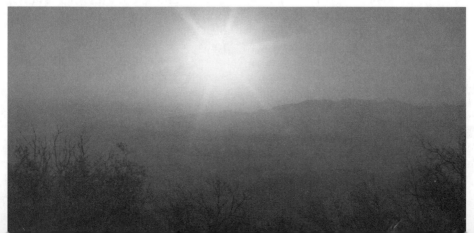

trip 2.9 Sunset Ridge

Distance	13–15 miles (one-way)
Hiking Time	7 hours
Elevation Gain	1500'
Difficulty	Strenuous
Trail Use	Cyclists
Best Times	September–May
Agency	Angeles National Forest (Mt. Baldy Visitor Center)
Recommended Map	Tom Harrison *Angeles High Country* or *Mount Baldy*, Glendora 7.5'

see map on p. 48

DIRECTIONS This is a one-way hike and is described in the mostly downhill direction. Position one vehicle at the end of the hike, and then take another to the start.

To reach the end from the 210 Freeway, exit on Foothill Blvd. Drive west 0.3 mile, then turn right (north) on San Dimas Canyon Rd. Follow it 2.0 miles to a stop sign at the corner of Golden Hills, then proceed 1.0 mile farther. Park at a wide spot in the road just above mile marker 1.40, shortly before reaching the top of the San Dimas Reservoir.

To reach the start, return the way you came to the 210 Freeway and drive east to Baseline Ave. Exit and drive west to the first intersection, Padua Ave. Turn right on Padua and travel north for 1.8 miles, until reaching Mt. Baldy Rd. Turn right and go up Mt. Baldy Rd. for 7 miles. On the outskirts of Mt. Baldy Village, turn left onto Glendora Ridge Rd. Travel 0.8 mile up the road to Cow Canyon Saddle. Park along the south side of the road (the lot on the north side is signed no parking). If the gate at the bottom of Glendora Ridge Rd. is closed, park outside the gate and hike the road.

Sunset Ridge is an island in the sky extending from Mt. Baldy Village to San Dimas Reservoir. A fire road runs the length of the ridge and makes for a good, long, and mostly downhill hike with views of Mt. Baldy, the San Gabriel Mountains, and the Inland Empire. In the spring after good winter rains, the chaparral slopes burst into color with wildflowers. For a more strenuous alternative with 4700 feet of elevation gain, take this trip in the opposite (uphill) direction.

The start from Cow Canyon Saddle has two options: a 3.6-mile dirt road or a much steeper 1.6-mile firebreak (see Trip 2.8). Both options lead to the top of Sunset Peak, a 1300-foot climb. Beyond, the fire road is almost all downhill.

The road leads south along the eastern edge of the San Dimas Experimental Forest. This 32-square-mile parcel of land is closed to public access and is used for scientific research, including the effects of erosion, air pollution, and fire in the chaparral ecosystem. In 3 miles, pass beneath the antenna farm called the Sunset Ridge Electronic Site.

To the west, Browns Flat is an unusual level clearing amidst the steep hills. The road descends, making large switchbacks.

ALTERNATIVE FINISH

Below the last switchback it is possible to take a shortcut by dropping down steep ridges into the upper reaches of the Claremont Wilderness Park or Marshall Canyon. The trail in this area mostly has vistas to the south, but look for a "window" on Sunset Ridge where you can peer onto the north side. A yellow box with a fire hydrant is located here. Just beyond, the narrow path can be found hidden among the bushes on the left (south) side of the fire road. It follows a slick firebreak down to the saddle at the northernmost point of the Wilderness Park, where the terminus is also hidden in brush. The USGS topographic map shows an old trail on this ridge. The lower part used to lead into Marshall Canyon, but now takes the more direct route into the Wilderness Park. Arrange to meet a vehicle at one of these trailheads.

The fire road continues west along the ridge above Marshall Canyon, and then switchbacks down to a point just above the reservoir. Beware of poison oak, which grows in large stands along the edge of the road. Pass a collapsed old water tank. Shortly beyond, at an elevation of 1700 feet, the road turns south. Look for a trail on the right, easy to miss, descending steeply westward. If you reach a large white water tank beside the road, you have gone 0.2 mile too far. Descend the trail for 0.3 mile to where your vehicle awaits.

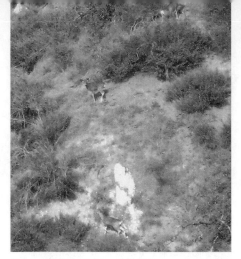

Deer grazing near Sunset Ridge

trip 2.10 Stoddard Peak

Distance	6 miles (out-and-back)
Hiking Time	3 hours
Elevation Gain	1000'
Difficulty	Moderate
Trail Use	Dogs
Best Times	All year
Agency	Angeles National Forest (Mt. Baldy Visitor Center)
Recommended Map	Tom Harrison *Angeles High Country* or *Mount Baldy* 7.5'

see map on p. 48

DIRECTIONS To reach the start from the 210 Freeway, exit on Baseline Rd. and drive west to the first intersection, Padua Avenue. Turn right on Padua and travel north for 1.8 miles, until reaching Mt. Baldy Rd. Turn right and go up Mt. Baldy Rd. In 2.7 miles, pass the turnoff on the right for Mountain Ave. (the sign is currently missing) Continue 3.7 miles. Just after passing over the dirt hogback blocking San Antonio Canyon, turn right on the Barrett-Stoddard Rd. and park in the small lot before crossing the bridge.

Stoddard Peak (4624') is located on the shoulder of Ontario Peak overlooking San Antonio Canyon. Despite its diminutive stature among the huge peaks circling the canyon, Stoddard offers excellent views of Mt. Baldy and is an enjoyable exercise hike or half-day excursion. The peak and nearby canyon were named for William Stoddard, who, in 1880, founded the first of many mountain resorts in this area. These resorts were immensely popular before the development of air conditioning. Ranchers sent their families up into the high country to escape the oppressive heat that blankets the Inland Empire during the summer months.

From the trailhead, hike east down the road, and cross the bridge over San Antonio

Mt. Baldy from Stoddard Peak

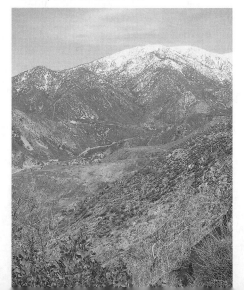

Creek. On the west side of the creek, you can see traces of the old Mt. Baldy Rd. that once ran along the creek before being washed out one too many times. Follow the Barrett-Stoddard Rd. past some private residences near Barrett Canyon and in 0.8 mile pass a gate. Continue, generally southward, past the mouth of Cascade Canyon and above the flat-topped Spring Hill where traces of an old farm can still be seen. In another 1.7 miles, cross a saddle to reach Stoddard Flat. Look to the right (west) for a trail chopped through the chaparral. Follow it up the hill, then along the rocky crest of a ridge. Hike 0.4 mile, passing two false summits before reaching the true summit of Stoddard Peak at the south end of the ridge. Return the way you came.

ALTERNATIVE FINISH

Alternatively, for a substantially longer adventure, it is possible to continue following the Cucamonga Truck Trail south from Stoddard Flat 5.6 miles down to Cucamonga Canyon and out to the top of Skyine Dr. in Alta Loma. At the time of this writing, some sections have been obliterated by flooding. Beware of poison oak along the route. Yet another option with a shuttle is to descend cross-country along Stoddard's south ridge over Peak 4324′ to the Lower San Antonio Fire Station on Mountain Ave. beside San Antonio Creek.

San Dimas, La Verne, Claremont, Upland

trip 2.11 Frankish Peak

Distance	4 miles (out-and-back)
Hiking Time	3 hours
Elevation Gain	1900′
Difficulty	Moderate
Trail Use	Dogs
Best Times	September–May
Agency	Angeles National Forest (Mt. Baldy Visitor Center)
Recommended Map	*Mount Baldy* 7.5′

see map on p. 48

DIRECTIONS From the 10 Freeway, exit north on Euclid Ave. Drive all the way to the north end of Euclid, following it as it curves west to join Mountain Ave. 5.3 miles from the freeway. Continue west 0.4 mile to a turnout on the right where the road begins to curve north at the San Antonio Dam. Park at the turnout.

While the Claremont Wilderness Park teems with hikers, nearby Frankish Peak rarely sees any visitors. It is steep and occasionally brushy in places, but offers an outstanding workout in a short distance and provides fabulous views over the valley on a clear day.

From the turnout follow the trail as it climbs a ridge to a dirt road in 0.6 mile. Turn right, proceed 0.1 mile, then turn left and head up 0.2 mile to the end of the road atop a small hill. From here, a trail climbs steeply. It turns right and levels out briefly before ascending an even steeper knife-edge dirt ridge. At the top, turn right and follow the use trail, faint in places, through low brush over a false summit. Continue east and join a fire road, which leads 0.2 mile on to the true summit. From here, enjoy the close-up views of Ontario Peak looming to the north and the expansive views of the Inland Empire spread out below.

ALTERNATIVE FINISH

If you would like a substantially longer trip, consider descending northeast from Frankish Peak on a fire road for 1.3 miles to

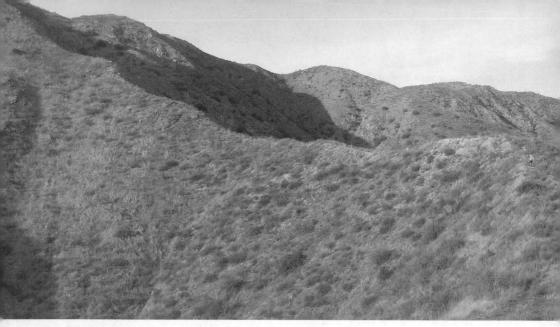

Frankish Peak "trail" atop ridge in foreground

the Cucamonga Truck Trail and following it 2.3 miles down Cucamonga Canyon, then turning right and hiking 1.1 miles to the edge of Alta Loma at the top of Skyline Dr.

This requires a car shuttle and a good map. Beware of washouts and poison oak on the Cucamonga Truck Trail.

trip 2.12 Etiwanda Falls

Distance	3.5 miles (out-and-back)
Hiking Time	2.5 hours
Elevation Gain	800'
Difficulty	Moderate
Best Times	All year, but hot in the summer
Agency	San Bernardino Special Districts
Recommended Map	Tom Harrison *Angeles High Country* or *Cucamonga Peak* 7.5' (locations of dirt roads not all accurate)

see map on p. 61

DIRECTIONS From the 210 Freeway, exit on Day Creek in Rancho Cucamonga. Drive north 1 mile, and then turn right on Wilson. Drive east 0.5 mile, then turn left on Etiwanda. Drive to the end of the road and park. Take care to avoid the no parking zone. This area is under construction and the driving directions are likely to change somewhat.

One of the Inland Empire's rare accessible waterfalls is hidden near the mouth of East Etiwanda Canyon just out of sight of millions of commuters. This moderate hike to the falls follows a good dirt road all the way. The route passes through the North Etiwanda Preserve. This land was set aside in 1998 to protect some of the last remaining alluvial fan sage scrub and other sensitive plants and animals that have been displaced as cities build up to the base of the foothills. The preserve is undergoing active improvement and new trails may exist by the time you hike here.

Begin hiking north on Etiwanda as it turns into a dirt road. Cross a power line road and pass a gate near a water tank; you are now entering the North Etiwanda

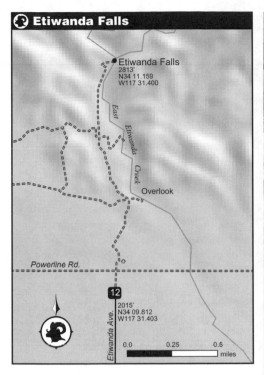

Etiwanda Falls

Etiwanda Falls
2813'
N34 11.159
W117 31.400

East Etiwanda Creek

Overlook

Powerline Rd.

12
2015'
N34 09.812
W117 31.403

Etiwanda Ave.

0.0   0.25   0.5
miles

Preserve. The path climbs steadily up the slope into the San Gabriel Mountains. In another 0.6 mile, arrive at a second crossroad. You may enjoy walking east for a few dozen yards to the top of a bluff overlooking East Etiwanda Creek, but the main path continues north. In another 0.5 mile, reach a four-way junction and continue straight. A sign indicates HABITAT SANCTUARY NO TRESPASSING, but foot traffic is nevertheless allowed. Pass another gate and continue on the flank of the deep wash. In 0.6 mile, the road ends at the top of the falls. Enjoy the overlook, but take care on the slick rock.

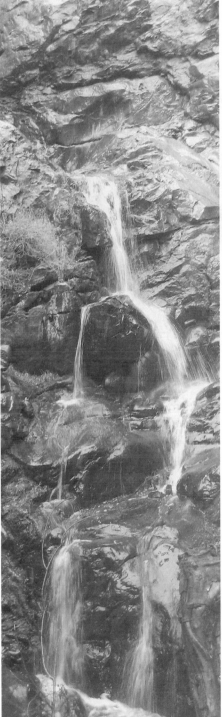

Etiwanda Falls

chapter 3

Western San Bernardino Mountains

The San Bernardino Mountains are part of California's unusual Transverse Ranges, running east to west rather than north to south. They have long attracted the attention of humans, at first for hunting, logging, and gold, but now most of all for recreation. The range is so large that trips for this area are divided into three chapters. This chapter describes the western end, especially around Lake Arrowhead and the alluring creeks at the interface of forest and desert. Chapter 4 focuses on the eastern end, where richly forested hills circle the jewel-like Big Bear Lake. Chapter 5 explores the steep and rugged San Gorgonio Wilderness on the southeast side of the range, cut off from Big Bear by the deep trench of the Santa Ana River.

The southern side rises abruptly from the endless concrete and asphalt of suburbia to the tall forests nearly a mile above sea level. This dramatic escarpment is the work of the infamous San Andreas Fault, which is likely to thrust the mountains even higher in the near geological future. The northern edge rolls off more gradually into the Mojave Desert. Numerous streams carve canyons on the north slopes and then flow together until they merge into the Mojave River and sink beneath the shifting sands. The hills and canyons are laced with a variety of mostly short trails.

The low western end of the San Bernardino Mountains is the most heavily populated, with significant communities at Lake Arrowhead, Crestline, Running Springs, Arrowbear, and Green Valley Lake. Lake Arrowhead was originally constructed as part of an ambitious project to divert the headwaters of the Mojave River southward to irrigate San Bernardino. The efforts began in 1892. After decades of effort and vast sums of money spent, the diversion project was defeated. A 1913 court ruling favored the desert residents who would have lost access to their water. However, the real estate and recreational value of the alpine lake became obvious, and mountain-goers have flocked to the region for a century now to enjoy its charms.

The western San Bernardinos have been hit by a succession of disastrous forest fires. Forests and chaparral have evolved to withstand naturally occurring fires from time to time. In a healthy environment, the mature trees generally survive these low-intensity fires, and in fact, chaparral needs periodic burns in order to reproduce. Fire plays an essential role in clearing out the undergrowth and keeping the ecosystem healthy. As the population in the forest increased during the 20th Century, the government began aggressively fighting fires to protect property. Years of fire suppression have led to overcrowded forests with large amounts of flammable debris on the forest floor. Ozone pollution and drought have further weakened the trees, rendering them susceptible to outbreaks of bark beetles that have killed many of the trees. The combination of heavily packed dead trees and dense ground cover has left the forest extremely vulnerable to high-intensity fires. The 1999 Willow Fire burned 64,000 acres north of Lake Arrowhead and was the largest fire in the San Bernardino National Forest in the past 80 years. Then, in October 2003, fourteen major fires simultaneously swept across California. The Grand Prix and Old Fires hit the Lake Arrowhead area, charring 59,000 acres and destroying 135 residences. The Cedar Glen area was particularly hard hit, with whole neighborhoods of cabins reduced to their foundations. The Slide Fire in October 2007 burned another 12,000 of the remaining acres and 272 homes around Running Springs and Green Valley Lake. Many of the trails in this chapter offer a sobering reminder of the power of wildfire and a fascinating glimpse into the ecological recovery process. The historic policy of fire suppression is obviously untenable and land managers are struggling to find a better approach and to reconcile the need for natural wildfires with people's desire to live in these fire-prone areas.

The best time to visit this area is in the fall or the late spring. Summers can be uncomfortably warm, although hiking early in the day or along shady creeks is still enjoyable. In the winter, access to higher trails is blocked by snow.

An extensive network of dirt roads has been carved through the San Bernardino Mountains, providing easy access to otherwise remote areas. These same roads draw throngs of ATV riders, especially on the northwestern slopes. The ceaseless roar of engines is not conducive to good hiking. Most of these trails are set back from the worst ATV traffic, but a few, especially around Holcomb Creek, can be a problem. Moreover, hunters flock to these hills in deer season (October and November), so it is prudent to dress brightly and stay especially alert to your surroundings in the fall.

Western San Bernardino Mtns

Moonrise over the burnt hills above Deep Creek

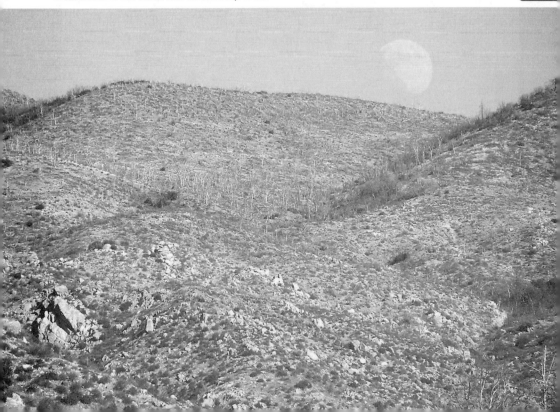

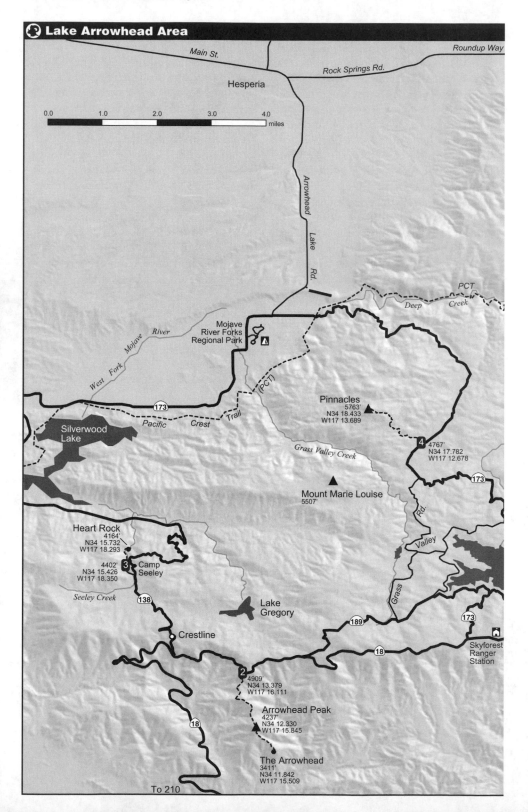

Lake Arrowhead Area

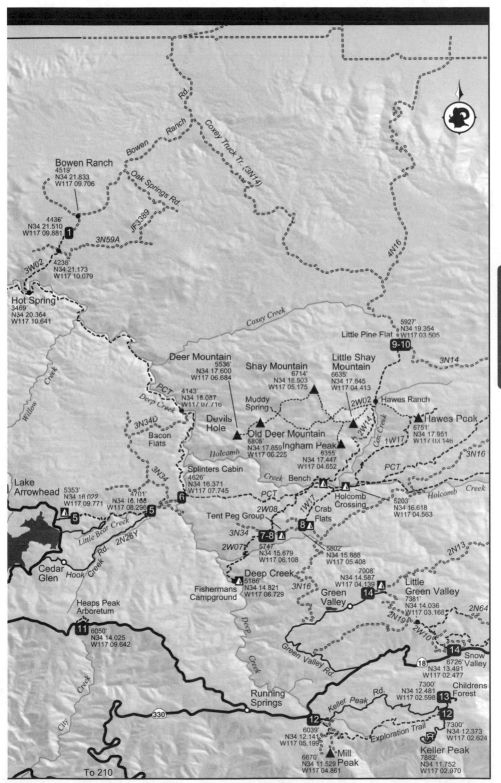

Bowen Ranch
4519'
N34 21.833
W117 09.706

Bowen Ranch Rd.

Coxey Truck Tr. (3N14)

Oak Springs Rd.

JF3389

4436'
N34 21.510
W117 09.881 **1**

3N59A

3W02

4238'
N34 21.173
W117 10.079

Hot Spring
3469'
N34 20.364
W117 10.641

Coxey Creek

4N16

5927'
N34 19.354
W117 03.505

Little Pine Flat **9-10** 3N14

Willow Creek

Deer Mountain
5536'
N34 17.600
W117 06.684

Shay Mountain
6714'
N34 18.503
W117 05.175

Little Shay
Mountain
6635'
N34 17.845
W117 04.413

PCT

4143'
N34 18.087
W117 07.716

Deep Creek

3N34D

Bacon
Flats

Devils
Hole

Muddy
Spring

2W02

Hawes Ranch

2W14

Cox Creek

Hawes Peak
6751'
N34 17.951
W117 03.146

Old Deer Mountain
6806'
N34 17.859
W117 06.225

Ingham Peak
6355'
N34 17.447
W117 04.652

1W17

PCT

3N16

Holcomb

Splinters Cabin
4626'
N34 16.371
W117 07.745

Creek Bench

Holcomb Creek

3N34

Lake
Arrowhead
5353'
N34 16.022
W117 09.771 **5**

4701'
N34 16.155
W117 08.296 **5**

4707'

6

PCT

Holcomb
Crossing

5203'
N34 16.618
W117 04.563

Little Bear Creek

2N26Y

Tent Peg Group

2W08

1W17

Crab
Flats

8

7-8

3N34

2W07

5747'
N34 15.679
W117 06.108

5802'
N34 15.888
W117 05.408

2N13

Cedar
Glen

Hook Creek Rd.

Deep Creek
5186'
N34 14.821
W117 06.729

Fishermans
Campground

3N16

7008'
N34 14.587
W117 04.139

Green
Valley

14

Little
Green Valley
7381'
N34 14.036
W117 03.168

2N64

2N19

2W10

Heaps Peak
Arboretum

6050'
N34 14.025
W117 09.642 **11**

Green Valley Rd.

14

(18)

Snow
6726' Valley
N34 13.491
W117 02.477

Deep Creek

330

Running
Springs

Keller Peak Rd.

7300'
N34 12.481
W117 02.598 **13**

Childrens
Forest

12

City Creek

12

6039'
N34 12.141
W117 05.199

6670'
N34 11.529
Mill Peak
W117 04.861

Exploration Trail

7300'
N34 12.373
W117 02.624

Keller Peak
7882'
N34 11.752
W117 02.970

To 210

trip 3.1 Deep Creek Hot Spring

Distance	4 miles (out-and-back)
Hiking Time	2 hours
Elevation Gain	900'
Difficulty	Moderate
Best Times	September–May
Agency	San Bernardino National Forest (Arrowhead Ranger Station)
Recommended Map	*Lake Arrowhead 7.5'*

see map on p. 64

DIRECTIONS From Interstate 15, 6 miles north of Cajon Pass in Hesperia, exit east on Main St. In 7.2 miles, bear left (east) on Rock Springs Rd. where Main Street curves south. Cross the dry bed of the Mojave River and follow Rock Springs Rd. east 2.8 miles to a junction where its name changes to Roundup Way. Continue east on Roundup Way for 4.4 miles, then turn right (south) onto the good dirt Bowen Ranch Rd. Stay right at a junction with Coxey Truck Tr. at 2.1 miles, and right again in 1.9 miles at a junction with Oak Springs Rd., then continue 1.4 miles to Bowen Ranch. Register at the ranch house and pay a modest use fee, then continue 0.5 mile through the ranch to the trailhead at the road's end on top of a hill.

High-clearance 4WD vehicles can reach an alternate trailhead a half mile closer, although the drive is slow enough that it is unlikely to save time. To reach this point, veer left onto Oak Springs Rd. at the junction mentioned above. In 1.4 miles, turn right onto a road signed JF3389 and pass through a gate. In 1.0 mile, stay right at a pair of junctions onto Forest Road 3N59A (marked JF3381 in some places). Drive 2.0 miles to a sign on the left for trail 3W02, which leads southwest to Deep Creek Hot Springs. 3N59A continues west and eventually joins an intricate maze of jeep trails that connect back to Bowen Ranch Rd., but navigation in this area is quite difficult.

Deep Creek Hot Spring

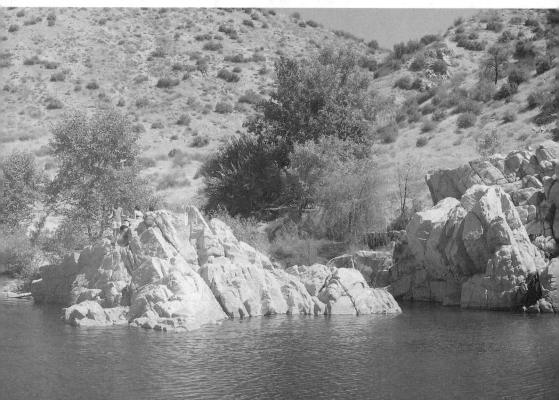

Deep Creek pours down a rugged canyon through the desert slopes of the San Bernardino Mountains before emptying into the Mojave River. The best hot spring in the range is found on the cliffs above Deep Creek; it pours through a series of pools down into the cool creek. This popular spot draws hikers to soak in the warm water during the winter and frolic in the creek on warmer days. Camping is allowed at the trailhead on Bowen Ranch but not at the hot spring. Do not bring glass, and take care to leave the place cleaner than you found it.

If you plan to do this hike in the summer, be aware that the trail leads across shadeless desert where temperatures commonly exceed 100°F. Bring plenty of water and remember that the return is all up hill. Avoid Deep Creek during thunderstorms because the narrow canyon presents a flash flood risk.

Follow the trail south, and then pass through a gate onto Forest Service land. In 0.5 mile, reach a junction with the 4WD road, 3N59A. This is the alternate starting point. Turn left, walk down the road 200 feet, and then turn right at another sign where trail 3W02 continues southwest. The next section of trail, nicknamed the Goat Trail, traverses onto a ridge that drops steeply down to Deep Creek. Turn left and walk upstream to a bend in the creek. There is a sandy beach on the north side, but you must ford the cold waters to reach the hot springs on the south side.

VARIATION

The hot springs can be reached from the Mojave River Forks Reservoir dam via a 6-mile hike up the Pacific Crest Trail (PCT). The dam is located 1 mile north of the junction of Arrowhead Lake Rd. and Highway 173 near Hesperia. The PCT crosses Deep Creek on an arched bridge, solving the problem of how to ford the cold, swift waters in the winter and spring.

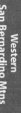

Western
San Bernardino Mtns

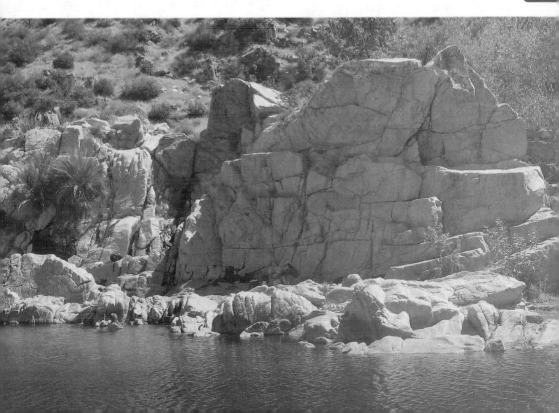

trip 3.2 Arrowhead Peak

Distance	4 miles (out-and-back)
Hiking Time	3 hours
Elevation Gain	1800'
Difficulty	Moderate
Trail Use	Dogs
Best Times	September–June
Agency	San Bernardino National Forest (Arrowhead Ranger Station)
Recommended Map	*San Bernardino North 7.5'*

see map on p. 64

DIRECTIONS From the 10 or 210 freeways in San Bernardino, exit north on Waterman Ave., which becomes the Rim of the World Highway (State Highway 18). As you drive through San Bernardino, you will see a signed historical marker on the right next to an athletic field. The marker offers a good view of the Arrowhead formation on the mountainside and an explanation of the legends behind the landmark. Continue up Highway 18 to the Crestline junction, then another 1.6 miles east. Park in a prominent turnout to the right of the highway at mile marker 19.45.

Looking north from San Bernardino, the outline of a huge arrowhead is emblazoned upon a hill called Arrowhead Peak. By further remarkable coincidence, the arrowhead points directly down to a hot spring at the foot of the mountains. Cahuilla Indian legend says that the arrowhead was shot from the sky by the God of Peace to point out a new homeland where the tribe could live safe from war-like neighbors. The pattern is created by a large area of granite rock just beneath the surface that prevents bigger plants from taking root. The small shrubs stand out in contrast to the greasewood and larger plants in the surrounding soil, giving the appearance of an arrowhead.

A series of health spas were built at the hot springs starting in the middle of the 19th Century. Today, the Campus Crusade for Christ owns the land and does not grant access to hikers. However, it is still possible to reach Arrowhead Peak from above by way of a trail coming down from Highway 18. The route is becoming overgrown, so long pants and sturdy boots are essential.

From the west end of the turnout, follow switchbacks down an eroded and overgrown old fire road to a saddle. The undulating trail veers right (west) through an oak grove to bypass a small hill, then continues right around the west shoulder of Peak 4422' overlooking Waterman Canyon. After another drop, the trail climbs steeply to the summit of Arrowhead Peak (4237'). Enjoy the view and return the way you came.

VARIATION

From the peak, adventurous hikers can descend the ridge to inspect the Arrowhead itself. This adds 0.7 mile and 800 feet of elevation change each way. A trail used to lead down this way, but few traces remain and the slopes are brushy in places. Hike cross-country to the south until you can follow a narrow ridge southeast to a prominent 3555-foot hill. The tip of the arrowhead is just below the hill. Unfortunately, the lower end of the trail is closed, so you must trudge back up the slope when you are through examining this geological oddity.

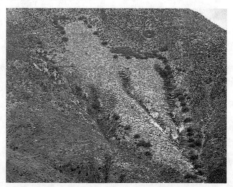

The Arrowhead

trip 3.3 Heart Rock

Distance	1 mile (out-and-back)
Hiking Time	1 hour
Elevation Gain	200'
Difficulty	Easy
Trail Use	Dogs, good for children
Best Times	All year, but waterfall is best in the spring
Agency	San Bernardino National Forest (Arrowhead Ranger Station)
Recommended Map	*Silverwood Lake 7.5'*

see map on p. 64

DIRECTIONS From the 10 or 210 freeways in San Bernardino, exit north on Waterman Ave., which becomes the Rim of the World Highway (State Highway 18). At the top of the ridge, exit onto Highway 138. Proceed north 1.2 miles to the stop sign in the middle of Crestline, and then continue 1.5 miles down to the Camp Seeley entrance road at mile marker 138 SBD 35.00. Turn left, then left again just outside the gate to Camp Seeley, and follow the narrow paved road across Seeley Creek to a gate, 0.4 mile from the highway. Park outside the gate on the right next to the 4W07 trail post.

The cool waters of Seeley Creek flow down the north slope of the San Bernardino Mountains beneath incense cedars and oaks. Through a fortuitous quirk of geology, they have carved a remarkable heart-shaped basin in the rock alongside a waterfall. Beyond, they rush down the granite slabs into an alluring pool. This short hike follows the bank of Seeley Creek to the Heart Rock overlook and the pool. The best times for this trip are in the spring when the waterfall is most dramatic and in the early summer when the water is tempting for a dip.

Follow the shady trail as it leads north from the parking area. Soon you will enjoy views of the creek as the trail follows above it. In 0.5 mile, look for an unmarked 3-way fork in the trail. From here, the route devolves into a maze of footpaths. To the right, descend a rocky path to a boulder overlooking Heart Rock and the waterfall. Keep a close eye on young children because the overlook is perched above a sheer cliff.

The path straight from the fork joins up with another path descending from the overlook to reach the base of the falls and a pleasant pool slightly farther downstream. This is a good place for a picnic. Unfortunately, thoughtless visitors leave their trash here; if you bring a garbage bag and pack out some of the litter, the site will be better for everyone.

The left fork leads back up to the paved road, which parallels the trail. However, the trail you arrived by is more scenic, so return the way you came.

Heart Rock

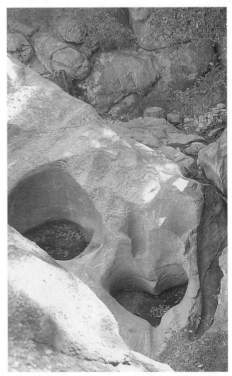

trip 3.4 The Pinnacles

Distance	3.5 miles (out-and-back)
Hiking Time	2.5 hours
Elevation Gain	1000'
Difficulty	Moderate
Trail Use	Dogs, good for children
Best Times	October–May
Agency	San Bernardino National Forest (Arrowhead Ranger Station)
Recommended Map	*Lake Arrowhead 7.5'*

see map on p. 64

DIRECTIONS From Lake Arrowhead, follow State Route 173 for 5 miles to the Rock Camp Forest Service Station, then continue 0.7 mile north to the Arrowhead Rifle Range. Park your vehicle off the highway on the east side.

The granite Pinnacles sit atop a hill on the desert slopes northwest of Lake Arrowhead. Rock climbers flock to the impressive boulders to test their skills. A trail leads to the high point, where you can scramble up some boulders for an outstanding view.

Walk through an opening in the fence and follow the southwest edge of the fenced rifle range. Then meander up a wash through chaparral and boulders until you can climb up the steep hill to the Pinnacles.

The most prominent tower to the north of the trail is called The Bong and features routes to challenge even the extreme rock climber (rated at 5.10–5.12). The trail continues to the summit boulder pile on the northwest end of the plateau. Some easy third-class scrambling is necessary to reach the airy perch.

Bong Rock *photo by Evan Harris*

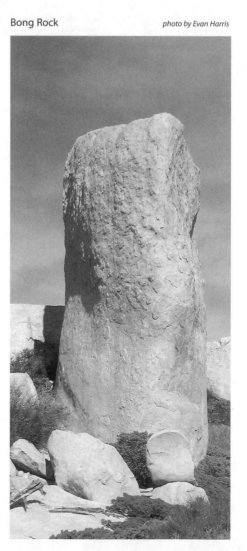

trip 3.5 Little Bear Creek

Distance	4 miles (out-and-back)
Hiking Time	3 hours
Elevation Gain	800'
Difficulty	Moderate
Trail Use	Dogs
Best Times	March–June, October–December
Agency	San Bernardino National Forest (Arrowhead Ranger Station)
Recommended Map	*Lake Arrowhead* 7.5' (inaccurate near North Shore Campground)

see map on p. 64

DIRECTIONS From State Highway 173, 2.8 miles northeast of the junction with Highway 189 at Lake Arrowhead Village, turn right (east) onto Hospital Rd. Follow the latter 0.25 mile to the North Shore Campground entrance, opposite the hospital. If you park in the campground you must pay the day-use fee. You can park for free in a small lot just outside the campground, but not in the hospital parking lot without permission. The campground amazingly escaped the 2003 Old Fire. As of this writing, the campground is open between May 1 and September 30.

If you wish to make an even shorter one-way trip with a car or bicycle shuttle, arrange a ride at the lower trailhead. (The bicycle shuttle involves significant elevation gain in both directions and is more strenuous than simply walking back up the trail.) To reach the lower trailhead, go back south on Highway 173 for 1.2 miles, then turn left (east) on Hook Creek Rd. Pass through the village of Cedar Glen for 2.3 miles to a gate at Forest Service Road 2N26Y. Continue 0.8 mile down the winding one-lane road and cross Hooks Creek. Look for a 3W12 trail marker on the left. If you reach a junction with 3N34 in 0.1 mile, you just missed the lower trailhead.

Little Bear Creek playfully rolls down the hill from Lake Arrowhead into Hooks Creek and onward into Deep Creek. It once cavorted beneath a delightful forest of pines, oaks, and incense cedars, but the 2003 Old Fire incinerated the entire canyon, along with countless cabins in Cedar Glen. Now, this hike is a sobering reminder of the power of wildfire and a fascinating opportunity to watch the forest regenerate itself.

The North Shore National Recreation Trail (3W12) begins at the far eastern end of the campground. It descends into a grove of black oaks, passing a spur leading over to a maintenance yard. In 0.1 mile, cross a dirt road and continue down along the north fork of Little Bear Creek. Follow the switchbacks down the hill and cross the tributary to reach a trail junction on the north bank of the main creek in 0.9 mile.

The right branch leads 0.1 mile to an alternate trailhead shaded under the cedars on Big Tree Dr., but this trip takes the left branch, which follows Little Bear Creek down the canyon past ghostly hulks of charred trees and through the manzanita, buckthorn, and other brush that comes first in the plant succession after fire. In 0.3 mile, climb 50 feet over a low ridge to bypass a bend in the creek. In another 0.7 mile, cross Little Bear Creek on a large log or some rocks and emerge at the 3W12 trailhead marker at the junction of Forest Roads 2N26Y and 3N34.

Return the way you came unless you have set up a car or bicycle shuttle.

Little Bear Creek

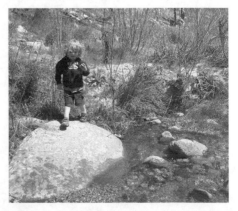

trip 3.6 Deep Creek

Distance	6 miles (out-and-back)
Hiking Time	3 hours
Elevation Gain	600'
Difficulty	Moderate
Trail Use	Dogs, suitable for backpacking
Best Times	March–June, October–November
Agency	San Bernardino National Forest (Arrowhead Ranger Station)
Recommended Map	*Lake Arrowhead, Butler Peak* 7.5'

see map on p. 64

DIRECTIONS From Highway 173 on the east shore of Lake Arrowhead, 1.6 miles northeast of the junction with Highway 189 at Lake Arrowhead Village, drive east on Hook Creek Rd through the village of Cedar Glen for 2.3 miles to a gate at Forest Service Road 2N26Y. Continue 0.8 mile down the winding one-lane road and cross Hooks Creek. Continue 0.1 mile on a good dirt road, then stay left at the junction with 3N34. Cross the creek again and make a right turn at 3N34C after 0.2 mile. Pass another gate and proceed 0.4 mile to the Splinters Cabin Trailhead where the hike begins. If the 3N34C gate is locked, park outside and walk from the gate, taking care not to block access.

Deep Creek carves a dramatic canyon through the desert slopes of the northern San Bernardino Mountains before emptying into the Mojave River. Although it flows through parched country, the creek and its many tributaries drain such a broad watershed that the water runs reliably year round. This hike follows a section of the PCT overlooking Deep Creek and then dips down to reach a pool.

The 2003 Old Fire wiped out the forest along the southern end of this hike and left only the chimneys of many cabins standing in Cedar Glen. A burning ponderosa pine fell and crushed the steel bridge across Deep Creek. The area is currently being rebuilt and the fire has not severely impacted the trail itself.

From the end of the road at the site of Splinters Cabin, look for a way to ford Hooks Creek to the north, then turn right and reach the PCT in 0.2 mile at the bridge over Deep Creek. Follow the PCT as it gently descends along the wall of the canyon. Pass the confluence with Holcomb Creek, and, in 3 miles, reach a jeep trail coming down

PCT Bridge over Deep Creek, still closed for repairs

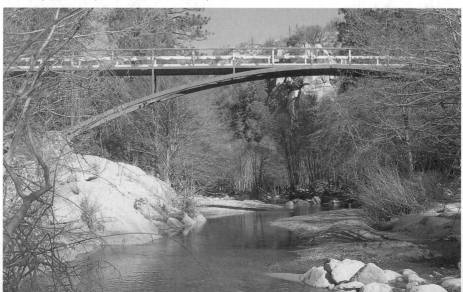

from Bacon Flats. Turn right and follow the path down to a large pool in Deep Creek.

ALTERNATIVE FINISH

Return the way you came. Alternatively, follow the jeep road (3N34D) up to Bacon Flats, then turn left and follow 3N34 back to the Splinters Cabin trailhead. This route is a mile longer but offers a change of scenery. Yet another option with a long car shuttle is to continue down the PCT 6.8 miles to Deep Creek Hot Springs and emerge at Bowen Ranch (see Trip 3.1).

VARIATION

If time permits, it is well worth visiting another beautiful nearby section of Deep Creek. Drive back to the junction of 3N34 and 2N26Y, then turn east on 3N34. The road is posted as 4WD, but the first part is usually passable by low-clearance vehicles. In 0.7 mile, reach a concrete bridge over Deep Creek and park on the far side. The section of Deep Creek leading upstream is one of the most rugged and beautiful streams in the San Bernardino Mountains, carving a course through granite cliffs. There is a fine sandy beach and you can explore along the ledges upstream for a short distance before the going gets difficult. 3N34 continues east, but promptly deteriorates into an extremely rocky and difficult jeep road with serious risk of body damage to stock SUVs.

trip 3.7 Fisherman's Camp

Distance	5 miles (out-and-back)
Hiking Time	3 hours
Elevation Gain	700'
Difficulty	Moderate
Trail Use	Equestrians, cyclists, dogs, suitable for backpacking
Best Times	March–November
Agency	San Bernardino National Forest (Arrowhead Ranger Station)
Recommended Map	*Butler Peak, Keller Peak 7.5'*

see
map on
p. 64

DIRECTIONS From the Rim of the World Highway (State Highway 18), 2.9 miles northeast of the intersection with Hwy 330 at the town of Running Springs and just past mile marker 018 SBD 34.50, turn left (north) onto Green Valley Rd. After 2.6 miles—just before you reach Green Valley Lake—turn left again onto Forest Road 3N16. Descend on this good dirt road toward Crab Flats Campground, passing several side roads and crossing Crab Creek (impassable in high water). Reach the junction with Big Pine Flat Rd. after 3.8 miles. Stay left on 3N34, passing Crab Flats Campground after 0.2 mile. Continue 1.1 mile along the deteriorating road to park at a clearing and large VISITORS TO DEEP CREEK sign near Tent Peg Group Camp.

Fisherman's Camp sits on the bank of Deep Creek in the rolling hills northwest of Green Valley. This trip involves an enjoyable tour of the backcountry roads and trails down to the rushing creek. It can be done as a day hike or an easy backpacking trip. Anglers should bring a rod and try their luck at coaxing the trout from their hiding spots. Note that all of Deep Creek is a Wild Trout Area (with a daily limit of two fish with a minimum size of 8 inches, and

use of bait and hooks with barbs is prohibited). As always, a valid California fishing license must be displayed by anyone fishing who is 16 years of age or older.

The Crab Creek Trail (2W07) leaves from the south side of the road. It passes through an area that was incinerated by the October 2007 Slide Fire. There is scarcely a trace of the Jeffrey and Coulter pines that once stood tall. The tough black oaks were also charred beyond recovery, but new green

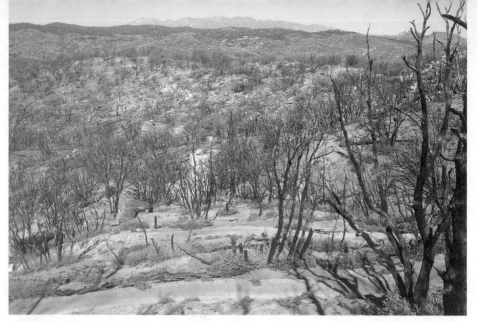
Aftermath of the Slide Fire at the Crab Creek Trail

shoots were already sprouting from the base of many oaks by the spring of 2008.

The trail climbs gently, and then contours west before switchbacking down the burnt slope. In 1.2 miles, the Crab Creek crossing marks the halfway point. Beyond, the trail becomes more gently graded and eventually reaches the bank of Deep Creek. Fisherman's Campground is a short distance upstream on the far side. Fording the stream can be dangerous during times of high water.

trip 3.8 Holcomb Crossing Trail Camp

Distance	5 miles (loop)
Hiking Time	3 hours
Elevation Gain	900′
Difficulty	Moderate
Trail Use	Equestrians, cyclists, dogs, suitable for backpacking
Best Times	March–June, September–November
Agency	San Bernardino National Forest (Arrowhead Ranger Station)
Recommended Map	*Butler Peak* 7.5′

see map on p. 64

DIRECTIONS From the Rim of the World Highway (State Highway 18), 2.9 miles northeast of the intersection with Hwy 330 in Running Springs and just past mile marker 018 SBD 34.50, turn left (north) onto Green Valley Rd. After 2.6 miles—just before you reach Green Valley Lake—turn left again onto Forest Road 3N16. Descend this good dirt road toward Crab Flats Campground, passing several side roads and crossing Crab Creek (impassable in high water). Reach the junction with Big Pine Flat Rd. after 3.8 miles. Stay left on 3N34, passing Crab Flats Campground after 0.2 mile, and park on the side of the road in another 0.3 mile.

The green forest meets the tawny desert on the north slopes of the San Bernardino Mountains. Holcomb Creek cuts a deep canyon through these slopes. This is an especially appealing part of the mountains, with tall pines, oaks, and cedars growing on the south side of Holcomb Creek. Growing on the sun-baked north side are pinyon pines, junipers, and desert scrub, while riparian woodland shades the stream bottom. Two trail camps are situated beneath shady pines on the banks of the creek. When the desert is sizzling and the high peaks are blanketed in snow, Holcomb Creek is an ideal destination for this hike or short backpacking trip. This area also attracts large numbers of offroaders and hunters, so the constant whine of engines and occasional crack of rifles interrupts the tranquility of the setting. Wear bright clothing so that you are easily visible.

This trip makes a loop, first following the dirt road west to Tent Peg Group Camp, then following a trail north down to the PCT. It then turns east on the PCT and follows Holcomb Creek to the trail camps before returning up a steep trail to where you parked. The return trail may not be obvious from the parking area, but don't worry—finding your vehicle will not be difficult.

Hike west along 3N34 for 0.8 mile to a large sign reading VISITORS TO DEEP CREEK near Tent Peg Group Camp. Look for the signed 2W08 trail leading north through the forest. Soon views open into the Holcomb Creek canyon below. The Willow Fire swept through this area in 1999 and evidence of the damage is still clearly visible.

In 1.5 miles, the trail ends at the PCT near the canyon bottom. Turn right (east) and walk upstream. In 0.6 mile, reach Bench Camp. In another 0.3 mile, pass ATV trail 1W17, leading back up to where you parked. Before taking it, however, continue another 0.3 mile on the PCT to Holcomb Crossing Trail Camp, shaded beneath the magnificent pines.

If time permits, consider exploring farther upstream along the PCT. When you are done, return to 1W17 and follow it southwest back to your vehicle.

Holcomb Creek

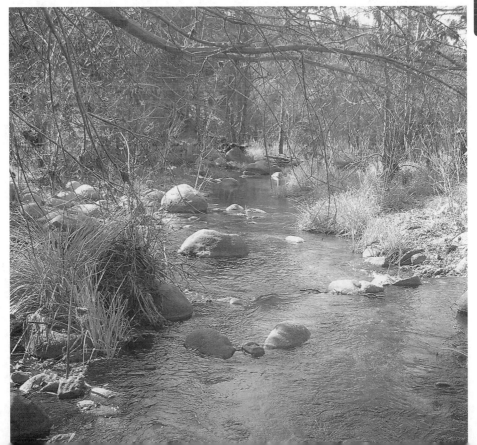

trip 3.9 Cox Creek

Distance	10 miles (out-and-back)
Hiking Time	5 hours
Elevation Gain	1100'
Difficulty	Moderate
Trail Use	Equestrians, dogs, suitable for backpacking
Best Times	September–May
Agency	San Bernardino National Forest (Arrowhead Ranger Station)
Recommended Map	*Butler Peak* 7.5'

see map on p. 64

DIRECTIONS From the Rim of the World Highway (State Highway 18), just past mile marker 018 SBD 34.50, turn left (north) onto Green Valley Rd. After 2.6 miles—just before you reach Green Valley—turn left again onto Crab Flats Rd (3N16). Descend on 3N16 for 3.8 miles, passing several small side roads and crossing Crab Creek, (impassable in high water) to a signed junction with 3N34. Stay right on 3N16 and proceed for 8.3 more miles northeast to Big Pine Flat, watching the transition from forest to desert vegetation. Then turn left (west) on the Coxey Truck Trail (3N14) and follow it 3.4 miles to Little Pine Flat. Turn left on Hawes Ranch Rd. (3N41) and park in the clearing outside the locked gate.

Alternatively, the trailhead can be reached from the north. From Interstate 15, 6 miles north of Cajon Pass, turn right (east) at the Hesperia exit. Follow Main Street east for 7.2 miles until it begins to curve south; then bear left (east) on Rock Springs Rd. Cross the Mojave River. In 3 miles, Rock Springs Rd. becomes Roundup Way. Continue 4.4 miles, then turn right (south) onto the good dirt Bowen Ranch Rd. In 2.1 miles, veer left at a BLM sign onto the good dirt Coxey Truck Trail (3N14). Follow this road as it climbs through the desert wonderland of Joshua trees and jumbo granite boulders, passing numerous side roads. In 9.3 miles, turn right on Hawes Ranch Rd. (3N41) and park in the clearing outside the locked gate.

The north slopes of the San Bernardino Mountains are visited more often by hunters and ATV riders than by hikers. However, this region offers seclusion and unique scenery in the transition zone between forest and desert. The drive to the trailhead is an enjoyable backroad experience in itself, exploring the maze of dirt roads that lace the range. An old path from Little Pine Flat leads past the defunct Hawes Ranch and down Cox Creek to its junction with Holcomb Creek. Two trail camps along Holcomb Creek make ideal destinations for an easy weekend backpacking trip. Be alert for hunters, especially during deer season in October and November. Large swaths of this area burned in the 1999 Willow Fire and this is a good place to watch nature regenerate. The trail is now unmaintained and starting to become overgrown in places because it receives little use, so long pants or gaiters may be helpful.

From Little Pine Flat, follow the gated jeep road south for 0.5 mile until it deteriorates into a trail. Continue along the upper reaches of Cox Creek and pass another stand of pines. Overhead you are likely to see numerous aircraft descending into the Los Angeles Basin because this trail is directly under Victor 283, one of the major airways used by jet traffic.

In another mile, descend a small slope and pass a clearing on your left where all

Hawes Ranch Trail

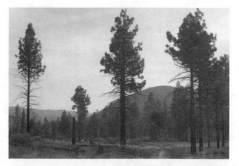

that remains of Hawes Ranch is a stone foundation and some barbed wire. Reach a signed junction 0.2 mile farther where Cox Creek begins to cut a deeper canyon. Trail 2W02 once led west toward Muddy Spring, but it has been obliterated by a jumble of downed trees left by the 1999 Willow Fire. Our route leads south on 2W14 (labeled 2W03 on the *Butler Peak* quadrangle).

The trail rounds the shoulder of Little Shay Mtn. and passes the bushy draw that marks Chipmunk Spring (no reliable water). Keep your eyes out for a small waterfall and some pools down in Cox Creek. In 2.6 miles, the trail crosses an ATV path, which is the best and most direct way down to Holcomb Creek. The former hiking trail, 2W14, turns west and contours above Holcomb Creek for some distance before descending, but it is overgrown and difficult to follow in places. On a warm day, Holcomb Creek invites you to relax in its cool waters. You can walk upstream to spend a night at the pleasant Holcomb Crossing Camp.

ALTERNATIVE FINISH

Just east of Holcomb Crossing Camp, another ATV trail climbs the ridge to Hawes Peak. If you choose to explore this route on your return, beware that the north and west sides of the peak have dense brush and trees, making for an awkward cross-country descent to Hawes Ranch or Little Pine Flat.

trip 3.10 Six Peaks of the Western San Bernardinos

Distance	15 miles (semi-loop)
Hiking Time	11 hours
Elevation Gain	5500′
Difficulty	Strenuous
Best Times	September–May
Agency	San Bernardino National Forest (Arrowhead Ranger Station)
Required Map	*Butler Peak* 7.5′

see map on p. 64

DIRECTIONS From the Rim of the World Highway (State Highway 18), just past mile marker 018 SBD 34.50, turn left (north) onto Green Valley Rd. After 2.6 miles—just before you reach Green Valley—turn left again onto Crab Flats Rd (3N16). Descend on 3N16 for 3.8 miles, passing several small side roads and crossing Crab Creek, (impassable in high water) to a signed junction with 3N34. Stay right on 3N16 and proceed for 8.3 more miles northeast to Big Pine Flat, watching the transition from forest to desert vegetation. Then turn left (west) on the Coxey Truck Trail (3N14) and follow it 3.4 miles to Little Pine Flat. Turn left on Hawes Ranch Rd. (3N41) and park in the clearing outside the locked gate.

Alternatively, the trailhead can be reached from the north. From Interstate 15, 6 miles north of Cajon Pass, turn right (east) at the Hesperia exit. Follow Main Street east for 7.2 miles until it begins to curve south; then bear left (east) on Rock Springs Rd. Cross the Mojave River. In 3 miles, Rock Springs Rd. becomes Roundup Way. Continue 4.4 miles, then turn right (south) onto the good dirt Bowen Ranch Rd. In 2.1 miles, veer left at a BLM sign onto the good dirt Coxey Truck Trail (3N14). Follow this road as it climbs through the desert wonderland of Joshua trees and jumbo granite boulders, passing numerous side roads. In 9.3 miles, turn right on Hawes Ranch Rd. (3N41) and park in the clearing outside the locked gate.

Six minor summits are clustered on the north slopes of the San Bernardino Mountains overlooking Holcomb and Deep Creeks and Little Pine Flat. These peaks are named Shay and Little Shay Mountains, Ingham Peak, Deer and Old Deer Mountains, and Hawes Peak. Shay and Little Shay are reportedly named for Art Shay, an early ranger at the Coxey Ranger Station. Hawes Peak was named for a 19th Century cattleman, possibly Francis Hawes, the founder of Hawes Ranch. Ingham Peak was named for Van Ingham, who worked for the Forest Service at the Fawnskin Ranger Station. It would hardly merit a name except that a forest fire happened on the peak in 1947 and the Forest Service needed a name for logistical purposes. Deer Mtn. is, of course, named for the plentiful mule deer that live in the vicinity. Peak 5805' was formerly called Deer Mtn. and is now informally known as Old Deer.

The region was badly burned in the 1999 Willow Fire and is presently littered with fallen dead trees. This is now a country of scrub oaks, yuccas, and beavertail cacti. Although this trip involves extensive cross-country navigation through difficult terrain to climb insignificant mountains, it is nevertheless rewarding to explore this remote corner of the mountains, enjoying solitude, expansive views, and a chance to watch the fire regeneration cycle in action. Visitors tend to love hiking here or hate it; few go away indifferent. The best time to come is in April or May when the wildflowers are in bloom. In deer season (October and November), beware of hunters who are drawn to these hills. The topographic map shows a number of springs in this area, but outside of the rainy season don't expect them to be running.

One way to visit all six peaks is to hike to the former site of Hawes Ranch, then climb Little Shay and Ingham Peaks. Return to a saddle northwest of Little Shay and follow the ridge to Shay Mtn. If you are feeling energetic, descend to a saddle near Muddy Springs, climb over Old Deer Mtn. to reach Deer Mtn., and fight your way back to Hawes Ranch. If you are still unsatisfied, climb the ridge to Hawes Peak before returning to Little Pine Flat. Many hikers will be satisfied by doing just one or a few of the summits. If you explore a different cross-country route than is mentioned here, you will find the going easier on the ridges than in the canyons because the ridges have less brush and fewer fallen trees.

Hikers returning toward Little Shay Mountain from Ingham Peak

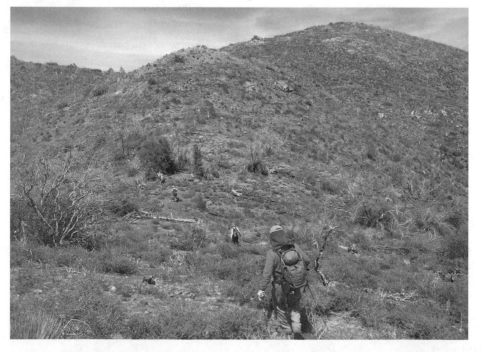

From Little Pine Flat, pass through the gate and hike south on an old jeep road. Several clusters of ponderosa and Jeffrey pines escaped the inferno and serve as a reminder of the former grandeur of the region. In 0.5 mile, the road deteriorates into a trail and passes another gate. It crosses some wetlands and more stands of pines. In 1.0 mile, descend a small slope and pass the site of Hawes Ranch in a clearing on your left. The ranch was founded around 1870. All that remains is a stone foundation and some barbed wire.

In 0.2 mile, reach a signed junction where Cox Creek begins to cut a deeper canyon leading south into Holcomb Creek. The unmaintained Hawes Ranch Trail (2W14) leads south to Holcomb Creek (see Trip 3.9). The Muddy Springs Trail (2W02) leads west, but it has been practically obliterated by fire and neglect.

To reach Little Shay Mtn., hike west on 2W02 for 0.1 mile. Leave the trail and hike cross-country 0.5 mile up the slope directly to the summit, following an old firebreak for much of the way.

To reach Ingham Peak from Little Shay, descend the west ridge 0.2 mile to a saddle. Turn left and hike 0.6 mile over two minor bumps to reach a third even less imposing bump, Ingham. Then return to the saddle.

Shay Mtn. is located to the northwest and can be recognized by the lone Coulter pine growing on the summit. To get there from the saddle west of Little Shay, follow the ridge west for 0.2 mile to another saddle. Trail 2W02 used to cross this saddle en route to Barrel and Muddy Springs. It was wiped out by fire, covered with downed trees, and is no longer maintained. Nature has completely reclaimed large swaths of the trail, but you may pick out a trace of it on the saddle. Continue northwest for 0.9 mile up the ridge to Shay Mtn.

Deer Mtn. is down in a hole near confluence of Deep and Holcomb creeks. Looking to the west from Shay Mtn., you can see a dirt airstrip at a ranch across Deep Creek.

The airstrip points directly at Deer Mtn. Study the scenery carefully to prepare for the cross-country route-finding. If you are ready for a tough slog through the burnt forest, follow the backbone of Shay Mtn. west for 0.7 mile until you can drop down a ridge on the south side for 0.5 mile directly to a rocky saddle where the Muddy Spring Trail once passed through. Climb southwest for 0.5 mile over two bumps studded with granite boulders, then up the ridge to Peak 5805′, informally known as Old Deer Mtn. Descend the ridge on the far side, taking care to stay left on the main ridge rather than getting lured down the face into the brush. Continue along the ridgeline 0.7 mile across another saddle and up to the summit of Deer Mtn.

Return to the rocky saddle. It was once possible to follow the Muddy Spring Trail 1.5 miles up to the saddle between Shay and Little Shay, then 1.1 miles down the canyon back to Hawes Ranch. The trail is in terrible condition and this route is now a tedious struggle through fallen trees and new brush. It is more straightforward to return to the summit of Shay Mtn. even though this involves more climbing. From Shay, it is possible to descend the east ridge to Hawes Ranch or choose a cross-country route northeast down the ridge to the Little Pine Flat Trailhead.

If you are still looking for more, continue on to Hawes Peak. The cleanest route climbs the west-northwest ridge from a point just south of Hawes Ranch. This involves fording Cox Creek and crossing an old barbed wire fence. Thread your way up the ridge through the scrub for 0.8 mile. An old fire break once led up the ridge, so the brush is not as dense. Just west of the summit, reach the dirt ATV track 1W17. Follow it east 0.2 mile to the summit. Then either retrace your steps to the trailhead or continue east along the ATV track for 0.2 mile to a point where you can pick a cross-country route directly back to Little Pine Flat, staying east of a row of low hills.

trip 3.11 Heaps Peak Arboretum

Distance	0.8 mile (loop)
Hiking Time	1 hour
Elevation Gain	100'
Difficulty	Easy
Trail Use	Good for children, handicapped accessible
Best Times	March–November
Agency	Rim of the World Interpretive Association
Optional Map	none

see map on p. 64

DIRECTIONS Heaps Peak Arboretum is located on the north side of Highway 18, 2 miles east of Highway 173 and 4.5 miles west of the junction with Highway 330 in Running Springs.

The Heaps Peak Arboretum is one of the best places to learn how to recognize trees commonly found in the San Bernardino Mountains. The handicapped-accessible trail makes a short loop through the forest, stopping at interpretive signs identifying Coulter and sugar pine, black oak, white fir, and incense cedar, and ending at a grove of giant sequoias. It is open year-round 24-hours a day, and is well worth a stop while driving between Lake Arrowhead and Big Bear. Volunteer staff are usually available on weekends from 11 A.M.–3 P.M. to answer questions.

Fred Heaps built a ranch near the site in the late 1800s. After a fire swept through the area in 1922, the Lake Arrowhead Women's Club and students from the elementary school replanted a diverse forest on the site. In the middle of the century, the land was abandoned and became an illegal dumping ground, but in 1982, volunteers led by George Hesemann restored the site and reestablished the arboretum. The 2003 Old Fire swept along the perimeter and thinned some of the seedlings, but left most of the trees healthier than ever.

Pamphlets available at the kiosk explain the numbered signs along the loop. Make a small donation if you choose to keep the pamphlet. The gently graded Sequoia Trail leads clockwise from the kiosk, passing the outhouse before making the pleasant loop.

trip 3.12 Exploration Trail

Distance	4.5 miles (one-way), or 9 miles (out-and-back)
Hiking Time	4 hours (out-and-back)
Elevation Gain	1300'
Difficulty	Moderate
Trail Use	Equestrians, cyclists, dogs
Best Times	April–November
Agency	San Bernardino National Forest (Arrowhead Ranger Station)
Recommended Map	*Keller Peak 7.5'*

see map on p. 64

DIRECTIONS From Highway 18 at a bend just east of Running Springs at mile marker 18 SBD 32.81, turn right (east) on Keller Peak Rd. and drive 0.1 mile. Park your vehicle at the signed Exploration Trail Trailhead on the right. If you want to make a one-way hike, leave another car or bicycle at the upper end of the trail, 4 miles up the paved Keller Peak Rd. The upper trailhead is on the right side just beyond a fork in the road; the left fork leads to the National Children's Forest Interpretive Trail (see Trip 3.13).

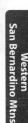

Western
San Bernardino Mtns

Conifer forest along the Exploration Trail

The Exploration Trail was completed in August 2005 as part of the Forest Service Centennial Project to celebrate the 100th birthday of the U.S. Forest Service. It parallels the Keller Peak Rd. through beautiful open oak and pine forest to the top of the road where the road meets the National Children's Forest Interpretive Trail. For an easier trip, follow the trail in reverse, downhill all the way. While you are in the area, consider visiting the historic Keller Peak Fire Lookout where volunteer firespotters may be able to give you a tour. The Keller Peak Rd. is an excellent route for cross-country skiing when the snow level is low enough.

Two trails depart from the lower trailhead; take the one on the right. The trail crosses Dry Creek, and then climbs alongside it for 0.6 mile through an open forest past huge granite boulders to a dirt road. Cross the road, then hike another 0.2 mile and cross a second road.

VARIATION

Mill Peak is located just south of this point, and you can make an easy detour up to the summit if you like. The jaunt adds a mile and 300 feet of elevation gain to your hike. To get there, turn right on the road, staying right at an immediate branch. In 0.4 mile, reach a gully on the north side of the peak, where you may see footprints. Hike up the last steep 0.1 mile to the top. The highest point is a boulder on the east lip of the peak. From here, you have expansive views down into the valley and out to the fire lookouts on Keller and Butler Peaks. Return the way you came.

The Exploration Trail continues climbing, roughly parallel to the Keller Peak Rd. but out of sight of traffic. It passes through fields of manzanita, then returns to open sugar pine forest and contours across the northwest slopes of Keller Peak to its upper terminus at the paved road.

trip 3.13 National Children's Forest Interpretive Trail

Distance	0.7 mile (semi-loop)
Hiking Time	30 minutes
Elevation Gain	100'
Difficulty	Easy
Trail Use	Good for children, handicapped accessible
Best Times	All year, but hot in summer
Agency	San Bernardino National Forest (Arrowhead Ranger Station)
Optional Map	none

see map on p. 64

DIRECTIONS From Highway 18, 1 mile east of Running Springs, consider stopping first at the Children's Forest Visitor Center, open Friday—Sunday, 9 A.M.–5 P.M. To reach the trailhead, continue east to a bend at mile marker 18 SBD 32.81, turn right (east) on the paved Keller Peak Rd., proceed 3.9 miles up the road, then turn left at a signed junction and go 0.1 mile to the Children's Forest parking area.

The National Children's Forest is home to youth programs in environmental education and leadership. It was established in 1970 after the Bear Fire burned 54,000 acres in the region. The Children's Forest has a staff of eight paid employees and over 200 volunteers who reach out to approximately 12,000 young people each year. The Interpretive Trail, redesigned by youth volunteers in 1993, is paved and accessible to wheel-chairs and strollers. The short loop, also called Trail of the Phoenix, leads through pines and manzanitas and offers views of the central San Bernardino Mountains.

The family-friendly and school class-friendly paved loop circles the chaparral and forest. A spur trail leads 0.2 mile up a gentle hill to a bench beneath a mature pine tree. Quiet and observant hikers are likely to encounter lizards, chipmunks, and birds.

Children's Forest Overlook

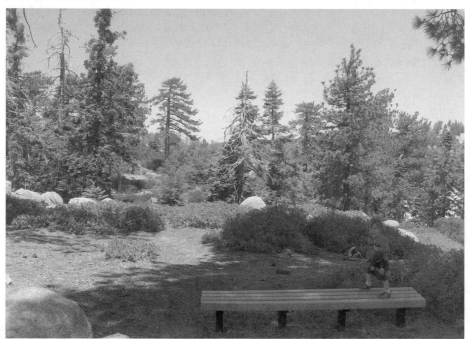

trip 3.14 Little Green Valley

Distance	2.5 miles (out-and-back)
Hiking Time	1.5 hours
Elevation Gain	700'
Difficulty	Moderate
Trail Use	Equestrians, cyclists, dogs
Best Times	April–November
Agency	San Bernardino National Forest (Arrowhead Ranger Station)
Recommended Map	*Keller Peak 7.5'*

see map on p. 64

DIRECTIONS Drive up the Rim of the World Highway (State Highway 18) to mile marker 038 SBD 37.24, 0.3 mile west of the Snow Valley parking area and 5 miles east of Running Springs. A dirt road forks left (north) to some cabins; turn up this road, then turn left immediately again and park in the clearing where you see the 2W10 GREEN VALLEY TRAIL sign.

Nestled on the ridge between Green Valley Lake and the Snow Valley Mountain Resort is a small meadow in Little Green Valley. The Little Green Valley Trail climbs from Highway 18 up to the meadow. Along the way, it passes an extensive network of roads and trails that are popular among mountain bikers and cross-country skiers. This short trip can be extended by returning via these trails or by continuing on to Green Valley Lake. This is a particularly beautiful area in the autumn when the black oaks are losing their leaves.

In October 2007, much of Southern California was up in flames. Twenty major fires raged across the state from Malibu to San Diego, fed by drought and unusually strong winds. The Slide Fire burned 12,000 acres and 200 homes in this area. It cleared the brush and some small trees

Lush forest along the Little Green Valley Trail

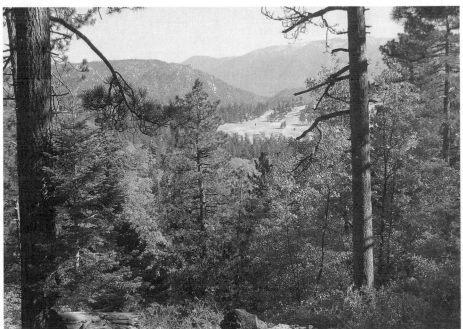

Western
San Bernardino Mtns

near Little Green Valley, but left most of the mature trees intact. Unfortunately, the same fire completely incinerated the forest farther north, including massive pines that had stood there since before the American Revolution.

Hike up the trail (2W10) northwest, crossing a small brook. In 0.2 mile, reach a dirt road. Turn right on the dirt road, go a few yards, then turn left and rejoin the trail on the other side. In another 0.4 mile, the trail crosses the road again. Beyond, the steepening trail follows switchbacks through the lightly burned zone.

In 0.4 mile, reach an unmarked and easily missed junction near some power lines. A bicycle trail forks off to the right and starts descending, while the main trail continues up along the power lines. This area might change as the Forest Service cleans up the fire damage; with luck the trail will become better marked.

Stay left and continue 0.1 mile up to the top of the ridge, where you reach Little Green Valley. This is a good spot to have a snack and enjoy the wildflowers. Beware of snakes in the tall grass. You have several options from here that are explained in the following paragraphs. You can return the way you came. You can continue on to Green Valley Lake. Or you can return on the bicycle trail.

ALTERNATIVE FINISH —————————————————

To reach Green Valley Lake, you cross the lower end of the meadow and the creek to reach Forest Road 2N19A. The path across the meadow can be indistinct, but the road picks up near the power lines. This road soon joins the main road, 2N19. Turn right and follow it 1.4 miles to the end of Meadow Lane in the resort town of Green Valley Lake. There are numerous unmarked roads forking off of 2N19, and the roads are changing because of logging. Try staying on what appears to be the main road, but navigation can be challenging.

A better option is to make a return loop on the south side of Little Green Valley. This is a popular area for bicycle races and you may be able to follow the arrows marking the racecourse. Return to the unmarked junction that you passed earlier just below Little Green Valley and turn east. The trail contours along the hillside, then crosses the North Fork of Deep Creek before reaching a hairpin turn on Forest Road 2N64 in 1.3 miles. Turn right on Forest Rod 2N64 and follow the road 0.8 mile down to Highway 18 by Lake View Point. Just before reaching the highway, turn right onto another single-track bicycle trail. This area is a maze with countless forks and variations, but as long as you pick a path that leads downhill and doesn't cross Highway 18, you'll eventually find your way back to the trailhead in less than 2 miles, making this a 5-mile loop. If you feel completely disoriented, hike downhill to the highway and follow it down instead.

chapter 4

Big Bear Lake Area

The San Bernardino Mountains are part of California's unusual Transverse Ranges, which run east to west rather than north to south. They have long attracted the attention of humans, at first for hunting, logging, and gold, but now primarily for recreation. The range is so large that trips for this area are divided the trails into three chapters. This chapter focuses on the eastern end, where richly forested hills circle the jewel-like Big Bear Lake. Chapter 3 describes the western end, especially around Lake Arrowhead and the alluring creeks at the interface of forest and desert. Chapter 5 explores the steep and rugged San Gorgonio Wilderness on the southeast side of the range, cut off from Big Bear by the deep trench of the Santa Ana River.

When ranchers, loggers, and miners first explored the San Bernardino Mountains, they found a long alpine meadow tucked between two ridges at the head of a creek. A seasonal lake, now called Baldwin Lake, sat at the east end of the valley. Benjamin Wilson and his posse stormed into the valley in 1845 in pursuit of Indians who had been rustling cattle from ranches in Riverside. Instead of locating the marauders, Wilson's gang discovered swarms of grizzly bears. He later wrote of the experience: "Twenty-two Californians went out in pairs, and each pair lassoed one bear, and brought the result to camp, so that we had at one and the same time eleven bears. That prompted me to give the Lake the name it now bears." Wilson's story didn't end here; he went on to become the first mayor of Los Angeles, a California state senator, and a wealthy philanthropist.

Big Bear Lake, as we know it, didn't exist at the time Wilson named it. In 1884, citrus ranchers in Redlands began to build a dam

Big Bear Lake

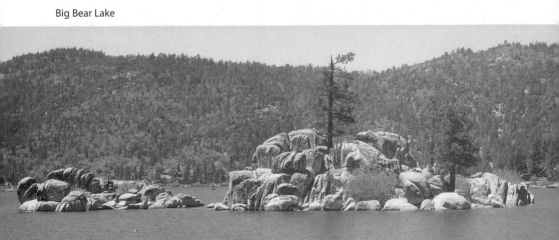

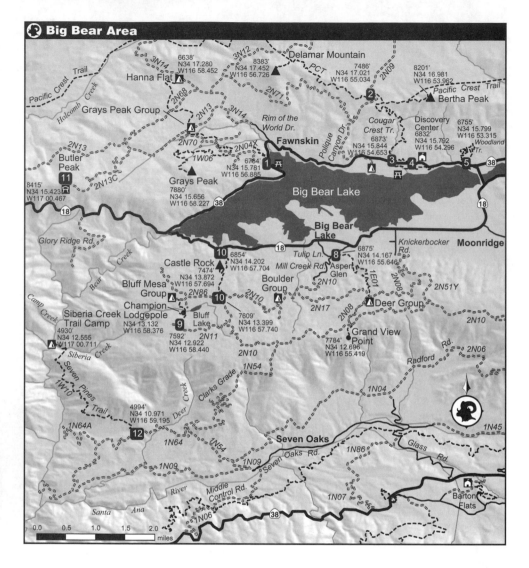

Big Bear Area

across the mouth of Bear Valley to create a reservoir. In 1910, the dam was expanded to its present height, forming, at the time, the world's largest man-made lake.

Hunters flocked to the San Bernardino Mountains in search of grizzly pelts. By 1906, the majestic beast was hunted to extinction in this range. In 1860, while tracking a wounded grizzly, Bill Holcomb discovered gold. Miners flocked to the valley north of Big Bear, which became known as Holcomb Valley, and soon a boomtown

of 2000 sprung up, becoming the most populous place in San Bernardino County. Within two years, it became evident that the visions of riches were overblown and the prospectors drifted away. The colorful Elias "Lucky" Baldwin started a second boom in 1874 at the nearby Gold Mtn., but it, too, proved disappointing.

Although gold prospectors were disappointed, entrepreneurs soon realized the economic potential in harvesting the rich forestlands for lumber. Approximately twenty-two sawmills were built in the vicinity of Big Bear. The intensive timber harvesting proved unsustainable and the environmental catastrophes that followed led President Roosevelt to establish a reserve in 1906 to protect the remaining forests in the San Bernardino Mountains.

In the first part of the 20th Century, winter sports enthusiasts began developing the slopes around the lake. By the 1950s and 1960s, skiing became a big business, and now Big Bear is best known among Southern Californians for the ski slopes. In the 1940s, developers pushed hard to establish a massive downhill ski area in the San Gorgonio wilderness south of Big Bear. Conservationists put up a fierce battle and ultimately prevailed when Chief Forester Lyle Watts ruled that the mountains had "a higher public value as a wilderness and a watershed than as a downhill ski area."

Threats of development continue to resurface from time to time.

Big Bear is now a popular mountain resort community. Skiers and snowboarders flock to the lifts during the winter, while boaters and anglers come in droves during the summer. The community of Big Bear Lake on the south side along Highway 18 offers every amenity that a visitor might desire. The ridges on all sides are laced with easy and moderate trails to tempt hikers up from the lake to the refreshingly cool ridges of the mountains.

Cross-country skiers enjoy the dirt roads around Big Bear in the winter. Some particularly suitable roads include 2N93 to Wildhorse Meadow, with great views of San Gorgonio, Polique Canyon Rd. (2N09) near Fawnskin, and the gently graded Van Dusen Canyon Rd. (3N09).

trip 4.1 Grays Peak

Distance	7 miles (out-and-back)	
Hiking Time	3 hours	
Elevation Gain	1200′	
Difficulty	Moderate	
Trail Use	Equestrians, cyclists, dogs	
Best Times	May–October	
Agency	San Bernardino National Forest (Big Bear Discovery Center)	
Recommended Map	*Fawnskin 7.5′*	

see map on p. 86

DIRECTIONS Follow State Highway 38 along the north shore of Big Bear Lake to the Grays Peak parking area just west of mile marker 038 SBD 56.41, 2.7 miles northeast of Big Bear Dam, or half a mile southwest of Fawnskin. There are restrooms and picnic tables here, and many spaces for parking.

Grays Peak is named for Alex Gray, who founded Gray's Landing on the north shore of Big Bear Lake in 1918. The 7952-foot summit is heavily forested, making for an enjoyable walk through the woods. This is one of the most popular moderate hikes in the Big Bear area and you should expect to have plenty of company on a pleasant summer day. The trailhead is in winter habitat for bald eagles and is closed from November 1 to April 1.

From the signed trailhead, follow the trail north overlooking the highway and Grout Bay. The trail soon begins switchbacking northwest up the Jeffrey pine, white fir, and black oak clad slopes. After cresting the low ridge, it abruptly turns left and reaches Forest Road 2N04X in 0.7 mile. Turn right. In 0.3 mile, turn right again at a T-junction with Forest Road 2N70.

In 0.1 mile, reach a sign on the left (south) for the Grays Peak Trail. Take this trail as it climbs through the forest. The Butler 2 Fire burned 14,000 acres on the northwest side of Big Bear Lake in September 2007. It singed the northwest side of Grays Peak and incinerated most of the forest around Hanna Flat and Butler Peak. You'll have occasional glimpses through the trees down to the lake below. After 2 miles of climbing, the trail circles around the summit and ends 100 feet below the top. You will have to scramble through buckthorns and over fallen logs if you wish to reach the true high point.

VARIATION

Grays Peak can also be reached from Grays Peak Group Camp. A 1.4-mile trail leads east from the camp to a point immediately northwest of the junction of the Grays Peak Trail with Forest Road 2N70. Pick up the Grays Peak Trail on the south side of 2N70 and follow the directions above for two miles to the summit.

A 1.5-mile trail also connects Grays Peak Group Camp to Hanna Flat Campground.

trip 4.2 Delamar Mtn.

Distance	5.5 miles (out-and-back)
Hiking Time	3 hours
Elevation Gain	1000'
Difficulty	Moderate
Trail Use	Dogs
Best Times	May–October
Agency	San Bernardino National Forest (Big Bear Discovery Center)
Recommended Map	*Fawnskin* 7.5'

see map on p. 86

DIRECTIONS From State Highway 38, 2 miles east of Fawnskin at mile marker 038 SBD 54.04, turn north onto the good dirt Polique Canyon Rd. (2N09). At a fork in 1.5 miles with 2N71, stay right on 2N09 toward Holcomb Valley. Continue 0.8 mile to the top of the divide, where you will see the signed Holcomb View Trail, part of the Pacific Crest Trail. Park here or on the side of the road where it becomes wider just beyond.

Delamar Mtn. (8398') is the high point on the ridge between Big Bear Lake and Holcomb Valley. The summit boulders stand clear of the dense forest, granting

Big Bear Lake and San Gorgonio Mtn. from Delamar Mtn.

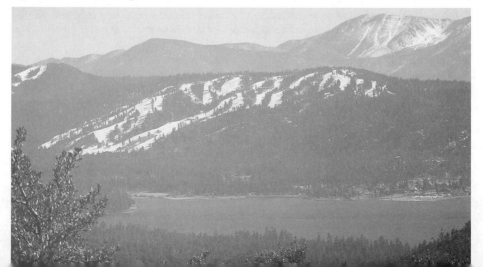

panoramic views in all directions. This trip reaches the mountain from the east by way of the Pacific Crest Trail (PCT).

Hike west along the PCT through the open forest of pines, oaks, and firs. In 1.5 miles, the trail crosses to the north side of the ridge, where snow may sometimes linger late in the spring. The trail continues for 0.5 mile, then begins a steady descent. At the point where the trail begins to descend, turn left and hike cross-country up the steep slope to the granite summit boulders. There is an even better view of Big Bear Lake from a lower summit 100 yards south. Return the way you came.

ALTERNATIVE FINISH

Alternatively, the PCT intersects Forest Road 3N12 just west of where you left the trail. With a car or bicycle shuttle, you can descend to the road and loop back to the start. From the junction of the PCT with 3N12, go west and then southwest 1.2 miles on 3N12. Turn left on 2N71 and follow it east around the south side of Delamar Mtn. for 4.2 miles back to Polique Canyon Rd. Turn left again and go 0.7 mile north to the initial trailhead.

---

trip 4.3 Cougar Crest (and Bertha Peak)

Distance	5 or 7 miles (out-and-back)
Hiking Time	2.5–4 hours
Elevation Gain	600' or 1400'
Difficulty	Moderate
Trail Use	Equestrians, dogs, good for children (to Cougar Crest)
Best Times	April–November
Agency	San Bernardino National Forest (Big Bear Discovery Center)
Recommended Map	Fawnskin 7.5'

see map on p. 86

Big Bear Lake Area

DIRECTIONS This trail starts half a mile west of the Big Bear Discovery Center on Highway 38 on the north shore of Big Bear Lake near mile marker 038 SBD 53.50.

A thousand-foot-tall forested ridge separates Big Bear Lake from Holcomb Valley to the north. The Cougar Crest Trail climbs from the north shore of Big Bear Lake up to a low point on this ridge, where it meets the Pacific Crest Trail. The Cougar Crest Trail offers a family-friendly hike through the forest, with occasional views down to the lake and across to the San Gorgonio Wilderness. It is extremely popular on the weekends, so do not expect to find solitude here. Peak baggers may choose to continue farther to Bertha Peak, though dense forest obscures the views from the summit and a cluster of antennas detracts from the natural ambience.

From the north end of the large parking lot, hike north up the wide trail (1E22) through a forest of pines, cedars, and western junipers. Small stands of manzanitas dot the open forest floor. Shortly after leaving the trailhead, pass a side trail leading east to the Big Bear Discovery Center (see Trip 4.4). The Cougar Crest trail climbs gradually but steadily. Look for the antenna-studded Bertha Peak to the north. In 2 miles, shortly before reaching the crest, look out for the best views back over the lake. Also, you can make out the fire lookout dramatically situated atop Butler Peak to the west. After crossing the first crest, the trail turns east and in another 0.3 mile reaches a signed junction with the PCT. There are some magnificent pinyon pines near this junction. Most hikers turn back here.

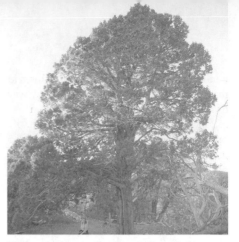

VARIATIONS

To reach Bertha Peak, turn right (east) and follow the PCT 0.5 mile to its junction with a road on the ridge. Continue east up this steep service road to the antennas atop Bertha Peak. This adds 800 feet of elevation gain and 1.3 miles each way.

Alternative trailheads for Bertha Peak include Polique Canyon Rd. (see Trip 4.2) and Van Dusen Canyon Rd. at their intersections with the PCT.

Western juniper on the Cougar Crest Trail

trip 4.4 Alpine Pedal Path

Distance	up to 4 miles (semi-loop)
Hiking Time	2 hours
Elevation Gain	200'
Difficulty	Easy
Trail Use	Dogs, cyclists, good for children, handicapped accessible
Best Times	April–November
Agency	San Bernardino National Forest (Big Bear Discovery Center)
Optional Map	*Fawnskin 7.5'*

see map on p. 86

DIRECTIONS This trail starts at the Big Bear Discovery Center on Highway 38 on the north shore of the lake just west of mile marker 038 SBD 53.00. The gate at the parking area closes early (5 P.M. in the summer), so park outside if you will not be back in time.

A flat trail along the north shore of Big Bear Lake links the Big Bear Discovery Center, popular Cougar Crest Trail, Serrano Campground, and Meadows Edge Picnic Area. Though this trail isn't much of a destination in itself, it makes for a pleasant excursion on foot or bicycle for those visiting the area. It is also accessible to strollers and wheelchairs.

The trail begins at the bicycle racks in front of the Discovery Center and leads west through a forest of Western junipers and pinyon pines for 0.5 mile to a junction with the Cougar Crest Trail (see Trip 4.3).

Sugarloaf Mtn. and the Big Bear ski areas from the Alpine Pedal Path

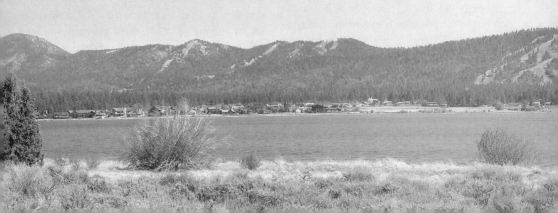

It descends to the Cougar Crest parking lot, and then crosses under Highway 38 to a junction in another 0.2 mile. Turn right to reach the Serrano Campground, but the main trail turns left (east) and leads 0.4 mile through more junipers and pines to the Meadows Edge Picnic Area on the shore of Big Bear Lake, where you can enjoy views of the ski areas on the ridge to the south and of Sugarloaf Mtn. to the southeast. It continues 1.2 miles along the shore of the lake to the eastern terminus at the Stanfield Cutoff bridge.

On the return, when you reach Meadows Edge, you can take a shortcut back by following the access road up to Highway 38 just west of the Discovery Center.

trip 4.5 Woodland Trail

Distance	1.7 miles (loop)
Hiking Time	1 hour
Elevation Gain	300'
Difficulty	Easy
Trail Use	Good for children
Best Times	April–November
Agency	San Bernardino National Forest (Big Bear Discovery Center)
Optional Map	*Fawnskin* 7.5' (trail not shown)

see map on p. 86

DIRECTIONS This trailhead is located on the north shore of Big Bear Lake off Highway 38 immediately opposite the East Boat Ramp. It is one mile east of the Big Bear Discovery Center at mile marker 038 SBD 52.11.

The Woodland Nature Trail tours a particularly fine portion of the forest on the north shore of Big Bear Lake in the transition region between the conifer and pinyon-juniper zones of the San Bernardino Mountains. The trail was constructed by volunteers in 1986, and features 20 numbered posts around the loop. Pick up a brochure at the trailhead, which provides historic, botanical, and geological information keyed to the sign posts. The Woodland Trail is ideal for families with young children looking for a good place to take a walk while visiting the Big Bear area.

The signed trail starts on the east side of the large parking area. It makes a counterclockwise loop. Watch for the Western juniper trees. Unlike their bush-like brethren common in the desert, the Western juniper stands tall and is sometimes confused with incense cedar. However, they are readily recognized as junipers by their characteristic needles. As you proceed, watch for oaks, stately 400-year-old Jeffrey pines, and pinyon pines. There are also good views of Big Bear Lake and the ski areas on the far side.

Boulders along Woodland Trail

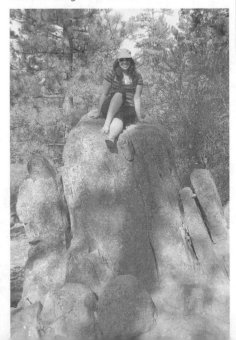

Big Bear Lake Area

trip 4.6 Sugarloaf Mtn.

Distance	7 miles (out-and-back)
Hiking Time	4 hours
Elevation Gain	1300'
Difficulty	Moderate
Trail Use	Equestrians, cyclists, dogs, suitable for backpacking (but no water available)
Best Times	May–October
Agency	San Bernardino National Forest (Big Bear Discovery Center)
Recommended Map	*Moonridge* 7.5'

[handwritten: 6.15 miles / strenuous (!) 3 miles of climb rock trail / marked trees]

DIRECTIONS From Redlands, drive east on State Highway 38 through Barton Flats to the beginning of Forest Road 2N93 near mile marker 038 SBD 35.7. The fair dirt road is easy to pass by, so keep a sharp eye out for it on your left (north) immediately past a small wash. Drive 5.5 miles up Forest Road 2N93 to Wildhorse Meadows. Continue up 2N93 0.6 mile beyond the meadow, to a fork on your left with a gated jeep road (again, easy to miss). Park your vehicle at the clearing on the east side of 2N93.

Alternatively, the trailhead can be reached from the north. From Highway 38, 3 miles southeast of Big Bear City near mile marker 038 SBD 45.75, drive 5.6 miles up 2N93 to a fork on your right.

The rounded Sugarloaf Mtn. (9952') is the tallest summit in the San Bernardino Mountains outside the San Gorgonio Wilderness. Located at the interface of two vegetation zones, it supports both the rich forests of Jeffrey pines and white firs common in the San Bernardino high country, and the juniper and pinyon pine woodland of the desert slopes. In late August and early September, lucky hikers may see the rare black swallowtail butterfly (*Papilo bairdi*). A forest service road leads high onto the shoulder of the mountain. This hike takes advantage of the road and follows the easiest path up the east ridge to the summit.

Hike west through a wooden gate immediately left of the gated road and follow

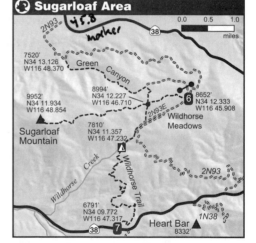

Sugarloaf Area

Sugarloaf Mtn. from the San Bernardino Divide

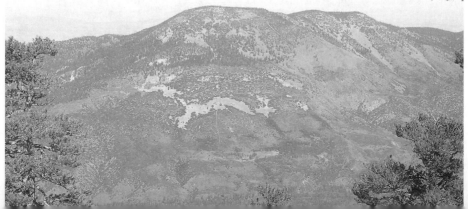

the ducked (ducks are rock piles marking the trail) path up onto the ridge. This area is home to some of the largest Western junipers in California. Unlike the bush-like California junipers found in the Mojave Desert, the Western junipers are mighty trees with reddish rope-like bark. The pines in this part of the forest are mostly ponderosas, rather than the similar looking Jeffreys, as you can tell by the smaller cones.

From the gated jeep road come to a trail junction in 0.9 mile. The right fork leads down Green Canyon to a lower trailhead on Forest Road 2N93 and the left fork leads down to Wildhorse Creek, but this hike continues straight along the ridge. In 1.5 miles, reach bump 9775′. Descend to a saddle, then climb again, reaching the cairn on top of Sugarloaf Mtn. in 1 more mile after the bump.

trip 4.7 Wildhorse Creek

Distance	8 miles (out-and-back)
Hiking Time	4 hours
Elevation Gain	1400′
Difficulty	Moderate
Trail Use	Equestrians, dogs, cyclists, suitable for backpacking
Best Times	April–October
Agency	San Bernardino National Forest (Big Bear Discovery Center)
Recommended Map	*Moonridge 7.5′*

see map on p. 92

DIRECTIONS From Redlands drive east on State Highway 38 to the turnoff of the Wildhorse Trail, on your left just before mile marker 038 SBD 33.40 and 0.2 mile before the Heart Bar Campground Rd. Turn left (north) and drive about 20 yards up a dirt road to a signed parking area.

Wildhorse Creek carves a canyon along a fault line down from the shoulder of Sugarloaf Mtn. The well-built Wildhorse Trail switchback takes you up to Wildhorse Creek Trail Camp, located at a spring near the top of the creek. This is an enjoyable backpacking trip or dayhike in the spring when San Gorgonio is clad in deep snow, and also in the summer when San Gorgonio permits are difficult to obtain.

The first mile of the Wildhorse Trail is an old logging road. It climbs through Jeffrey pines, pinyons, and junipers. The trail switchbacks take you onward for 2 miles and views steadily improve as you ascend. The last mile passes around a bump on the ridge and descends into the richly forested Wildhorse Creek, where you will find the trail camp in a clearing beside the stream beneath Jeffrey pines. Water is usually available in the creek.

Wildhorse Trail Camp

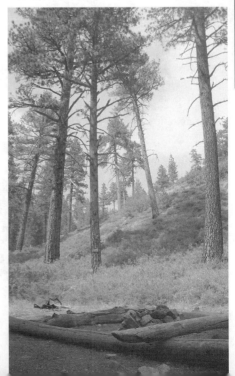

Big Bear Lake Area

If you want a longer hike or a side trip after camping, the Wildhorse Trail continues up the canyon on the opposite side of the creek. You can take it to Wildhorse Meadow or all the way to Sugarloaf Mtn. This part of the trail is steep, but your efforts are rewarded by wild roses, Indian paintbrush, spectacular Western juniper trees, and the meadow full of ferns and corn lilies. In 0.7 mile, the trail reaches an old closed jeep track (2N93E) that follows the west side of Wildhorse Meadow. In another 0.2 mile up the road, a trail on the left is marked with a sign reading Sugarloaf Mountain. This trail climbs 0.4 mile to the four-way junction on the Sugarloaf Trail. From here, you can turn left and hike another 2.5 miles to the summit.

Return the way you came. An old trail once descended Wildhorse Creek, but it crossed private property. The Forest Service has closed the trail and allowed it to return to nature.

trip 4.8 Grand View Point

Distance	6.5 miles (out-and-back)
Hiking Time	3 hours
Elevation Gain	1100'
Difficulty	Moderate
Trail Use	Dogs, cyclists; equestrians permitted but not recommended
Best Times	May–October
Agency	San Bernardino National Forest (Big Bear Discovery Center)
Recommended Map	*Big Bear Lake* 7.5' (not all trails and roads shown)

see map on p. 86

DIRECTIONS From the west end of Big Bear Lake Village at mile marker 018 SBD 47.45, where a sign points to Mill Creek Rd. and picnic grounds, turn south onto Tulip Lane. Proceed 0.5 mile to the Aspen Glen Picnic Area on your right.

Grand View Point, high on the ridge above Big Bear Lake, offers an unobstructed view across the Santa Ana River Canyon to the tall summits of the San Gorgonio Wilderness. A somewhat confusing network of trails leads up from the Aspen Glen picnic area to the point. Go on a clear day when you can fully appreciate the

Hikers approaching Grand View Point

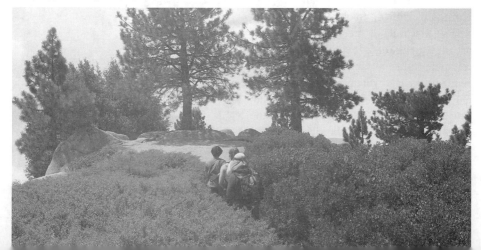

vistas. This whole ridge south of Big Bear is popular among mountain bikers.

Follow the Pineknot Trail (1E01) from the east end of the parking area. In 100 yards, stay left at a fork and follow the trail over a rise and down into a willow-choked draw. Stay right at a second trail junction and follow the broad path up the draw, then across the creek, beneath the shade of the Jeffrey pines, white firs, and black oaks.

After crossing Forest Road 2N08, the trail levels out, passes Deer Group Camp, and parallels 2N08 to reach Forest Road 2N10 at the top of the ridge. Cross the road and follow the signed trail 0.3 mile southeast to the open summit of Grand View Point.

Return the way you came, or pre-position mountain bikes on 2N10 for an exhilarating ride down the dirt roads.

trip 4.9 Champion Lodgepole

Distance	0.6 mile (out-and-back)
Hiking Time	30 minutes
Elevation Gain	50'
Difficulty	Easy
Trail Use	Dogs, equestrians, cyclists, good for children
Best Times	June–October
Agency	San Bernardino National Forest (Big Bear Discovery Center)
Optional Map	*Big Bear Lake 7.5'*

see map on p. 86

DIRECTIONS From the west end of Big Bear Lake Village at mile marker 018 SBD 47.45, a sign points to Mill Creek Rd. and picnic grounds, turn south onto Tulip Lane. Proceed 0.4 mile, then turn right on Mill Creek Rd., which becomes good dirt Forest Service Road 2N10 in 0.7 mile. Proceed 3.8 miles, then turn right on 2N11 at a sign pointing to Champion Lodgepole. Proceed 1.0 mile to a signed parking area on the right for the Lodgepole Pine Trail (1W11).

Lodgepole pines (*Pinus contorta*) are so named because saplings were used by Native Americans to build their dwellings. Also known as tamarack pines, they are common in the Sierra Nevada and also live above 8000 feet in the cool upper reaches of the San Gorgonio Wilderness. Lodgepole pines are easily recognized by their thin gray scaly bark, golf ball-sized cones, and pairs of needles. A small stand of lodgepoles, likely left over from a colder bygone era, can be found perched on Bluff Mesa at about 7600 feet. One of these, a double-trunked behemoth, is the largest known lodgepole in the world. It stands 110 feet tall and is 20 feet in circumference. Biologists estimate that the Champion germinated in 1560, four years before Shakespeare's birth. It is reached by way of a scenic drive on a good dirt road followed by a short nature walk.

Champion Lodgepole Pine

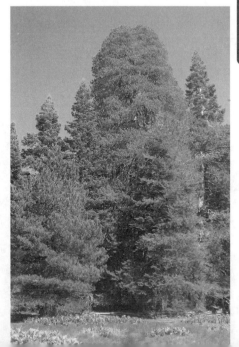

Look for an interpretive pamphlet at the trailhead. Fourteen numbered posts point out features along the route that are explained in the pamphlet. The trail (1W11) leads down along a seasonal creek through a forest of white firs and Jeffrey pines. It then curves left and comes to a fork in 0.3 mile. The left fork is the Siberia Creek Trail, which once led 7 miles down to Siberia Creek Trail Camp (see Trip 4.12), but which has not been maintained in some time. Stay right and promptly arrive at the Champion Lodgepole beside a lush meadow. The Forest Service has fenced off the tree; keep your distance so that the Champion is not loved to death.

Return the way you came.

VARIATIONS

Alternatively, you can explore the trail as it continues north 0.4 mile to Forest Road 2N86A just east of Bluff Mesa Group Camp, or you can wander west along the Siberia Creek Trail until it drops off the edge of Bluff Mesa at Gunsight Notch.

trip 4.10 Castle Rock

Distance	1.6 mile (out-and-back)
Hiking Time	1.5 hours
Elevation Gain	700'
Difficulty	Moderate
Trail Use	Dogs, good for children
Best Times	May–October
Agency	San Bernardino National Forest (Big Bear Discovery Center)
Recommended Map	*Big Bear Lake* 7.5' (note: this map incorrectly shows the trail climbing west of Castle Rock)

see map on p. 86

DIRECTIONS From State Highway 18 across from mile marker 018 SBD 45.50, 1.2 miles east of Big Bear dam, or 3 miles west of Big Bear Lake Village, the marked trail 1W03 starts up a forested gully. Park 100 yards east of the trailhead in a clearing on the north side of the highway.

The ridge south of Big Bear Lake is studded with granite outcrops. Castle Rock is the largest and most interesting, regularly drawing rock climbers to its steep walls. A scrambling route around the backside leads agile hikers to the summit. Castle Rock offers some of the most spectacular views of Big Bear Lake because it towers above the trees that obstruct views from most points around the lake.

The steep and rocky trail climbs through a lush forest of Jeffrey pines and white firs.

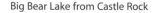
Big Bear Lake from Castle Rock

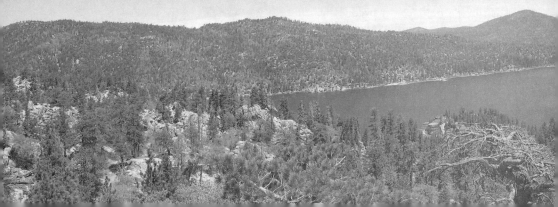

Watch for old false trails and take care not to cut switchbacks. In 0.6 mile, it reaches Castle Rock. Be sure to stay on the main trail rather than veering off on some of the climber's trails that lead up to the steep walls of the rock. The main trail curves around the south side of the outcrop and crosses a dry creek bed. On the far side of the creek, the main trail starts leading south up the hill away from Castle Rock, but an access trail heads back north across the creek to the west end of the rock. Follow this access trail around to the north side of the rock and look for an obvious notch on the north side of the rock west of the highest point.

Scramble up boulders toward the notch, but before reaching it, turn left up a gigantic "stairway" that leads to the eastern summit. This involves third class climbing and those uncomfortable with rock scrambling will prefer to stop at the base. After enjoying the view, return the way you came.

VARIATION

Alternatively, the Castle Rock Trail (1W03) continues south from Castle Rock 0.6 mile through beautiful open forest dotted with boulders and manzanita patches to a signed trailhead on Forest Road 2N86 near its junction with 2N10.

trip 4.11 Butler Peak

Distance	0.3 mile (out-and-back)
Hiking Time	15 minutes
Elevation Gain	100′
Difficulty	Easy
Trail Use	Good for children
Best Times	May–October
Agency	San Bernardino National Forest (Big Bear Discovery Center)
Optional Map	*Butler Peak 7.5′*

see map on p. 86

see map on p. 86

Big Bear Lake Area

DIRECTIONS From Highway 38 in Fawnskin, turn northwest at the sign for Butler Peak onto Rim of the World Dr., which becomes 3N14. In 1.3 miles, turn left on 2N13 at a sign pointing to the lookout. Go 2.1 miles, and then turn left on the fair dirt road 2N13C, which climbs 2.5 miles to a parking area below the Butler Peak fire lookout. 2N13C may be gated when the lookout is closed. It crosses a creek that may only be passable in high clearance vehicles during high water.

Butler Peak (8531′) is one of a network of mountaintops in the San Bernardino National Forest hosting historic fire look-outs. Other lookouts include Keller Peak, Strawberry Peak, Morton Peak, Red Mtn., Black Mtn., and Tahquitz Peak. The 360°

views from Butler Peak are among the most impressive, encompassing Big Bear Lake to the east, San Gorgonio to the southeast, the Santa Ana River Canyon and Keller Peak to the south, Lake Arrowhead to the west, and Holcomb Creek and the desert slopes to the north. The hike to the summit is very short, but is steep and rocky and not suited for those unsteady on their feet. The tower is open 9 A.M.–5 P.M. on weekends, holidays, and some weekdays from Memorial Day to Labor Day. However, the high summit may be snowbound until June in wet years.

In September 2007, the Butler 2 Fire burned 14,000 acres northwest of Big Bear Lake, including Butler Peak itself. Vast sections of the forest in this area have been incinerated. This is an interesting place to watch nature's process of regeneration after the devastation. **The area was temporarily closed in 2008 because of fire dam-**

age. Before your visit, call the Big Bear Discovery Center to check if the road has reopened.

From the parking area, follow the trail that switchbacks up to the fire lookout, which is precariously perched on the rocky summit outcrop. Along the way, keep your eyes out for burnt stumps of trees that were blasted by lightning. Climb two flights of steep stairs to the lookout.

The tower was constructed in 1931 by the Civilian Conservation Corps (CCC) and was staffed for decades by the Forest Service. It is now staffed by trained volunteer fire lookouts, who are also happy to show visitors the sights and explain how the fire lookout works. If you are interested in becoming a fire lookout volunteer, contact the Arrowhead Ranger Station or ask the volunteers at the lookout for more information.

Butler Peak Fire Lookout

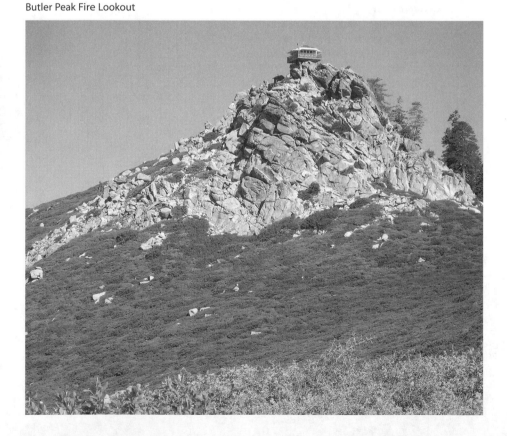

trip 4.12 Siberia Creek Trail Camp from Seven Pines

Distance	8 miles (out-and-back, with a possible overnight camp)
Hiking Time	4 hours
Elevation Gain	1300'
Difficulty	Moderate
Trail Use	Dogs, suitable for backpacking
Best Times	October–April
Agency	San Bernardino National Forest (Big Bear Discovery Center)
Recommended Map	*Big Bear Lake* and *Keller Peak* 7.5'

see map on p. 86

DIRECTIONS From Redlands drive 19 miles east on State Highway 38 to the town of Angelus Oaks. At a dirt turnout just beyond the north end of town, turn left (north) and descend Middle Control Road (1N06), a good dirt road. (If it is closed for the winter, continue east to the paved Glass Rd., follow Glass Rd. down to Seven Oaks Road, then backtrack to the bottom of Middle Control Road.) In 0.5 mile, you pass a waterfall at a bend in the road. Continue down to reach the Santa Ana River Road (1N09), 3.8 miles from the highway. Turn left (west) and drive 0.2 mile to a junction with the fair dirt Clarks Grade Road (1N54). Turn right and ascend Clarks Grade 1.8 miles to a junction with Forest Road 1N64. Turn left (west) and descend. Past Clarks Ranch Camp, cross two fords of Deer Creek that may be impassable in high water. After 1.7 miles, you will arrive at the Siberia Creek Trailhead (1W10) on the right. Park in a turnout on the right just beyond.

Siberia Creek Trail Camp is a small campsite nestled in the forest at the confluence of Siberia and Bear Creeks southwest of Big Bear Lake. It is accessed by three trails, one from Snow Valley, a second from Champion Lodgepole Pine above Big Bear, and a third from Seven Pines on the Santa Ana River to the south. At the time this book went to press, the trail from Champion Lodgepole (1W04) was completely overgrown below Gunsight Notch and the other two routes are brushy and washed out in places. Long pants, long sleeves, gaiters, and even a garden pruner are recommended if the trail has not been recently maintained. However, this trip is an enjoyable adventure for intrepid souls willing to brave the dirt roads and the brush to see a little-visited corner of the San Bernardino Mountains.

The trail cuts west through the dense south-facing chaparral, especially scrub oak, manzanita, sage, buckthorn, and yucca. This section can be brutally hot in summer months. In 1.3 miles, the trail rounds the bend and turns north on the slopes overlooking Bear Creek. The west-facing chaparral is subtly different in character,

but possibly even denser. The bare slopes of Slide Peak across the canyon are impressive to behold. If you are watchful, you may notice an abandoned mine shaft adjacent to the trail. Old mine shafts are extremely dangerous. Some hikers asphyxiated while exploring this one.

An oak clings precariously to the rocky hillside.

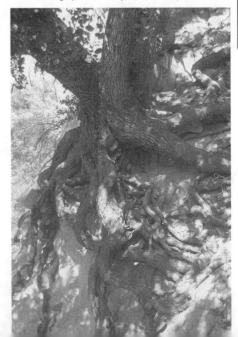

Big Bear Lake Area

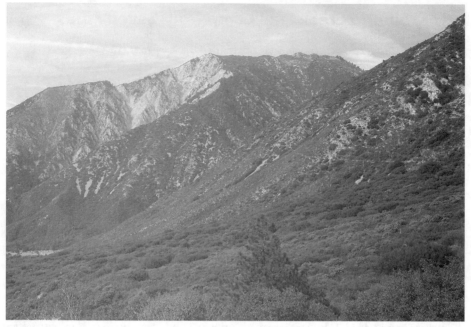

Slide Peak

In another 1.7 miles, pass a junction with the overgrown Siberia Creek Trail (1W04) coming from the Champion Lodgepole tree above Big Bear. Your trail drops abruptly, enters a splendid forest, crosses Siberia Creek, and arrives in a mile at Siberia Creek Trail Camp, a small clearing above the roaring Bear Creek. The last part of the trail before the camp can be hard to find in the autumn because of the fallen leaves. However, cross-country travel in the canyon is difficult, so it is worth searching out the correct trail.

After enjoying the creek and possibly spending a night at the secluded camp, return the way you came.

chapter 5

San Gorgonio Wilderness

The San Bernardino Mountains are part of California's unusual Transverse Ranges, running east to west rather than southeast to northwest. They have long attracted the attention of humans, at first for hunting, logging, and gold, but now most of all for recreation. The range is so large that trips for this area are divided into three chapters. This chapter explores the steep and rugged San Gorgonio Wilderness on the southeast side of the range, cut off from Big Bear by the deep trench of the Santa Ana River. Chapter 3 describes the western end, especially around Lake Arrowhead and the alluring creeks at the interface of forest and desert. Chapter 4 focuses on the eastern end, where richly forested hills circle the jewel-like Big Bear Lake.

San Gorgonio Wilderness, located in the southeast portion of the San Bernardino Mountains, is home to California's tallest mountains south of the Sierra Nevada. The biggest peaks are located along the 7-mile crest of the Great San Bernardino Divide stretching from San Gorgonio Mtn. to San Bernardino Peak. This divide drops below 10,000 feet at only one point, Dollar Lake Saddle, and separates the Santa Ana River Canyon and Big Bear areas to the north from Mill Creek, the Yucaipa Ridge, and the eastern Los Angeles Basin to the south. This section also describes hikes on the nearby Yucaipa Ridge and Santa Ana River even though they are outside the Wilderness area proper.

The San Bernardino Mountains were once of interest only to a handful of miners and loggers, but by the 1920s had become a center of Southern California recreation. Nearly 100,000 people visited the range each year and roads were cut across many of the slopes. Soon, winter sport interests were calling for a ski resort on the north face of San Gorgonio Peak. Conflicts between developers and conservationists raged for decades. In 1964, the Wilderness Act was passed by Congress, setting aside untrammeled wild areas for the benefit of present and future generations. The 58,969-acre San Gorgonio Wilderness is one of these areas.

The peaks of San Gorgonio Wilderness hold distinguished roles in the history of Southern California. In 1852, Colonel Henry Washington established the first survey point in Southern California to begin surveying the newly admitted state. He selected San Bernardino Peak because it was prominently visible from much of the Los Angeles basin. He led a crew of 12 sturdy men up the arduous, trailless, chaparral-clad north slope and established a 24-foot-tall survey marker half a mile west of the true summit. Measurements were distorted by the heat waves rising off the valley, so enormous fires were lit on the mountain and at various other points in the valley so that surveying could be performed at night. Baseline Rd. in the Inland Empire still essentially follows the east-west line designated by the survey.

In 1872, Watson Goodyear of the California Geological Survey and Mark Thomas of San Bernardino claimed the first recorded ascent of San Gorgonio Mtn., known as Old Grayback at the time. There is some

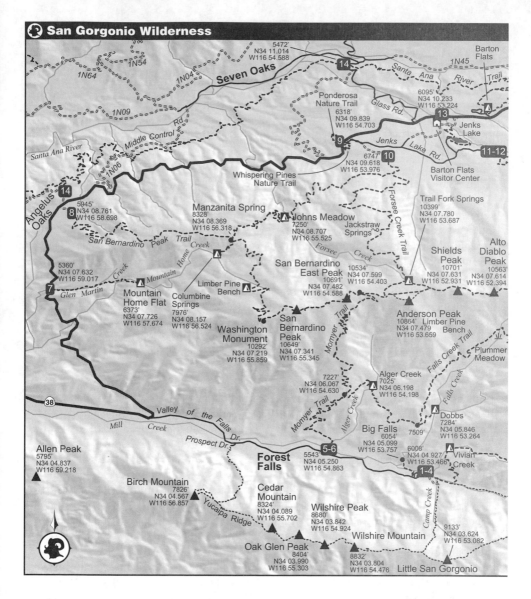

San Gorgonio Wilderness

controversy about whether this party reached the correct summit, but numerous other parties climbed the mountain in the subsequent decade.

The most heavily used routes to the top of San Gorgonio Mtn. are the steep Vivian Creek Trail from the south and the long South Fork Trail from the north. The long traverse across the ridge is a three-day rite of passage for many Boy Scouts and successful trekkers proudly wear their "I Climbed the Nine Peaks" patch. Aspen Grove is also a great place to watch the leaves changing in the fall. However, there are many other lesser-traveled trails and cross-country routes on the mountain where the intrepid hiker can find solitude and beauty.

Access to the mountains in this area is a growing issue. The Falls Creek Trail from Mill Creek was built in 1898 by John Dobbs and was used by the public for a century, but it was closed because of complaints

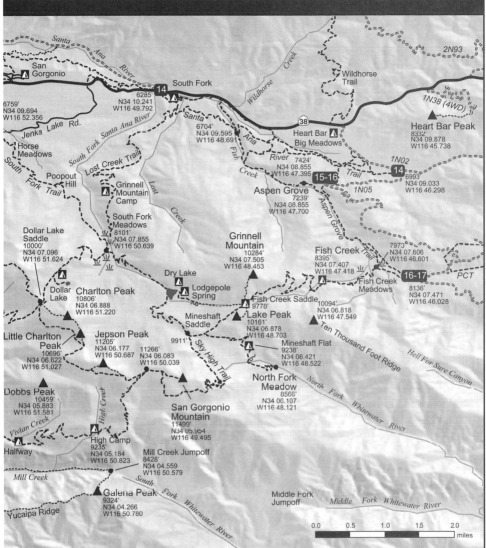

from a landowner, adding 3 miles each way to the climb to Dollar Lake Saddle. The Banning Water District and the Morongo Indians have also recently closed southern access to the San Gorgonio Wilderness. When the Southern Pacific Railroad laid tracks through Banning Pass, it received every other section of land for several miles on both sides of the tracks as incentive to build. Southern Pacific sold much of the land to finance construction. Now, more

than a century later, the Yucaipa Ridge is still a checkerboard of public and private land as a result of this grant. No fewer than three dirt roads and three trails once served the ridge, but not a single one remains accessible now that private landowners have forbidden access to hikers.

A wilderness permit is required to enter the San Gorgonio Wilderness. It can be obtained at no charge from the Mill Creek Ranger Station. Permits for some trails can be self-issued. Permits for the most popular routes can be obtained at the station while it is open. Advanced reservations can be made by mail or fax. The largest number of hikers and campers flock to the Wilderness on summer weekends and quotas for the popular trails are reserved weeks in advance. If you find yourself unable to get a permit for Vivian Creek or South Fork, consider Fish Creek as a great alternative. The fall is a better time to seek seclusion. Hardy mountaineers equipped with skis, snowshoes, or crampons venture into the high country in the winter and spring.

Summer also brings a pattern of afternoon thundershowers, especially in July and August. Moisture from the ocean is forced upward by the prevailing westerly breezes as it hits the wall of mountains. Heated by the afternoon sun, towering cumulus clouds build over the summit and dump their contents in violent storms. Hikers typically have advanced warning as the clouds gather and the sky darkens before the storm hits. On these days, it is best to be off the exposed ridges before noon to avoid lightning strikes. Hikers aiming for a single-day ascent of San Gorgonio in the summer should plan on a very early start.

There are many fine camping sites scattered throughout the Wilderness. Many of the higher sites are dry; plan ahead and fill your water bottles at the last dependable source. Bears are active in some of these areas and have learned to steal food hanging from tree branches, so bear canisters are recommended. Canisters can be purchased or rented from the Mill Creek Ranger Station. Campfires are not allowed in the Wilderness at any time.

San Gorgonio Wilderness is served by a large and active volunteer group called the San Gorgonio Wilderness Association (SGWA), which works with the grievously underfunded US Forest Service to provide visitor information, patrol and maintain trails, and protect the Wilderness. They have an information-packed web site (including current trail conditions and water reports) at www.sgwa.org and also welcome new volunteers each year.

For further reading about this area, see John Robinson's books: *The San Bernardinos* and *San Gorgonio—A Wilderness Preserved.*

San Gorgonio from the south

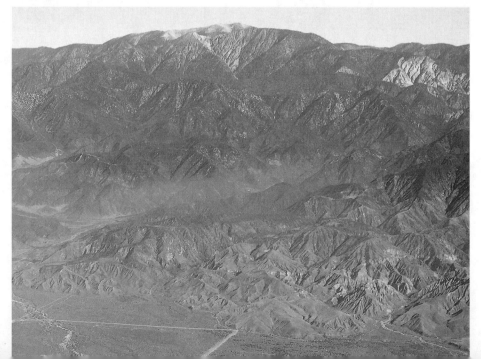

trip 5.1 San Gorgonio via Vivian Creek

Distance	17 miles (out-and-back)
Hiking Time	9 hours
Elevation Gain	5500'
Difficulty	Strenuous
Trail Use	Dogs, suitable for backpacking
Best Times	June–October
Agency	San Bernardino National Forest (Mill Creek Ranger Station)
Recommended Map	Tom Harrison *San Gorgonio Wilderness* or *Forest Falls, San Gorgonio Mtn.* 7.5'
Permit	San Gorgonio Wilderness Permit Required

see map on p. 102

DIRECTIONS From Redlands drive east on State Highway 38 to the huge hairpin turn at mile marker 038 SBD 15.00. Turn right on Valley of the Falls Dr. and proceed 4.5 miles to its end. Turn left and park at the Vivian Creek Trailhead.

At 11,499 feet, San Gorgonio Mtn. is the tallest summit in Southern California and is an obligatory climb for serious local mountaineers. The Vivian Creek Trail was the first established route to the summit of San Gorgonio. At the behest of Thomas Aker, owner of the Forest Home resort in Mill Creek, the trail was hacked up the steep and brushy mountainside under the direction of Albert Vivian of Yucaipa in 1898. Now that there are numerous excellent trails on the mountain, many hikers still believe Vivian Creek is the best. It is steep and direct, offers fantastic views, and passes three fine trail camps en route. If you plan to hike this route on a summer weekend, request your permit long in advance

because the quotas frequently fill 2–4 weeks ahead of time. Vivian Creek is also a good but demanding snow route in the spring; snowshoes, ice axe, and crampons may be required, depending on the conditions.

From the signed Vivian Creek Trailhead at the east end of the parking area, hike east along an old dirt road, ignoring forks that lead to nearby cabins. In 0.5 mile, the Vivian Creek Trail turns north and crosses Mill Creek (occasionally hazardous at times of very high water).

The trail then switchbacks steeply northward through the forest of oaks until, in 1 mile, it rounds a corner and enters a hanging valley carved by Vivian Creek. There is scenic camping here beneath the incense

San Gorgonio summit

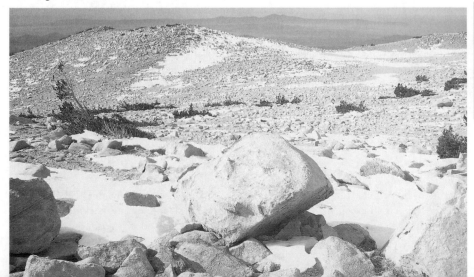

San Gorgonio Wilderness

cedars, white firs, and Jeffrey pines, though it is too low to be a practical campsite for summit-goers. In late spring, you will likely enjoy hundreds of lilies in full bloom.

The trail turns east and follows Vivian Creek up the valley for 1.3 miles to Halfway Camp before making broad switchbacks up the next ridge and turning a corner in 2.3 miles to High Camp, situated on High Creek, which tumbles down the south wall of San Gorgonio. This site, at 9400 feet amidst the hardy lodgepole pines, can be bitterly cold even on summer nights, but is most convenient for those backpacking the mountain.

Beyond High Camp, the trail makes some gratuitously long switchbacks as it climbs east to the next ridge, then turns north and follows the ridge up to treeline. San Gorgonio Mtn. is one of Southern California's few summits above treeline, earning its nickname of "Old Grayback" for the bare sandy soil on the summit ridge. Reach a T-junction 2.4 miles from High Camp. Turn right (east), proceed 0.2 mile to another junction with the Sky High Trail, stay left, and continue 0.4 mile to the wind-swept summit boulders.

Some backpackers spend a night on the summit. This site is fully exposed to the elements, but offers solitude and spectacular views. Return the way you came, or if you've arranged a shuttle, descend any of the other trails described in this chapter.

trip 5.2 Little San Gorgonio Peak

Distance	5 miles (out-and-back)
Hiking Time	6 hours
Elevation Gain	3100'
Difficulty	Strenuous
Best Times	March–November
Agency	San Bernardino National Forest (Mill Creek Ranger Station)
Required Map	Tom Harrison *San Gorgonio Wilderness* or *Forest Falls* 7.5'

see map on p. 102

DIRECTIONS From Redlands drive east on State Highway 38 to the huge hairpin turn at mile marker 038 SBD 15.00. Turn right on Valley of the Falls Dr. and proceed 4.5 miles to its end. Turn left and park at the Vivian Creek Trailhead.

Little San Gorgonio Peak (9133') is the second highest point on the Yucaipa Ridge and is the most difficult summit to reach. An insidiously direct cross-country route leads up Camp Creek, gaining 3000 feet in 1.3 horizontal miles, for an astonishing average grade of 23 degrees. Despite the short distance, the trip is only suited to experienced cross-country climbers with strong route-finding skills. If in doubt, try the significantly easier Galena Peak first (see Trip 5.3). Camp Creek is also a natural avalanche chute and accumulated snow in the north-facing gully can linger into early summer. This is an excellent snow climb in early spring when continuous well-consoli-dated snow covers the talus, waterfalls, and bushes. Be careful to assess the avalanche risk before venturing up. By late spring, the snow bridges over the creek have thinned, and present a falling hazard, but reveal delightful waterfalls. The creek dries up later in the season. An ice axe and crampons are necessary in early season and a helmet is prudent any time of year. Any time of year that you visit, your exertions are rewarded with solitude and stunning views of the peaks along the San Bernardino Divide and Yucaipa Ridge.

From the signed Vivian Creek Trailhead at the east end of the parking area, hike east along an old dirt road, ignoring forks

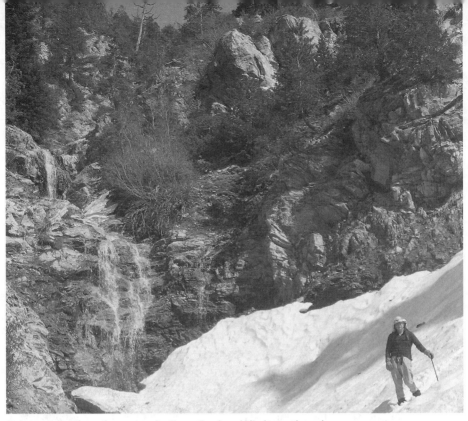
Stairstep Falls, where the route exits Camp Creek and climbs southward

that lead to nearby cabins. In 0.2 mile, look for the narrow gravel wash of Camp Creek crossing the trail in a grove of incense cedars. It comes down from the first prominent canyon you pass along the hike. Turn right and ascend the creek (dry later in the season). In 0.1 mile, cross a dirt road. The forest opens, revealing impressive views up the canyon. The shattered rock ridges on both sides are extremely unstable.

In another 0.3 mile, the canyon narrows. In another 0.1 mile, stay left in the main canyon at a fork with a tributary. 0.1 mile beyond that, reach a waterfall that can be bypassed by climbing the slope to the west, then traversing back above.

In yet another 0.1 mile the canyon veers left (southeast) and you reach the second waterfall, actually a series of falls stairstepping up the canyon. Although it is possible to pick a path around the falls, the recommended route is to depart Camp Creek at this point and climb south directly to Yucaipa Ridge.

Hike up the steep slope until it is convenient to veer slightly left and gain a ridgeline. As you climb the relentless slopes, the ponderosa pines and incense cedars give way to lodgepole pines; white firs and sugar pines also keep you company nearly all the way to the ridge. Views across Mill Creek toward San Bernardino Peak and San Gorgonio steadily improve as you get higher. After 0.8 mile of strenuous climbing, reach the crest of Yucaipa Ridge about 0.2 mile east of an antenna site. Take a moment to identify where you are so you can find the same point for your descent later on.

The Oak Glen Divide Trail once ran along this ridge and traces of it are still visible threading through the chinquapin. Turn left (east) and hike 0.5 mile to the summit of Little San Gorgonio Peak. Enjoy the dramatic views, and then return the way you came. For a very strenuous alternative, follow the ridge east or west to climb more peaks (see Trip 5.19).

trip 5.3 Galena Peak

Distance	8 miles (out-and-back)
Hiking Time	6 hours
Elevation Gain	3400'
Difficulty	Strenuous
Trail Use	Suitable for backpacking
Best Times	May–November
Agency	San Bernardino National Forest (Mill Creek Ranger Station)
Recommended Map	Tom Harrison *San Gorgonio Wilderness* or *Forest Falls* and *San Gorgonio Mountain 7.5'*

see map on p. 102

DIRECTIONS From Redlands drive east on State Highway 38 to the huge hairpin turn at mile marker 038 SBD 15.00. Turn right on Valley of the Falls Dr. and proceed 4.5 miles to its end. Turn left and park at the Vivian Creek Trailhead.

At 9324 feet, Galena Peak is the tallest and most dramatic summit on the long Yucaipa Ridge. Its north face has been carved into soaring buttresses and forbidding ravines. After a fresh coat of snow in the spring, Galena Peak looks like it could have been transported to Southern California from the Swiss Alps. Moreover, Galena Peak provides fantastic views of San Gorgonio Mtn. The steep and crumbling rock on the north face is too dangerous to climb directly, so the peak is best reached from the Mill Creek Jumpoff via the northeast ridge. Even so, this is a strenuous and challenging cross-country hike. It follows Mill Creek's channel for several miles, so the route is best avoided during times of high water.

From the signed Vivian Creek Trailhead at the east end of the parking area, hike east along an old dirt road, ignoring forks that lead to nearby cabins. In 0.5 mile, the Vivian Creek Trail turns north and crosses Mill Creek but our route continues east. In 0.1 mile, the trail disappears entirely and you must hike east up the creek bed. The best route may change as flash floods churn up the channel, but at the time of this writing, staying in the bed near the south bank avoided the worst of the boulder hopping.

After about 2 miles, the channel narrows and you come to two waterfalls. Adept rock scramblers can pass the waterfalls on the slabs and steep dirt immediately to the right, but an easier way is to climb out of the riverbed on the right and follow a use trail for 0.1 mile past the falls and back down into Mill Creek.

Beyond, the canyon steepens, and then abruptly rises to the infamous and phenomenally loose Mill Creek Jumpoff. This saddle is best climbed by scrambling up the center on loose tan scree, left of the even

North face of Galena Peak

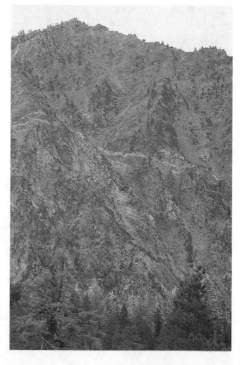

looser gray rock and sand. Near the top, traverse right on more loose scree above the gray rock and below the manzanita. Rockfall is almost inevitable, so large groups should take special care here; helmets would be prudent. The top of the jumpoff is 3.2 miles from the trailhead.

From Mill Creek Jumpoff, you can see the east summit of Galena Peak to the south. Follow a use trail up the ridge. The trail avoids all of the nasty brush and offers some stunning views into the abyss of Galena's northwest face. It was once easy to follow, but was badly eroded during thunderstorms in the summer of 2007. The distance is only 0.5 mile, but the climbing is steep and strenuous.

Galena has east and west summits. The east summit where the trail ends is the official peak and is where the climbing register can be found. If you have time and energy remaining, consider taking the 10-minute walk along the ridge to the west summit, which is 15 feet taller. The west summit also offers breathtaking views along the jagged Yucaipa Ridge toward Little San Gorgonio Peak.

Return the way you came. Do not be lured down the loose and dangerous cliffs of the north face.

trip 5.4 Big Falls

Distance	0.6 mile (out-and-back)
Hiking Time	30 minutes
Elevation Gain	100'
Difficulty	Easy
Trail Use	Dogs, good for children
Best Times	All year
Agency	San Bernardino National Forest (Mill Creek Ranger Station)
Optional Map	Tom Harrison *San Gorgonio Wilderness* or *Forest Falls* 7.5'

see map on p. 102

DIRECTIONS From Redlands drive east on State Highway 38 to the huge hairpin turn at mile marker 038 SBD 15.00. Turn right on Valley of the Falls Dr. and proceed 4.3 miles to the Big Falls parking area on the left. If you reach the Vivian Creek Trailhead, you went 0.2 mile too far.

Mill Creek cuts a deep swath through the loose rocks south of San Gorgonio Mtn. There are numerous waterfalls along the lateral streams pouring down the steep faces into Mill Creek. Falls Creek has the most impressive waterfall, uncreatively named Big Falls. It is hidden behind the mouth of the canyon, but can be viewed from this short hike.

Bring sandals and a swimsuit. The creek and pools along the way are popular for water play on a warm day. However, be careful in the spring or during other times of high water when Mill Creek can be hazardous to cross. Also, do not try to climb the rocks adjacent to Big Falls; they are

Big Falls

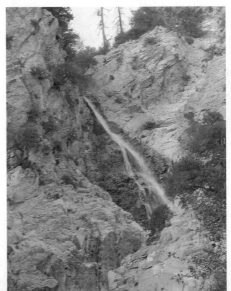

San Gorgonio Wilderness

extremely loose and hikers have gotten into trouble here in the past.

From the north edge of the Big Falls Trailhead parking lot, look for a trail marker and follow the trail west along the bank of Mill Creek. Falls Creek Canyon is the first canyon on the north to the west of the parking area. As you approach, cross Mill Creek (the trail is washed out here every spring) and follow the Big Falls Trail into the mouth of Falls Creek Canyon and up the slope to a viewing platform with a metal railing.

trip 5.5 Alger Creek or Dobbs Trail Camps

Distance	7 or 11 miles (out-and-back)
Hiking Time	4–6 hours
Elevation Gain	2100' or 2800'
Difficulty	Moderate
Trail Use	Dogs, suitable for backpacking
Best Times	June–November
Agency	San Bernardino National Forest (Mill Creek Ranger Station)
Recommended Map	Tom Harrison *San Gorgonio Wilderness* or *Forest Falls* and *San Gorgonio Mountain* 7.5'
Permit	San Gorgonio Wilderness Permit Required

see map on p. 102

DIRECTIONS From Redlands drive east on State Highway 38 to the huge hairpin turn at mile marker 038 SBD 15.00. Turn right on Valley of the Falls Dr. and proceed 2.9 miles to the Momyer Trailhead on the left. If you reach the fire station, you have gone 100 yards too far.

The southern face of the San Bernardino Divide is rarely visited. Tucked away half way up the slopes are two splendid trail camps, located alongside rushing creeks and shaded beneath towering incense cedars. Backpackers looking for solitude can find it here. In the summer when popular trails are reserved weeks in advance, these camps are usually available.

The Momyer Trail, named for Joe Momyer, who was instrumental to the protection of San Gorgonio Wilderness, departs the northwest corner of the parking area. It crosses the boulder-strewn bed of Mill Creek to reach a sign on the north side. Beyond the sign, turn right and follow the trail parallel to the creek through the forest before turning back north. Climb out of the forest and begin switchbacking through the sun-baked chaparral with great views of the steep Yucaipa Ridge to the south across the valley. At the first major switchback, you may see traces of the old trail coming up from Torrey Pines Rd. Soon, you climb back

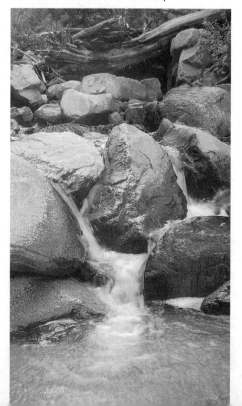

Falls Creek below Dobbs Trail Camp

into the oak forest, where squirrels busily scamper about, stocking up their winter supply of acorns. At 2.5 miles, cross the Wilderness boundary, and 0.15 mile farther, come to a signed junction

Turn right (east) and contour along the slope for 0.8 mile, passing a spring and then switchbacking steeply down into the canyon cut by Alger Creek. On the west bank is the Alger Creek Trail Camp.

VARIATION

For those seeking a taste of history and an even more remarkable camp, cross Alger Creek and continue southeast 1.5 miles to a junction at the south end of a long ridge. Follow the trail that descends northeast, switchbacking down for 0.5 mile to the confluence of two forks of Falls Creek. At the end of the 19th Century, the mountain man John Dobbs built his cabin immediately above the two streams on a flat clearing beneath the mighty cedars. Now, scarcely a trace of the dwelling remains, but the Dobbs Trail Camp is one of the most scenic in all of Southern California.

Return the way you came. The Falls Creek Trail, built by John Dobbs in 1898 and used by the public for a century, once shortcut 3 miles each way off the hike to Dobbs Camp, but now it has been closed by the Forest Service because of complaints by a private landowner.

trip 5.6 Momyer to Falls Creek Loop

Distance	20 miles (loop)
Hiking Time	10 hours
Elevation Gain	5900'
Difficulty	Strenuous
Trail Use	Dogs, suitable for backpacking
Best Times	June–October
Agency	San Bernardino National Forest (Mill Creek Ranger Station)
Recommended Map	Tom Harrison *San Gorgonio Wilderness* or *Forest Falls, Big Bear Lake, Moonridge,* and *San Gorgonio Mountain* 7.5'
Permit	San Gorgonio Wilderness Permit Required

see map on p. 102

DIRECTIONS From Redlands drive east on State Highway 38 to the huge hairpin turn at mile marker 038 SBD 15.00. Turn right on Valley of the Falls Dr. and proceed 2.9 miles to the Momyer Trailhead on the left. If you reach the fire station, you have gone 100 yards too far.

Few hikers venture up the unrelenting switchbacks on the enormous southern wall of the San Bernardino Divide. But those who do are rewarded with solitude, a unique perspective on the mountain, and a first-rate workout. This trip climbs the Momyer Trail, which is the shortest and steepest route to the crest. It follows the flat ridge top east to Dollar Lake Saddle, and then descends the Falls Creek Trail to form a great loop. This route is handy when the more popular trailheads book up in the summer or as a speedy way to the ridgeline for avid peak baggers. It also tours a diverse forest featuring many species of pines (Jeffrey, limber, lodgepole, sugar, and even Coulter) and oaks (black, live, and scrub), white firs, incense cedars, and, of course, endless chaparral. The upper Momyer Trail is seldom maintained and long pants are helpful, but the worst of the brush is still cut back from the trail.

The Momyer Trail departs the northwest corner of the parking area and crosses the boulder-strewn bed of Mill Creek to reach a sign on the north side. Beyond the

San Gorgonio Wilderness

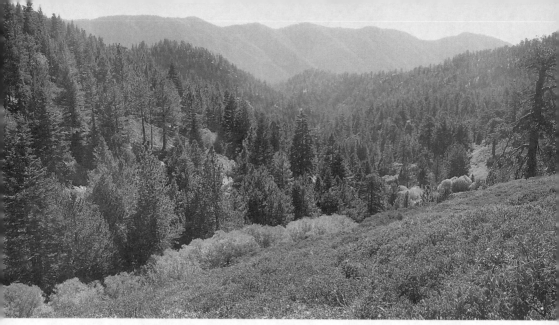

Falls Creek Trail near Plummer Meadow

sign, turn right and follow the trail parallel to the creek through the forest before turning back north. Climb out of the forest and begin switchbacking through the sun-baked chaparral with great views of the steep Yucaipa Ridge to the south across the valley. At the first major switchback, you may see traces of the old trail coming up from Torrey Pines Rd. Soon, you climb back into the oak forest, where squirrels busily scamper about. At 2.5 miles, cross the Wilderness boundary, and 0.15 mile farther, come to a signed junction. Stay left up the Momyer Trail toward San Bernardino Peak; you will later return to this point on the Falls Creek Trail from Dollar Lake Saddle and Alger Creek.

The Momyer Trail climbs through a zone where the trees have been devastated by bark beetles and the path can be hard to follow at times when it is covered with debris of downed firs and pines. At about 8500 feet, the forest yields to a vast field of manzanita, buckthorn, chinquapin, and other chaparral. On a clear day, you can see over the Yucaipa Ridge to Perris Lake (with a distinctive island), saddle-backed Santiago Peak, and even the Pacific Ocean. At 10,000 feet, the trail crosses the south ridge of San Bernardino East Peak and gradually

climbs to the east, then switches back to meet the crest at a signed junction east of the peak, 6.8 miles and 4800 feet up from the trailhead.

Turn right and follow the trail east through the fine lodgepole forest atop the San Bernardino Divide. Stay on the main trail; don't be lured down the Forsee Creek Trail. Along the way, pass Anderson Peak, Shields Peak, and the formidable Alto Diablo Peak. Enjoy the views north across the Santa Ana River Canyon to Big Bear Lake, which looks like a sapphire floating in the sky. Northwest of Alto Diablo is a cirque littered with avalanche debris, which has two terminal moraines left over from the last ice age when a glacier hung on the north face of the ridge. Also, pass trail camps at Anderson Flat, Shields Flat, High Meadow Springs, and Red Rock Flat. After 3.6 miles, arrive at the four-way junction of Dollar Lake Saddle.

Turn right (southwest) and descend toward Plummer Meadows. This is a fine place to compare pinecones in the fall. The tall lodgepole produce deceptively tiny cones. The supple limber pines, found slightly lower, produce somewhat larger cones. After crossing the two forks of Falls Creek, enter stands of Jeffrey pines (with 6″

shapely cones) and sugar pines (with the world's longest pine cones). Observant hikers may note the enormous widow-maker cones of the Coulter pine farther down near the trailhead. Cross another fork of Falls Creek, and then follow the east side of a long ridge to a trail junction, 4.1 miles down from the saddle. Consider a brief tour east to Dobbs Camp (see Trip 5.5), but the main trail turns west.

At a prominent bend in the trail is the junction with the old Falls Creek Trail, built by John Dobbs in 1898 and used by the public for a century as the most popular route into San Gorgonio Wilderness high country. The trail is now closed because of complaints by a private landowner. Instead, veer north, cross a small creek, then descend into the deep canyon carved by Alger Creek. On the west side is a fine trail camp shaded beneath the cedars, 1.5 miles from the Dobbs turnoff. Switchback up to the north, then contour southwest 0.8 mile back to the junction with the Momyer Trail. Turn left and follow it back to the trailhead.

trip 5.7 Mountain Home Flats

Distance	3.5 miles (out-and-back)
Hiking Time	2.5 hours
Elevation Gain	1100'
Difficulty	Moderate
Trail Use	Dogs, suitable for backpacking
Best Times	April–November
Agency	San Bernardino National Forest (Mill Creek Ranger Station)
Required Map	Tom Harrison *San Gorgonio Wilderness* or *Big Bear Lake* 7.5'

see map on p. 102

DIRECTIONS From Redlands drive east on State Highway 38. Take the huge hairpin turn at the mouth of Mill Creek Canyon, and then continue 3.4 miles to a bridge over Glen Martin Creek at mile marker 038 SBD 18.44. There is very limited parking just south of the bridge, and more at a turnout 0.25 mile north. Do not mix up this trailhead with Mountain Home Creek, which is 1.5 miles farther south.

N estled among the firs, pines, and cedars in a sheer canyon beneath San Bernardino Peak is a trail camp perched on a small flat. Though it is less than 2 miles from the highway, few visitors make the steep climb and you are likely to have the spot to yourself. This is an enjoyable destination for a picnic or short backpacking trip.

A narrow trail starting at the south end of the bridge leads east into Glen Martin Canyon beneath the shady oaks. It soon drops down to the floor of the creek and briefly crosses to the north side. The creek soon divides and the trail follows the south fork. This part of the forest is home to many Coulter pines, with their enormous "widow maker" pine cones, which are uncommon

Mountain Home Flats Trail Camp

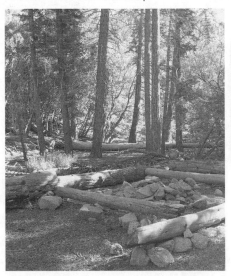

higher up in the San Bernardino Mountains.

The trail soon veers right and switchbacks up to the south ridge of the canyon. There are several poor use trails splitting off where hikers missed a switchback; take care to stay on the main trail because it is the easiest. In 1.0 mile, cross the ridge into the forested upper reaches of Mountain Home Creek. The trail claims your attention as it clings to the edge of a decomposing cliff,

then descends to the creek, crossing just above a series of pools connected by a small waterfall. The trail then switchbacks steeply again up before leveling out in another 0.7 mile near the trail camp at Mountain Home Flats.

There are several good tent sites under the stately trees. You can make a short but steep descent to Mountain Home Creek directly north of camp to fetch water. Return the way you came.

trip 5.8 San Bernardino Peak

Distance	16 miles (out-and-back)
Hiking Time	8 hours
Elevation Gain	4700′
Difficulty	Strenuous
Trail Use	Dogs, suitable for backpacking
Best Times	June–October
Agency	San Bernardino National Forest (Mill Creek Ranger Station)
Recommended Map	Tom Harrison *San Gorgonio Wilderness* or *Big Bear Lake* and *Forest Falls* 7.5′
Permit	San Gorgonio Wilderness Permit Required

see maps on pp. 102 & 123

DIRECTIONS From Redlands drive east on State Highway 38 to Angelus Oaks. Follow signs for the San Bernardino Peak Trail (1W07). First turn right from Highway 38 on Manzanita Rd. toward the fire station at mile marker 038 SBD 20.00. Then make an immediate left and drive for 0.1 mile, passing the station. Make a right onto a fair dirt road past the station at a sign indicating 1W07. Stay right at two forks and go 0.3 mile to a large dirt parking area with the signed SAN BERNARDINO PEAK TRAILHEAD.

San Bernardino Peak anchors the west end of the great San Bernardino Ridge. The rolling ridge continues east to San Gorgonio Mtn. and beyond, generally maintaining an altitude in excess of 10,000 feet until abruptly plummeting into Hell for Sure Canyon. From the western parts of the Inland Empire, San Bernardino Peak is the most prominent portion of the ridge. On a clear winter day, its white summit towers proudly above the valley cities. San Bernardino Peak is also noteworthy because Southern California was first surveyed from a vista near the summit. This strenuous hike from the hamlet of Angelus Oaks to the summit of San Bernardino Peak offers ever-expanding views and a tour of many

of the vegetation zones of San Gorgonio Wilderness.

The San Bernardino Peak Trail begins steadily switchbacking up the ridge through a forest of pines, oaks, and white firs. After 2 miles and nearly 1600 feet of elevation gain, you pass a sign marking the San Gorgonio Wilderness boundary. Soon after, the grade abruptly eases as you reach a long bench covered in chaparral. Near the east end of the bench, in another 2.3 miles, a side trail to the right leads down to Manzanita Spring, then on to Columbine Springs Trail Camp; water is available in early summer at the first spring and usually through midsummer at the second.

The main trail begins climbing again. In 1.4 miles and 1000 feet of gain, reach

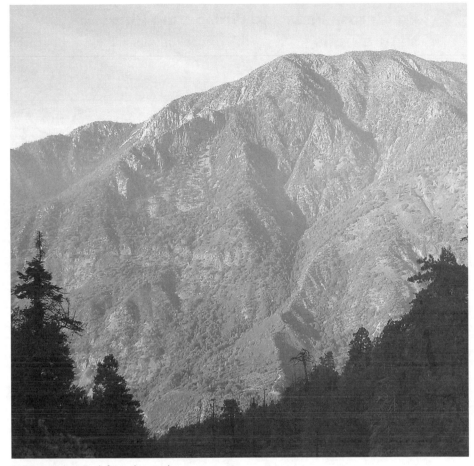

San Bernardino Peak from the south

Limber Pine Bench Trail Camp. This is a large and popular site for those backpacking the mountain, and water is usually available from a spring near the next major switchback on the trail. On a clear night, there are breathtaking views of the city lights laid out below.

The trail continues through an open forest of lodgepole pine, switchbacking up to gain the west ridge of San Bernardino Peak in 1.5 miles. Once you reach the ridge, keep your eyes open for a side trail marked by a plaque leading to Washington Monument, 50 feet off the main trail. This large rockpile marks the site from which Colonel Henry Washington established the initial point for surveying Southern California in 1852.

Heat waves distorted the measurements, so bonfires were built at each triangulation point and the surveys were completed at night. Baseline Avenue still follows the east-to-west line established in the survey.

The main trail continues up the ridge. In another 0.7 mile, it passes along the north side of San Bernardino Peak. A side trail climbs the short distance to the 10,649-foot summit, where you can enjoy views of the San Bernardino Ridge, Mill Creek, the Yucaipa Ridge, San Jacinto, Baldy, and beyond.

Return the way you came. Or, with a shuttle, descend the Momyer Trail (see Trip 5.6), the Forsee Creek Trail, or any of the other fine trails farther along the great ridge.

San Gorgonio
Wilderness

trip 5.9 Ponderosa Vista and Whispering Pines Nature Trails

Distance	0.7 mile each (loops)
Hiking Time	30 minutes
Elevation Gain	200′, 150′
Difficulty	Easy
Trail Use	Dogs, good for children
Best Times	April–November
Agency	San Bernardino National Forest (Mill Creek Ranger Station)
Optional Map	*Big Bear Lake 7.5*

see map on p. 102

DIRECTIONS From Redlands drive east on State Highway 38. Just before mile marker 038 SBD 25.51 and Jenks Lake Rd., pull off on the side of the road. The Ponderosa Vista Trailhead is on the north side and the Whispering Pines trailhead is on the south.

These two nature trails are conveniently located for families camping in the Barton Flats Area or driving the back way to Big Bear.

The Whispering Pines Trail (1E33) was constructed in 1969 for an episode of the television show, *Lassie*, in which a blind girl followed Lassie and a ranger around the trail to learn about the forest. The trail winds counterclockwise through the oaks and pines up a gradual hill. In the late spring, this can be a good place to see wildflowers. Woodpeckers have perforated the tall trees atop the hill. There are ten signs along the path and a booklet describing the sights at each sign is usually available at the trailhead for a fee.

The Ponderosa Vista Nature Trail (1E19) makes a counterclockwise loop to a scenic overlook with views across the Santa Ana River Canyon to the dramatic face of Slide Peak and beyond to the San Gabriel Mountains. Signs explain some of the sights along the way. There was once a 0.3-mile short loop that returned directly from the overlook, but it has been obliterated by downed trees and lack of use; the longer 0.7 mile loop is presently the only option.

Examining tree rings on the Ponderosa Trail

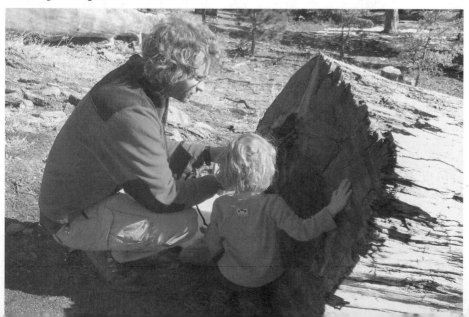

trip 5.10 Johns Meadow

Distance	6 miles (out-and-back)
Hiking Time	3 hours
Elevation Gain	800'
Difficulty	Moderate
Trail Use	Dogs, suitable for backpacking
Best Times	May–November
Agency	San Bernardino National Forest (Mill Creek Ranger Station)
Recommended Map	Tom Harrison *San Gorgonio Wilderness* or *Big Bear Lake* 7.5'
Permit	San Gorgonio Wilderness Permit Required

see map on p. 102

DIRECTIONS From Redlands drive east on State Highway 38 to Jenks Lake Rd., just before mile marker 038 SBD 25.51. Turn right (southeast). After 0.3 mile stay right again onto a fair dirt road where a sign reads FORSEE CREEK TRAIL. Drive 0.5 mile to the large parking area at the trailhead.

Unlike most of the long and steep trails climbing into San Gorgonio Wilderness, the Johns Meadow trail offers a moderate hike, which samples the pleasures of the woods and creeks. Though there is scarcely any meadow any longer, the trail ends at a pleasant camp shaded beneath the white fir on a bench above Forsee Creek. The trail was built by hardy San Bernardino Boy Scouts starting in 1969. The meadow was named in honor of John Surr of San Bernardino, a charter member of Defenders of the San Gorgonio Wilderness, who died in 1971 while hiking on San Bernardino Peak. This is a popular destination for a picnic or easy backpacking trip and often attracts Boy Scout groups. Quiet hikers will likely hear birds calling to one another and scolding interlopers; squirrels and lizards are also common and the forest's larger denizens are sometimes sighted. In the summer, the wild berries and flowers along the creeks add to the trip's delights.

The first part of the trail is one of the steepest, climbing the slopes beneath white firs, ponderosa pines, incense cedars, and black oaks. In 0.3 mile, pass the San Gorgonio Wilderness Boundary sign, then in another 0.1 mile, reach a fork. The Forsee Creek Trail continues straight toward the San Bernardino Divide, but this trip turns right toward Johns Meadow.

The trail becomes fairly level as it contours along the slope. Majestic sugar pines shade parts of the trail and you may see their long cones heavily loading the branches or fallen on the ground below. The trail crosses a seasonal creek, rounds a hill, and descends to another seasonal creek before climbing to a small saddle overlooking Forsee Creek. It is worth making the very short scramble up the nearly bald hill northwest of the saddle for some of the best views of the trip into the Santa Ana River Canyon and to the surrounding mountains.

Descend from the saddle and cross Forsee Creek. A mammoth avalanche swept down the creek in 2005 and you can still see the shards of trees scattered about like broken matchsticks. Up the hill on the far side, reach the spacious campsites in the soft duff, 3 miles from the trailhead.

Sugar pine cones

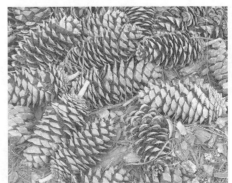

San Gorgonio Wilderness

If you would like a longer jaunt, an unmaintained trail continues up to Manzanita Spring The trail picks up on the far (southwest) side of the campsites and crosses a tributary creek. Beyond the creek, it immediately forks; both branches have faint sections, and both rejoin in 0.3 mile at a switchback. The trail then climbs up the hill and is in remarkably good condition for the remainder of the way. Pass stands of manzanitas and buckthorns, and then reach lodgepole pines just before arriving in 1.9 mile at the San Bernardino Peak Trail. This option adds another 1000 feet of elevation gain. Beyond the Manzanita Spring trail junction, it is possible to continue south for 0.5 mile, dropping 300 feet to the seasonal Columbine Springs, where there is another trail camp.

Another option from Manzanita Spring is to climb San Bernardino Peak (see Trip 5.8) and descend the Forsee Creek Trail past Jackstraw Springs back to your vehicle. This excellent loop involves a total of 18.5 miles and 4000 feet of elevation gain.

trip 5.11 South Fork Meadows

Distance	9 miles (out-and-back)	
Hiking Time	4 hours	
Elevation Gain	1400'	see map on p. 102
Difficulty	Moderate	
Trail Use	Dogs	
Best Times	May–November	
Agency	San Bernardino National Forest (Mill Creek Ranger Station)	
Recommended Map	Tom Harrison *San Gorgonio Wilderness* or *Moonridge* 7.5'	
Permit	San Gorgonio Wilderness Permit Required	

DIRECTIONS From Redlands drive east on State Highway 38 to Jenks Lake Rd., 50 yards before mile marker 038 SBD 25.51. Turn right (southeast) and follow Jenks Lake Rd. 2.5 miles to the new, well-marked South Fork Trailhead. There is a vast paved parking area with restrooms on your left.

South Fork Meadow is tucked away on the north side of San Gorgonio Wilderness in a forested valley beneath the tall peaks. It is one of the few places where hikers can venture into the Wilderness without grueling climbs up the steep slopes. In the summer, the trail is dotted with wildflowers and a quiet brook bubbles through the ferns in the meadow. There are so many springs bursting forth that the meadow was once known as Valley of the Thousand Springs. In the winter, backcountry skiers test their mettle on the trail and sometimes on the open slopes above. (A hardy group of Pomona College students made the first ski ascent of San Gorgonio on February 3, 1931.) The meadow was once a popular campsite, but has suffered from overuse and is now closed; Dry Lake, 1.8 miles farther up the trail, is a reasonable alternative.

The South Fork Trail (1E04) leads south from the trailhead through a stately forest of Jeffrey pines and white firs. In 1.5 miles, it passes through Horse Meadow; 1.0 mile beyond, it reaches the Wilderness boundary, 1000 feet up from the start. Look for a sign pointing out a short trail to the east leading up Poopout Hill to a vista of San Gorgonio framed by the trees. (Poopout Hill got its name in the 1930s, when youth groups coming up from camps near Barton Flats would turn around here.)

Return to the main trail and continue southeast. In 1.8 miles, pass a junction with

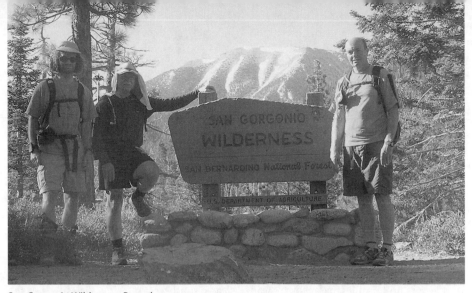

San Gorgonio Wilderness Boundary

the Lost Creek Trail coming in from the north via Grinnell Ridge. 0.3 mile beyond, arrive at the lush South Fork Meadows, where you can enjoy a picnic and admire some of the most spectacular wildflowers in the San Bernardino Mountains. The trail forks here, with one branch leading to Dollar Lake and the other to Dry Lake (see Trip 5.12), but this trip ends here and returns the way you came.

trip 5.12 San Gorgonio via Dollar and Dry Lakes

Distance	23 miles (loop)
Hiking Time	11 hours
Elevation Gain	4700′
Difficulty	Strenuous
Trail Use	Dogs, suitable for backpacking
Best Times	June–October
Agency	San Bernardino National Forest (Mill Creek Ranger Station)
Recommended Map	Tom Harrison *San Gorgonio Wilderness* or *Moonridge* and *San Gorgonio Mountain* 7.5′
Permit	San Gorgonio Wilderness Permit Required

see map on p. 102

DIRECTIONS From Redlands drive east on State Highway 38 to Jenks Lake Rd., 50 yards before mile marker 038 SBD 25.51. Turn right (southeast) and follow Jenks Lake Rd. 2.5 miles to the new, well-marked South Fork Trailhead. There is a large paved parking area with restrooms on your left.

This loop up and over San Gorgonio from the north is longer than the Vivian Creek approach, but is arguably even more scenic. It features a fine forest, scenic meadows with wildflowers, an extended traverse at and above treeline, and visits to both of the tiny lakes in San Gorgonio Wilderness. This trip can be done as a long dayhike or as a 2–3 day backpacking trip. If you are backpacking, check www.sgwa.org for the latest information on availability of water. This side of the mountain can hold its snowpack into the early summer, so check conditions and bring appropriate gear.

The South Fork Trail (1E04) leads south, climbing gradually but steadily through the forest of Jeffrey pines and white firs. In a good summer, it passes fields of

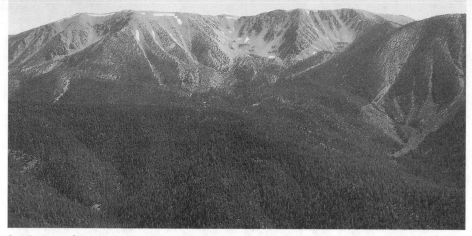
San Gorgonio from the north

wildflowers. In 1.5 miles, pass Horse Meadows. In another 1.0 mile, reach the Wilderness boundary. Take a short side trail to the left (east) to a worthwhile viewpoint on Poopout Hill where San Gorgonio Mtn. is framed between the trees, then return to the main trail.

Continue 2.1 miles to South Fork Meadows, where several springs and creeks converge to support a lush fern-filled bog. In the later summer and fall, this may be the last convenient reliable source of water. The trail forks, with one branch to Dry Lake and the other to Dollar Lake. Take the left (southeast) fork toward Dry Lake. As you climb, the diverse forest gives way to pure stands of lodgepole pines. In 1.8 miles, reach the outlet of Dry Lake, where you can enjoy another fine view of the mountain ahead. By midsummer, the lake is usually a boggy meadow. Deer can frequently be seen here, grazing and drinking. The Dry Lake and Lodgepole Spring campsites are located along the east side of the lake, but the main trail leads south along the west side, then switchbacks up, arriving at Mine Shaft Saddle in 2.2 miles, where the Fish Creek Trail comes in from the east.

Continue on to the right up Sky High Trail as it spirals around the mountain to gain the last 1500 feet of elevation on a gradual slope. The trail passes limber and lodgepole pines, which become shorter and more weather-beaten until being reduced to stunted krummholz at treeline. It initially leads southeast, offering views across the north fork of the Whitewater River (see Trip 5.17) to the Ten Thousand Foot Ridge, which drops down into Hell for Sure Canyon. Pass the wreckage of a C-47 transport plane that splattered against the mountainside in 1952 en route from Tucson to March Air Force Base during a December blizzard. Then climb eight switchbacks and traverse around to a junction west of the summit in 3.8 miles. Finally, turn right and hike the last 0.4 mile to the top of San Gorgonio Mtn. Hardy backpackers may pitch their tents on the wind-swept summit for a magical night beneath the stars.

To complete the loop, return to the junction west of the summit and continue west. In 0.2 mile, pass another junction where the Vivian Creek Trail comes up from the south. Continue west for 3.2 miles around Jepson, Little Charlton and Charlton Peaks to a four-way junction at Dollar Lake Saddle, where you dip below 10,000 feet for the first time since Mineshaft Saddle. Descend the Dollar Lake Trail 0.5 mile to a turnoff for tiny Dollar Lake, which was formed when a terminal moraine dammed a small valley as the last glaciers retreated from San Gorgonio's north face. Another trail camp is located near the lake. Continue down the main trail 1.8 miles to South Fork Meadows, go left on the South Fork Trail and finally grind out the last 4.6 miles back to the trailhead.

trip 5.13 Jenks Lake

Distance	3 miles (semi-loop)
Hiking Time	2 hours
Elevation Gain	600'
Difficulty	Easy
Trail Use	Dogs, equestrians, cyclists, good for children
Best Times	May–October
Agency	San Bernardino National Forest (Mill Creek Ranger Station)
Required Map	Tom Harrison *San Gorgonio Wilderness* or *Big Bear Lake* 7.5'

see map on p. 102

DIRECTIONS From Redlands drive east on State Highway 38 to the Barton Flats Visitor Center at mile marker 038 SBD 26.84. Park in the visitor center lot or in the wide turnout alongside the highway. Note the visitor center closes at 4:30 P.M., so park outside if you won't be back in time.

Captain Lorin Shaw Jenks built a trout pond in the 1870s, using a small dam and diverting water from the South Fork of the Santa Ana River along a 1.5-mile ditch. He raised fish and sold them in San Bernardino. Capt. Jenks also founded a resort by the lake and was renowned for regaling his guests with tall tales, but the business failed because the three-day burro ride from town was too long for most visitors. His lake, nestled beneath the tall mountains and surrounded by splendid forest, is now a popular destination for anglers, youth groups, and families. It is stocked with bluegill, sunfish, large mouth bass, and rainbow trout. Unfortunately, the water is now closed to swimming. While the lake can be reached from the paved Jenks Lake Rd., it

is more enjoyable to take the short hike up from Barton Flats Visitor Center, and then saunter around the lake before returning the way you came.

The Barton Flats Visitor Center is normally open 7:30 A.M.–4:30 P.M., Thursday–Sunday from May through October. It was closed in the 1970s by the understaffed Forest Service, but reopened in 1986 and has been operated ever since by volunteers from the San Gorgonio Wilderness Association. If you are camping nearby, inquire here about nature walks and interpretive programs. The flats got their name from Dr. Ben Barton, who raised sheep in Redlands in the 1860s and drove them each summer to graze in the mountain meadows. Barton Flats is now the site of 25 youth camps, the

Jenks Lake

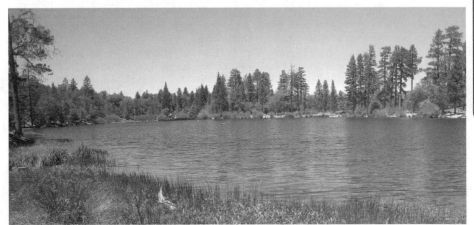

San Gorgonio Wilderness

densest collection of camps in any National Forest. Over 30,000 children a year spend time at these camps.

The trail, marked with a sign reading RIO MONTE PANORAMA, starts next to the gate at the east end of the Barton Flats Visitor Center. It leads east between Highway 38 and Frog Creek through a forest of incense cedars, black oaks, ponderosa pines, and white firs. In 0.2 mile, reach a signed Jenks Lake Trail marker. The entrance to Camp Arbolado is across the highway and this is an alternative starting point. Just beyond the marker, the trail turns right onto a dirt Forest Service road. Immediately after this turn, stay on the dirt road and pass another spur road leading along some power lines. In another 0.2 mile, cross Frog Creek at a lovely spot shaded beneath incense cedars. Then, in another 0.2 mile, turn left onto another dirt road at a trail marker; the main road continues up to private cabins. The

trail makes two more switchbacks before arriving at Jenks Lake near the outlet and a wooden pier.

Turn left and make a clockwise loop around the lake. You are likely to see ducks, squirrels, and butterflies along the way. The first part of the trail is paved and passes a picnic ground and outhouse. At the end, continue around the lake on a dirt access road to reach the southeast corner, where you may meet youth groups launching boats. A narrow dirt footpath continues along the south side of the lake. Hikers unsure of their footing will want a walking stick or helping hand along this stretch. Unfortunately, inconsiderate visitors leave quite a bit of litter along this beach; if you bring a trash bag and carry some out, you'll make the lake more enjoyable for everyone. Reach the parking area at the west end of the lake and circle back to the trail you came up.

trip 5.14 Santa Ana River Trail

Distance	38 miles (one-way)
Hiking Time	2–5 days
Elevation Gain	2800′ gain, 7800′ loss
Difficulty	Moderate–Strenuous Backpack
Trail Use	Dogs, equestrians, cyclists, suitable for backpacking
Best Times	March–November
Agency	San Bernardino National Forest (Mill Creek Ranger Station)
Required Map	*Moonridge, Big Bear Lake, Keller Peak, Yucaipa* 7.5′ (trail not depicted fully)

see maps on pp. 102 & 123

DIRECTIONS This lengthy hike is divided into several segments. The driving directions for each trailhead are given below, starting on Highway 38 in Redlands.

Big Meadows: Drive up State Highway 38 to the Heart Bar Campground turnoff just past the 038 SBD 33.48 mile marker. Turn right (south) and follow Forest Service Road 1N02 for 1.3 miles to a junction with 1N05. Park in a dirt clearing next to this junction.

South Fork Campground: Drive up State Highway 38 to a paved trailhead parking area on your left (north) just past mile marker 038 SBD 30.74, and 100 feet before the South Fork Campground turnoff to the right.

Glass Rd.: Drive up State Highway 38 to Glass Rd., between Jenks Lake Rd. and Barton Flats near mile marker 038 SBD 26.54. Turn left (north) on Glass Rd. and descend 2.1 miles to the signed Santa Ana River Trailhead. If you reach an intersection on the canyon bottom, you went 0.1 mile too far.

Angelus Oaks: Drive up State Highway 38 to Angelus Oaks. Just past mile marker 20.00, turn left (west) into the parking area for The Oaks Restaurant. Stay right through the parking area and pass the post office, then turn left on the dirt Forest Road 1N12. Immediately stay right at a sign for Thomas Hunting Grounds and pass through a gate. In 0.2 mile, park at the signed trailhead.

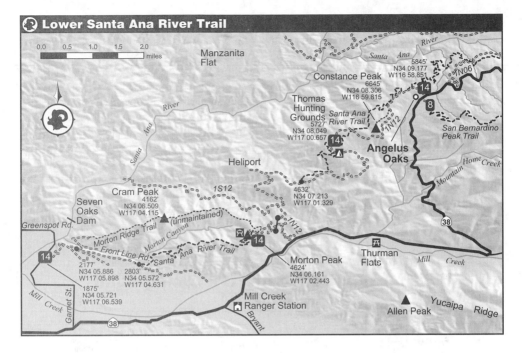

Lower Santa Ana River Trail

Thomas Hunting Grounds: Drive up State Highway 38 to Angelus Oaks. Just past mile marker 20.00, turn left (west) into the parking area for The Oaks Restaurant. Stay right through the parking area and pass the post office, then turn left on the dirt Forest Road 1N12. Immediately stay right at a sign for Thomas Hunting Grounds and pass through a gate. Follow the road 3.5 miles to a junction where the Santa Ana River Trail crosses the road, marked by a small sign. Many fine yellow-post campsites are scattered about this area.

Morton Peak Fire Lookout: A high clearance vehicle is recommended. From State Highway 38, 0.1 mile east of mile marker 038 SBD 10.50, turn left (north) onto the fair dirt Forest Road 1N12. Drive 1.2 miles up the road to a junction. A gated road turns left up to the Morton Peak Fire Lookout. If the gate is open, turn left and drive 1.4 miles to the lookout. Otherwise, leave the vehicle at the junction.

Seven Oaks Dam: From Redlands drive east on State Highway 38 to Mentone. 0.4 mile east of mile marker 038 SBD 05.00, turn left (north) on Garnet St., which crosses Mill Creek on a narrow bridge, makes two sharp turns, and becomes Greenspot Rd. Drive 2.5 miles to the unmarked Front Line fire road, on your right (east). Park here outside the locked gate; do not block the gate. If you reach a second bridge over the Santa Ana River near the Seven Oaks Dam, you have gone 0.3 mile too far.

The Santa Ana River is fed by snowmelt and alpine springs flowing down from the north face of San Gorgonio and from Big Bear Lake. As the river gathers strength, it carves a deep canyon between San Gorgonio and Big Bear, plunging down to the Seven Oaks Dam before joining with Mill Creek and flowing past Redlands and San Bernardino en route to the sea. The Santa Ana River Trail (2E03) follows the wild upper portion of the river to the point where the river is tamed by the dam. According to

the Santa Ana Watershed Project Authority, this trail will become the top portion of a 110-mile Crest to Coast Trail, which has been under sporadic construction since the 1960s. A paved bikeway will follow the river from Seven Oaks Dam to the sea.

It is hard to say whether the Santa Ana River Trail is an underused gem-in-the-rough or a sad mistake in trail planning. The river is rarely in sight of the trail, and only comes in direct contact with the trail at South Fork Campground. Some portions are poorly marked. Several miles of the route above Morton Peak follow a dirt road rather than trail. On the other hand, the trail offers good views as it traverses conifer and oak forests, riparian zones, a meadow, and chaparral-clad hillsides. Its length is exceeded in the Inland Empire only by the Pacific Crest Trail. And traveling the full distance gives a unique perspective into one of the regions major watersheds.

The top segment from Big Meadows to South Fork Campground is most popular among hikers and equestrians because it is conveniently located near many campgrounds and offers a loop option. The next two segments from South Fork Campground to Angelus Oaks are heavily used by serious mountain bikers. The trail is exposed, narrow, and uneven. Some cyclists consider this to be one of the best rides in Southern California. The lower segments receive sparse use and offer solitude and sweeping views. The long trail has strong promise for backpacking or extreme trail running, and the periodic road crossings make caching water or food easy.

trip 5.14 *Segment A:*
Big Meadows to South Fork Campground

Distance	5.5 miles (one-way), or 11 miles (out-and-back, or loop)
Hiking Time	3 hours (one-way)
Elevation Gain	200′ gain, 800′ loss (one-way)
Required Map	Tom Harrison *San Gorgonio Wilderness* or *Moonridge* 7.5′ (trail not depicted accurately on either map)

see map on p. 102

This segment can be done as a one-way hike with a car or bicycle shuttle, as an out-and-back hike, or as a loop returning along a poorly marked parallel trail. The trail system in this area is evolving rapidly and there are presently a number of unmarked side trails that can be confusing.

The trail starts at a large Santa Ana River Trail sign on the west side of the road opposite the parking area at the junction of 1N02 and 1N05. In 0.3 mile, pass a junction on the right leading back to 1N02 near the Wild Horse Equestrian Campground. In another 0.6 mile, pass a junction on the left marked ASPEN GR/FISH CR, which climbs steeply up to the Aspen Grove Trailhead. Pass above the aptly named Big Meadows. Although it is hard to see, another trail runs parallel at the edge of the meadow and several side trails drop down to it. In 1.2 miles, pass an unmarked trail on the left, which climbs up to Fish Creek below Aspen Grove. In 0.3 mile, pass the top of a closed jeep road. The trail continues contouring through the forest, then descends into the Fish Creek drainage. In 0.7 mile, reach a hairpin turn. An unmarked trail at this turn also leads left up Fish Creek to Aspen Grove (see Trip 5.15). But our trail heads downstream for 0.1 mile, and then turns left. The right fork leads down to a defunct camp. The trail has been rerouted around here and is not indicated properly on current maps. Look for signs reading 2E03 marking the correct route. The Santa Ana River Trail generally contours along the mountainside, winding in and out of various drainages. The forest is characteristic of the northern San Gorgonio region, including a mixture of ponderosa and Jeffrey pines, white firs, and black oaks. In 1.5 miles, reach a junction with the Lost Creek Trail (1E09) on the left, which makes a long climb to South Fork Meadows, but our trail turns right and descends.

In 0.6 mile, reach the paved entrance to South Fork Campground. This is a good turnaround point for a loop trip (see below). If you are making a one-way trip, the lower

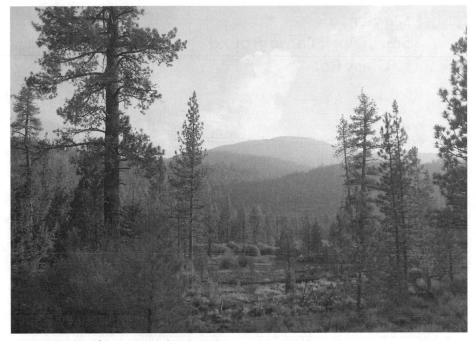

Near Big Meadow after a summer thunderstorm

trailhead parking is located directly across Highway 38. However, a more pleasant alternative to braving the busy road is to cross the campground entrance road to a trail sign, and then veer left under a highway bridge alongside the Santa Ana River. Then follow the edge of the river beneath beautiful incense cedars. In the summer, expect to see red-tipped Indian paintbrush and other wildflowers. Reach the trailhead parking at another large sign.

ALTERNATIVE FINISH

If you don't have a vehicle waiting, the least confusing option is to return the way you came. If you feel more adventurous, return to the trail sign at the entrance of South Fork Campground. Follow an intermittent trail east between the river and the edge of the campground. After passing the end of the campground, the trail continues alongside the river. In 0.6 mile, reach a fuel tank alongside the trail. The trail soon vanishes at a defunct camp, so a better choice is to ford the river and pick up another path leading east between the river and the highway. Pass the gated access road at the mouth of the camp and continue close to Highway 38. Immediately before reaching another paved road leading southeast from the highway, turn right and follow the trail back across the river. The trail then leads southeast and soon follows the edge of Big Meadows. Various short spurs lead south back up to the main Santa Ana River Trail. This area is a maze of equestrian trails and requires good navigational skills.

VARIATION

It is possible to make a fine long loop by following the Lost Creek Trail to South Fork Meadows, then continuing up to Dry Lake and taking a faint path up to Fish Creek Saddle. Descend the Fish Creek Trail to Fish Creek Meadow. Follow the Aspen Grove Trail down, and then take the Santa Ana River Trail back to the trailhead. This route requires a San Gorgonio Wilderness Permit. This route is approximately 20 miles, depending on the exact path selected.

San Gorgonio Wilderness

trip 5.14 *Segment B:*
South Fork Campground to Glass Rd.

Distance	6 miles (one-way)
Hiking Time	3 hours
Elevation Gain	300′ gain, 1100′ loss
Required Map	*Big Bear Lake 7.5′*

see map on p. 102

This segment descends along the upper reaches of the Santa Ana River Canyon. This segment and the next traverse a steep hillside with infrequent opportunities for camping. The trail is popular among mountain bikers.

From the signed Santa Ana River Trailhead parking northwest of the South Fork Campground entrance, walk west through a conifer forest along a Forest Service road, which crosses the South Fork of the Santa Ana River. In 0.1 mile, a signed trail begins on the left side of the road. The slope starts to drop away as you contour above the head of the river canyon. Sugarloaf Mtn. looms to the north, forming the opposite wall of the canyon. In 0.6 mile, reach a signed spur trail on the left leading up to High-

way 38 across from Jenks Lake Rd. East. Dispersed camping is allowed along this spur trail in the East Flat area north of the highway. The plant communities change as the slope becomes steep and sun-baked, giving way to live oaks, then manzanitas, and even prickly pear cacti. In another 2.4 miles, reach a signed four-way junction. The left fork climbs 1 mile up to Barton Flats and San Gorgonio Campgrounds. The right fork once led down to the river and Forest Road 1N45, but it has not been maintained recently and is blocked with fallen trees and washouts, so it is not recommended. The main trail continues west, gradually descending into the river canyon, and reaches a signed junction with Glass Rd. in another 3 miles.

Santa Ana River Canyon

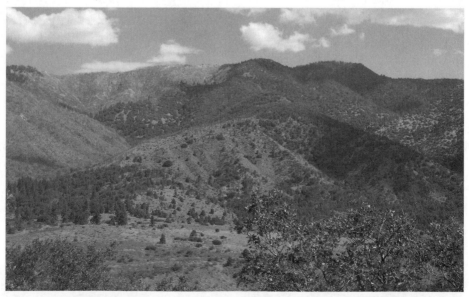

trip 5.14 *Segment C:*
Glass Rd. to Angelus Oaks

Distance	8 miles (one-way)
Hiking Time	5 hours
Elevation Gain	1200' gain, 800' loss
Required Map	*Big Bear Lake 7.5'*

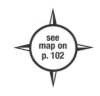

see map on p. 102

This segment follows the edge of the Santa Ana River Canyon past the resort community of Seven Oaks before climbing back up to cross Middle Control Rd. and on to Angelus Oaks. The undulating trail curves in and out to cross numerous tributary creeks, where wildflowers, firs, oaks, and a variety of pines can be found. Camping opportunities are limited. Mountain bikers use this trail heavily, but a fall on some of the steep slopes could be serious.

Starting from the trailhead at Glass Rd., hike west along the Santa Ana River Trail (2E03). In 0.5 mile, cross Barton Creek. In another 0.8 mile, an unmarked trail drops down toward the resorts. In 1.2 miles, reach an overlook where you can gaze west over the river canyon to the dramatic slope of Slide Peak. Keller Peak Fire Lookout stands on the high point just above Slide Peak. In 0.4 mile, cross Forsee Creek, where tasty blackberries ripen in late summer.

In 0.3 mile, reach a rutted dirt road. Follow the road downhill; it soon narrows back down to a trail following the path of the old road cut. In 0.9 mile, reach a junction. The right fork ends in 0.25 mile at Middle Control Rd. at a 2E03 sign. But this trip takes the left fork to stay on the main trail. Cross Schneider Creek, then in 0.9 mile cross Kilpecker Creek and arrive at Middle Control Rd. (1N06) at another 2E03 sign. (This junction is 2.0 miles down Middle Control Rd. from Highway 38.)

The trail resumes on the west (right) side of the road and follows another old road cut. In 1.1 miles, cross the jumbled granite blocks of Cold Creek Canyon. In another 0.5 mile, the trail begins switchbacking upward in earnest. Stay on the main trail, passing a faint side path leading right at the first switchback. In another 1.7 miles, reach the end of a logging road. A side trail to the left leads 0.2 mile up to the Santa Ana River Trailhead at Angelus Oaks, while the main trail continues southwest. Dispersed dry camping is feasible in this area.

Slide Peak from Santa Ana River Trail

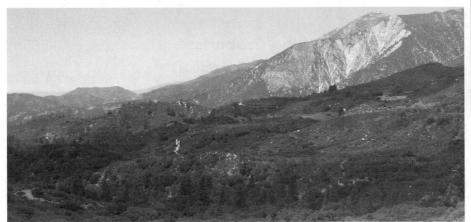

trip 5.14 *Segment D:*
Angelus Oaks
to Thomas Hunting Grounds

Distance	4 miles (one-way)
Hiking Time	2 hours
Elevation Gain	400′ gain, 500′ loss
Required Map	*Big Bear Lake, Keller Peak 7.5′*

see
maps on
pp. 102
& 123

This short segment winds along the west shoulder of Constance Peak, with dramatic views into the deep Santa Ana River Canyon and to the mountains beyond.

If you are starting at the Angelus Oaks Trailhead described in the driving directions, hike 0.2 mile down to meet the main trail at a logging road. Turn left and hike southwest on the trail. In 1.3 miles, cross another logging road. Hike through a forest of pines, firs, and oaks. Enjoy the expansive views over the Santa Ana River up Bear Creek, over Manzanita Flat, and out to Slide Peak. From here, you can see the fire lookouts atop both Butler and Keller Peaks.

The forest gives way to chaparral as it crosses the west side of Constance Peak. In 1.9 miles, cross Forest Road 1N12 at an unsigned point west of the peak. Follow a spur road, which soon ends at a signed clearing where the trail resumes. In 0.7 mile, reach 1N12 again, where this segment terminates. This beautiful area is called Thomas Hunting Grounds and several fine yellow-post campsites can be found in the open woodland. The origin of the place name is uncertain, but John Robinson speculates that it was named for Mark Thomas of San Bernardino, who guided W. A. Goodyear of the California Geological Society on the first claimed ascent of San Gorgonio in 1872.

Approaching Thomas Hunting Grounds

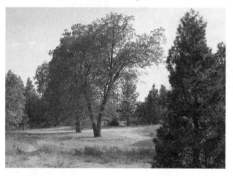

trip 5.14 *Segment E:*
Thomas Hunting Grounds
to Morton Peak Fire Lookout

Distance	7.5 miles (one-way)
Hiking Time	4 hours
Elevation Gain	700′ gain, 1800′ loss
Required Map	*Keller Peak, Yucaipa 7.5′*

see
map on
p. 123

This segment follows a short stretch of trail, and then joins a dirt road. Some maps such as the Fine Edge San Bernardino Mountains Recreation Topo show the trail leading all the way to Morton Peak, but chaparral has reclaimed the lower part. The trail is exposed to the merciless sun and can be unpleasantly hot on a summer

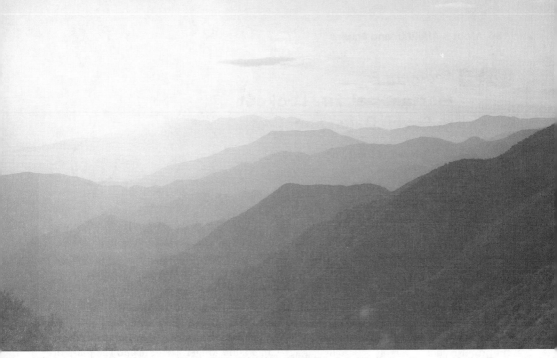

Sunset over the San Bernardino and San Gabriel Mountains

afternoon; bring plenty of water. During the fall hunting season, wear bright colors and be particularly alert for the first half mile.

For a truly unusual and romantic finish, consider renting the Morton Peak Fire Lookout for an evening. Plan to arrive before the lookout host departs at 5 P.M. This is a spectacular place to watch sunset, sunrise, and the lights of the Inland Empire. Guests bring their own sleeping bags, water, and camp stove. The lookout sleeps 3 adults and rents for $75/night. Call 1(800) 424-4232 or visit www.bigbear.com for reservations.

From Thomas Hunting Grounds find the small sign at the trailhead on Forest Road 1N12 and hike west on the Santa Ana River Trail. In 0.2 mile reach an unmarked junction with a dirt road. The trail follows the road for 50 yards, then splits off to the left at a sign reading NO MOTOR VEHICLES. Pass above some yellow post campsites and near another dirt road before switchbacking down a steep slope. In 1.5 miles, reach a notch in the ridge where the trail meets 1N12 again. Instead of crossing the road, take the trail that continues west on the

north side of the ridge. In 0.8 mile, the trail terminates at the road.

Turn right and descend 1N12. A mountain bike ride is particularly appealing for travel on this segment. Pass a spur road on the right at a switchback in 1.1 miles, and then a second spur on the right in another 1.9 miles. In another 0.6 mile, reach a junction with a road on the right labeled 2E03 leading up to the Morton Peak Fire Lookout. The gate is locked when the lookout is closed.

If you are not planning to visit the lookout, you can meet a vehicle here or descend 1N12 another 1.2 miles to Highway 38. To reach the lookout, hike west up the road for 1.2 miles to a junction. A signpost beside a trail on the left reading PLEASE STAY ON EXISTING ROADS AND TRAILS marks the continuation of the Santa Ana River Trail. However, it is worth continuing up the road for 0.2 mile to the lookout on Morton Peak, where you can enjoy spectacular views in all directions. The lookout is normally staffed by volunteer fire lookout hosts from May through October; these volunteers enjoy sharing their wealth of knowledge with visitors.

trip 5.14 *Segment F:*
Morton Peak Fire Lookout to Seven Oaks Dam

Distance	6.5 miles (one-way)
Hiking Time	3.5 hours
Elevation Gain	2800′ loss
Required Map	*Yucaipa* 7.5′

see map on p. 123

The final segment of the Santa Ana River Trail descends a ridge overlooking Morton Canyon. It then follows the dirt Front Line Rd. down to the paved Greenspot Rd beneath Seven Oaks Dam. This is the lowest and hottest section of the trail and is not recommended in the summer. The south side of the ridge was incinerated in the August 2006 Emerald Fire, which was started by illegal and negligent target shooting. This chaparral is growing back rapidly, and this is a good place to watch the process of regeneration.

From the top of Morton Peak, descend the access road east for 0.2 mile. Look for an old road cut on the left. This was once the Morton Ridge Trail that led to Cram Peak and down to Seven Oaks Dam, but it has not been maintained in years and is badly overgrown with chaparral; the route is not particularly enjoyable today.

About 20 feet beyond the road cut, a trail on the right side is marked with a sign reading PLEASE STAY ON EXISTING ROADS AND TRAILS. This is the continuation of the Santa Ana River Trail, although the signage currently gives no clue of this fact. The good trail descends switchbacking to the south before following the ridge west. An excessive number of trail markers warn mountain bikers to stay in control. At a point south of Cram Peak, the trail makes several more switchbacks to drop off the toe of the ridge and join Front Line Rd. (1S14) at a gap in the fence, 4.4 miles down. This junction is marked with another PLEASE STAY ON EXISTING ROADS AND TRAILS sign but no Santa Ana River Trail marker.

Turn right and follow Front Line Rd. west along a low ridge. In 1.2 miles, pass a road coming in sharply from the left above old orchards. Just after, another road descends right into Morton Canyon. (This road meets the Morton Ridge Trail on the north side of the canyon.)

Beyond this point, the USGS topographic map is no longer accurate and the maze of dirt roads can be confusing. Your goal is to get down to the paved Greenspot Rd. to the west. In 0.2 mile, turn left (south) and descend to another dirt road. Turn right and follow the road northwest above more orchards. In 0.1 mile, turn left. In another 0.3 mile, pass a junction on the left leading east into the orchards, but stay on the main road, which leads another 0.2 mile west to the unsigned terminus of the Santa Ana River Trail at Greenspot Rd.

Morton Peak Fire Lookout

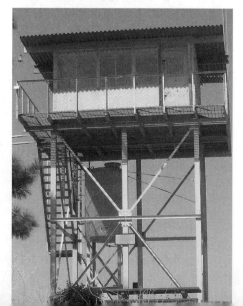

trip 5.15 Aspen Grove

Distance	1.8 miles (out-and-back)
Hiking Time	1 hour
Elevation Gain	350'
Difficulty	Easy
Trail Use	Dogs, good for children
Best Times	October
Agency	San Bernardino National Forest (Mill Creek Ranger Station)
Recommended Map	Tom Harrison *San Gorgonio Wilderness* or *Moonridge* 7.5'
Permit	San Gorgonio Wilderness Permit Required

see map on p. 102

DIRECTIONS From Redlands drive east on State Highway 38 to the Heart Bar Campground turnoff just past the 038 SBD 33.48 mile marker. Turn right and follow Forest Service Road 1N02 for 1.3 miles, passing the campground entrance. At a junction, turn right on 1N05, a fair dirt road, and proceed 1.6 miles to the signed Aspen Grove Trailhead at a hairpin turn in the road.

In October each year, quaking aspens (*Populus tremuloides*) leaves turn bright yellow for a few short weeks, and then drop from the trees. Aspen Grove is one of only two places in California outside the Sierra Nevada where the splendid trees can still be seen. This hike follows Fish Creek through four groves of aspens. The willows in the creek also change colors, adding to the festive display beneath the evergreen firs and pines. Call the Mill Creek Ranger Station for current foliage information. Neither of the recommended maps is quite accurate at portraying the maze of trails around Big Meadows, but the main trail from the Aspen Grove Trailhead is clearly marked.

From the trailhead, walk south 0.3 mile down to Fish Creek. Cross the creek and immediately reach a trail junction in a dense grove of aspen. It can be hard to get a perspective on the trees because you are right beneath them. Trails lead north and south from this junction along the west side of Fish Creek (note: trail repeatedly crosses creek). The naming of the trails is somewhat confusing. The Aspen Grove Trail leads south to join the Fish Creek Trail beyond Lower Fish Creek Meadow (see Trip 5.16). An unnamed trail leads north to join the Santa Ana River Trail. The best groves of aspen are actually found to the north.

Turn right (north) and follow the trail downstream along the creek. The forest is unusual because it consists predominantly of white firs, though Jeffrey pines are also plentiful. In 0.25 mile, pass a second grove of aspens mixed with willows and cross back to the east side of the creek. In another 0.15 mile, look for a stately grove of aspens lined up on the far side of the creek. In another 0.2 mile cross Fish Creek three more times and reach a fourth grove of aspens.

VARIATION

Return the way you came. If you would like a longer walk, consider continuing down Fish Creek to the junction with the Santa Ana River Trail (see Trip 5.14), then east along the river trail to either of two unmarked junctions where you can loop back. This is only recommended if you are familiar with the area and comfortable navigating; the trails are not properly indicated on the recommended maps.

Aspen Grove

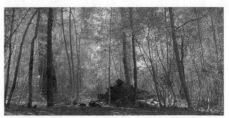

San Gorgonio Wilderness

trip 5.16 Fish Creek Meadows

Distance	4 miles (out-and-back)
Hiking Time	2 hours
Elevation Gain	650'
Difficulty	Easy
Trail Use	Dogs
Best Times	May–November
Agency	San Bernardino National Forest (Mill Creek Ranger Station)
Recommended Map	Tom Harrison *San Gorgonio Wilderness* or *Moonridge* 7.5'
Permit	San Gorgonio Wilderness Permit Required

see map on p. 102

DIRECTIONS From Redlands drive east on State Highway 38 to the Heart Bar Campground turnoff just past the 038 SBD 33.48 mile marker. Turn right and follow Forest Service Road 1N02 for 1.3 miles, passing the campground entrance. At a junction, turn right on 1N05, a fair dirt road, and proceed 1.6 miles to the signed Aspen Grove Trailhead at a hairpin turn in the road. If you plan to do a one-way hike, leave another vehicle 4.7 miles farther up 1N05 at the Fish Creek Trailhead. Along the way, stay right at three forks, not all of which are marked.

Fish Creek defines the northeastern boundary of San Gorgonio Wilderness. This pleasant hike up the valley leads to a small meadow. A short detour to the north leads to several stately groves of aspens.

From the Aspen Grove Trailhead, walk south 0.3 mile and cross Fish Creek to reach a fork. The trail to the right leads down to Aspen Grove (see Trip 5.15), but this trip turns left. Hike south along the west bank of the creek through a forest of tall white firs. In 1.2 miles, cross to the east side of the creek and stay right at an unmarked fork. (The left fork passes along the east edge of Lower Fish Creek Meadow and leads to the Fish Creek Trailhead in 1.1 miles.) Shortly beyond, Lower Fish Creek Meadow comes into view beside the trail and in 0.6 mile,

reach a signed trail junction with the Fish Creek Trail.

VARIATION

At this point, you can retrace your steps to the trailhead. If you would like to visit more of Fish Creek Meadows, turn right (west) at the junction and proceed 0.5 mile to Upper Fish Creek Meadow, where you may find columbine, Indian paintbrush, and corn lilies.

ALTERNATIVE FINISH

Alternatively, for a one-way hike, turn left (east) and go 0.6 mile to the Fish Creek Trailhead at the end of 1N05. This requires a 4.7-mile car or bicycle shuttle; mountain bikers should beware that there is uphill travel in both directions.

Lower Fish Creek Meadow

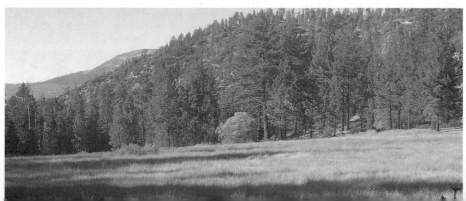

trip 5.17 San Gorgonio via Fish Creek

Distance	19 miles (out-and-back)
Hiking Time	10 hours
Elevation Gain	3600'
Difficulty	Strenuous
Trail Use	Dogs, suitable for backpacking
Best Times	June–October
Agency	San Bernardino National Forest (Mill Creek Ranger Station)
Recommended Map	Tom Harrison *San Gorgonio Wilderness* or *Moonridge* and *San Gorgonio Mountain* 7.5'
Permit	San Gorgonio Wilderness Permit Required

see map on p. 102

DIRECTIONS From Redlands drive east on State Highway 38 to the Heart Bar Campground turnoff just past the 038 SBD 33.48 mile marker. Turn right and follow Forest Service Road 1N02 for 1.3 miles, passing the campground entrance. At a junction, turn right on 1N05, a fair dirt road, and proceed 6.3 miles, staying right (on the main road) at three forks, to the signed Fish Creek Trailhead at the end of the road.

Fish Creek drops down the northeast slopes of San Gorgonio Mtn. A long dirt road leads high up into its headwaters. The Fish Creek Trail, completed in 1971, is the easiest route to the summit, and is also one of the most lightly used, so you are likely to be able to get a permit when the more popular Vivian Creek and South Fork Trail have reached their quotas. The forests, meadows, and wide-ranging views are magnificent and this route would likely see as much travel as the others if the trailhead were closer to the highway. Fish Creek also provides backpackers access to excellent camping at Mineshaft Flats.

The Fish Creek Trail (1W07) leads west from the southern end of the parking area into a forest of Jeffrey pines and white firs. In 0.6 mile, come to a junction near Lower Fish Creek Meadow. The right fork leads to Aspen Grove (see Trips 5.15–5.16), while the Fish Creek Trail continues straight. Stay on Fish Creek Trail, cross two trickling forks of Fish Creek, and hike alongside the bushy Upper Fish Creek Meadow.

In 1.2 miles, reach Fish Creek Trail Camp at the bottom of a draw, with tent sites cleared beneath the towering firs. Great forested slopes rise on three sides, with Ten Thousand Foot Ridge to the south and Grinnell Mtn. to the west. Water might

be available from the draw just up the trail; check conditions in advance before depending on it.

The trail follows the draw, then soon crosses it and begins long switchbacks up the east slope of Grinnell Mtn. The mountain was named for Joseph Grinnell, a zoologist from the University of California who made the classic study of animals in the eastern San Bernardino Mountains from 1905–07. Lodgepole pines begin appearing, with their distinctive flaky bark and small cones, and soon crowd out all the other trees. After 3 miles of steady climbing, reach Fish Creek Saddle, where there is yet more dry camping. (An unmaintained and faint trail leads west down the draw to Lodgepole Spring, just above Dry Lake, where you may find water.) Continue southwest for 0.8 mile, through a ghost forest of dead lodgepoles on the north slopes of Lake Peak, to a saddle with a trail junction leading 1.2 miles down to Mineshaft Flat overlooking the Whitewater River's North Fork.

VARIATION

Mineshaft Flat is a great destination for a backpacking trip if you don't care to hike all the way to San Gorgonio. This round trip is 14 miles with 3000 feet of elevation gain. You'll beat the crowds and find plenty

San Gorgonio Wilderness

of camping on soft ground beneath the lodgepoles under Gorgonio's steep slopes. Tremendous avalanches sweep down these slopes in the winter every few decades, laying waste to all trees in their path. Watchful and lucky hikers may see the herd of desert bighorn sheep that roam the ridges and canyons where humans rarely visit. Mineshaft Flat was the site of an unsuccessful mining operation early in the 20th Century. Water is usually available from a spring below the trail 0.4 mile below the flats where the trail crosses the Whitewater River. You might choose to continue another 0.8 mile down the canyon to North Fork Meadows where there was once camping beside Big Tree. The flat sites are now overgrown and not recommended presently, but it is a quiet destination for lunch and peaceful contemplation.

From Fish Creek Saddle pass along the south side of a hill, locally known as Zahniser Peak, for 0.2 mile to a second junction at Mineshaft Saddle. Take the Sky High Trail to the left (south), which spirals around the mountain to gain the last 1500 feet of elevation on a gradual slope. It passes limber and lodgepole pines, which become shorter and more weather-beaten until being reduced to isolated shrubs at treeline. At about 10400 feet, pass the wreckage of a C-47 transport plane that splattered against the mountainside on a stormy night in 1952. Then climb eight switchbacks and traverse around to a junction west of the summit in 3.8 miles. Finally, turn right and hike the last 0.4 mile to the top of San Gorgonio Mtn. Hardy backpackers may pitch their tents on the wind-swept summit for a magical night beneath the stars.

VARIATION

Dedicated peak baggers might choose to hike Lake Peak and/or Grinnell Mtn. from Fish Creek Saddle on the return. To reach Lake Peak, hike south up to the ridge, then turn right and follow the ridge to the boulder pile that forms the summit. This adds 400 feet of gain and 0.3 mile each way. To reach Grinnell Mtn., hike north along the ridge, bypassing some obstacles on the left. You may find traces of a use trail along the way. The summit is broad, flat, and forested, but the true high point is marked by a cairn near the east side. This adds 500 feet of gain and 0.6 mile each way.

North Fork of the Whitewater River from Mineshaft Flat

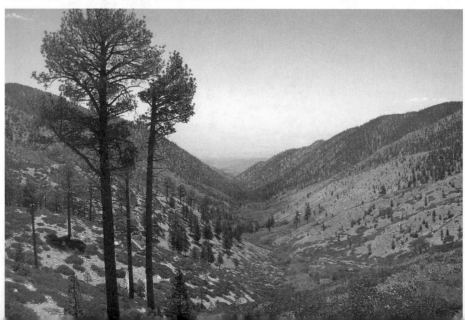

trip 5.18 San Gorgonio Nine Peaks Challenge

Distance	25 miles (one-way)
Hiking Time	14 hours
Elevation Gain	8000'
Difficulty	Very strenuous
Trail Use	Dogs, suitable for backpacking
Best Times	June–October
Agency	San Bernardino National Forest (Mill Creek Ranger Station)
Required Map	Tom Harrison *San Gorgonio Wilderness* or *Forest Falls, San Gorgonio Mountain, Moonridge,* and *Big Bear Lake* 7.5'
Permit	San Gorgonio Wilderness Permit Required

see map on p. 102

DIRECTIONS There are many variations on where to start and end this trip. This version assumes you start at the Vivian Creek Trailhead and end at the San Bernardino Peak Trailhead. To drop a vehicle at the San Bernardino Peak Trailhead, follow State Highway 38 to Angelus Oaks. Look for signs for the San Bernardino Peak Trail (1W07). From Highway 38, first turn right on Manzanita Rd. toward the fire station at mile marker 038 SBD 20.00. Then make an immediate left and drive for 0.1 mile, passing the station. Make a right onto a fair dirt road past the station at a sign indicating 1W07. Stay right at two forks and go 0.3 mile to a large dirt parking area with the signed SAN BERNARDINO PEAK TRAILHEAD. To reach the Vivian Creek Trailhead, descend State Highway 38 heading southwest toward Redlands to the huge hairpin turn at mile marker 038 SBD 15.00. Turn right on Valley of the Falls Dr. and proceed 4.5 miles to its end. Turn left and park at the Vivian Creek Trailhead.

The great San Bernardino Divide forms the backbone of San Gorgonio Wilderness and is the highest ridge in California south of the Sierra Nevada. The west end is anchored by San Bernardino Peak, while the east end culminates above treeline on the towering summit of San Gorgonio Mtn. A well-built trail, constructed by the Forest Service in 1938, runs the length of the gently undulating crest, passing seven other minor peaks along the way. A worthwhile challenge is to climb all nine of these summits; the undertaking has become so popular that the San Gorgonio Wilderness Association sells an "I Climbed the Nine Peaks" arm patch to commemorate the deed. Boy Scout troops do the hike as a 3-day backpacking trip. Experienced mountaineers can do it in one long day. This trip is recommended for those who already know the area well because it usually involves some hiking before dawn and/or after dark. Good navigation skills are required to locate the minor peaks on the ridge. Although this is a very strenuous route, it is easier than the other Nine Peaks challenges around Mt. Baldy and the Desert Divide.

Carefully study the map and choose the route you would like to take. This description assumes a start up the Vivian Creek Trail to San Gorgonio Mtn. followed by an east-to-west traverse ending at Angelus Oaks. It has the advantage of doing the hardest climb in the morning while you are fresh and being mostly downhill thereafter. Another alternative is to start up the Fish Creek Trail; this route has less elevation gain but a much longer car shuttle. If only one vehicle is available, it is possible to ascend Vivian Creek, descend the Momyer Trail, then hike or cycle Valley of the Falls Dr. 2 miles back to the Vivian Creek Trailhead.

Many of the peaks along the ridge were named by a young surveyor named Donald McLain in 1920 as he spent the summer roaming and mapping the high country. Those honored by place names include Willis Jepson, the University of California botanist who wrote *Manual of the Flowering Plants of California*; Rushton Charlton, McLain's boss and the Supervisor of Angeles

San Gorgonio Wilderness

National Forest, who ironically opposed wilderness protection for San Gorgonio; Leila Shields, manager of Camp Radford on the Santa Ana River; and Lou Anderson, the Barton Flats ranger.

Climb the Vivian Creek Trail (see Trip 5.1) 8 miles to the trail junction on the crest. Just above this junction is a vista point with a fine view west along the entire San Bernardino Divide. Turn right (east) and proceed 0.6 mile to the summit of San Gorgonio. At this point, you have completed two-thirds of the elevation gain but only one third of the distance. Return to the junction and hike west past the junction of the Vivian Creek Trail. As the trail descends near Jepson Peak, hike cross-country to the summit, then descend to rejoin the trail. Follow the trail around Jepson Peak to a bend north of the peak. Hike cross-country from here up Little Charlton and Charlton Peak, and then descend to Dollar Lake Saddle.

Follow the trail northwest as it passes the insignificant rock pile, which has been informally dubbed Alto Diablo Peak, and scramble to the top. The crux of this climb is to identify the summit, which is marked on the Tom Harrison map but not on the USGS topo. It is the first high point reached after climbing up from Dollar Lake Saddle. If you begin switchbacking down toward Shields Flat, you just missed it.

The trail then follows the north side of the ridge. The tall lodgepole pines and fine views more than compensate for your fatigue. Make similar short excursions to the summits of Shields Peak, Anderson Peak, San Bernardino East Peak, and finally San Bernardino Peak, 9 miles from San Gorgonio. Then descend the last weary 8 miles to Angelus Oaks (see Trip 5.8).

VARIATION

Extraordinarily ambitious peak baggers can scale even more summits in this beautiful high country. For example, at least two mountaineers have dayhiked all 17 named peaks: Grinnell, Ten Thousand Foot Ridge, Lake, Zahniser, Bighorn, Dragon's Head, San Gorgonio, Jepson, East Dobbs, Dobbs, Little Charlton, Charlton, Alto Diablo, Shields, Anderson, San Bernardino East, and San Bernardino. This 38-mile loop with 12,000 feet of elevation gain can be done without a car shuttle by starting at the South Fork Trailhead and descending the Forsee Creek Trail.

San Bernardino Divide

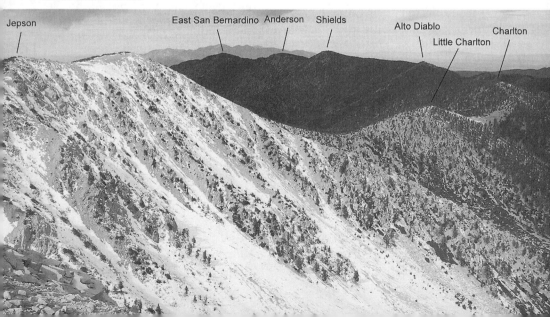

trip 5.19 Seven Peaks of the Yucaipa Ridge

Distance	13.5 miles (one-way)
Hiking Time	13 hours
Elevation Gain	6100'
Difficulty	Very strenuous
Best Times	May–November
Agency	San Bernardino National Forest (Mill Creek Ranger Station)
Required Map	Tom Harrison *San Gorgonio Wilderness* or *Forest Falls, San Gorgonio Mountain 7.5'*

see map on p. 102

DIRECTIONS The hike requires a 3-mile shuttle between trailheads. From Redlands drive east on State Highway 38 to the huge hairpin turn at mile marker 038 SBD 15.00. Turn right on Valley of the Falls Dr. In 1.4 miles, after crossing the bridge over Mill Creek, turn right on Prospect Dr. Leave a vehicle 0.1 mile up the road, taking care not to park on private property or block traffic. Return to Valley of the Falls Dr. and continue 3.1 miles to its end. Turn left and park at the Vivian Creek Trailhead.

The Oak Glen Divide or Yucaipa Ridge, running parallel to and south of the San Bernardino Divide, separates Mill Creek Canyon from Oak Glen and Yucaipa. The ridge tapers from a jagged knife-edge at the east end to a rounded series of humps on the lower west end. This trip follows the crest all the way from Galena Peak to Birch Mtn., visiting Little San Gorgonio Peak, Wilshire Mtn., Wilshire Peak, Oak Glen Peak, and Cedar Mtn. along the way. It involves cross-country travel nearly the entire way, and has some extremely steep and loose sections; despite the relatively short distance, the trip is only suitable for highly experienced navigators who are comfortable moving quickly on difficult terrain. The USGS topographic maps are strongly advisable because they have far more detail than can be shown on a larger scale map. The trip's difficulty can be reduced somewhat by only doing the section from Galena Peak to Little San Gorgonio Peak, or from Little San Gorgonio Peak to Birch Mtn., but both of these options are still serious undertakings.

Long pants and gaiters are strongly recommended because some patches of brush are inevitable. A hiking pole or work gloves are also handy on the unstable terrain. Large parties may want helmets because rock fall is almost certain. The USGS 7.5' maps are indispensable for cross-country navigation. They show the Oak Glen Divide Trail along the top of the Yucaipa Ridge, but it has not been maintained in years and is scarcely visible. Access to the ridge from all directions has also been severely curtailed by private property owners.

The hike begins at the Vivian Creek Trailhead and ends on Prospect Dr. in Forest Falls. Start by climbing Galena Peak by way of Mill Creek Canyon and the Mill Creek Jumpoff (see Trip 5.1). Hike over to the west summit and inspect the route to the west. Little San Gorgonio Peak is the high point visible 2.3 miles away and is lower than Galena, but the next stretch to reach it is more demanding and time consuming than the entire climb to Galena Peak. Rick Kent describes the traverse in the summit register as "a wickedly diabolical route!" The route follows the knife-edge ridge studded with rocky gendarmes and dotted with brush. Most of the terrain is class two, but there are a few third class moves along the way. Along the way, savor the some of the finest viewpoints of the four Saints: San Gorgonio, San Bernardino, San Jacinto, and San Antonio.

The crux of the traverse is to descend the first part of the ridge to the saddle between Peak 9164' and Peak 8868'. The easiest path tends to follow the crest, or just below on the south, but occasionally has to dip farther down on the south to escape brush or to veer onto the crumbling north face to bypass obstacles. Beyond the saddle, the ridge becomes less steep and a use trail can occasionally be found. There are many large patches of brush that can be circumvented with careful route finding. Climb over Peak 8868´, then down to the next saddle, and then up over the rocky top of Peak 9240´+, then down into the saddle at the top of Camp Creek. Finally, hike up the open slopes to the summit of Little San Gorgonio Peak.

The remainder of the Yucaipa Ridge loses its knife-edge character and is much easier to follow. Moreover, the Oak Glen Divide Trail once followed the crest and traces of it are still visible, guiding you past patches of brush. From Little San Gorgonio Peak, descend west to a saddle, then climb to a hill with a communications tower. If you need to escape the ridge because of a shortage of time or energy, the best way down begins about 0.2 mile east of the tower and descends northward onto a ridge that drops into Camp Creek (see Trip 5.2). Otherwise, follow the dirt service road west down and then gently up to Peak 8832´, which is called Wilshire Mtn. by the Sierra Club. When the service road turns left (south) and begins to descend, leave it and hike to the nearby flat wooded summit.

Descend northwest, and then hike back up southwest to Wilshire Peak. Wilshire Peak is named for Joe Wilshire, a pioneer apple grower in Oak Glen. The old trail is marked by single rock cairns in places and tends to follow the crest. It is convenient when you can locate it, but not worth too much effort to precisely follow because it has been completely obliterated in places. Descend the steep northwest ridge of Wilshire Peak, then take the easy hike over nearby Oak Glen Peak to Cedar Mtn. Sadly, no cedars are to be found on the summit.

Just 0.1 mile west of the summit is a sign marking the junction of the Oak Glen Divide Trail with a trail climbing up from Oak Glen, though both trails are scarcely visible any longer.

Hike northwest, passing on the south side of two bumps on the ridge, to the Birch-Cedar Saddle. The Oak Glen Divide Trail may be found contouring around the north slope of Birch Mtn., but it is easier to hike directly up the ridge to the summit of Birch Mtn. The complete traverse from Little San Gorgonio Peak involves 4.8 miles and 1100 feet of elevation gain. Again, there are no birches on the summit. Birch Mtn. was apparently named for Birch Creek, which itself was named for misidentified trees.

The most practical, though unpleasant and difficult, descent to Forest Falls begins at the Birch-Cedar Saddle. From the east end of the saddle, hike east into the canyon between Oak Creek and Bridal Veil Creek. It is convenient to aim for the ridge east of the canyon where the walking is unobstructed, but rock

Gnarled tree on the Yucaipa Ridge

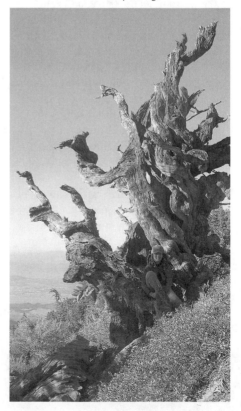

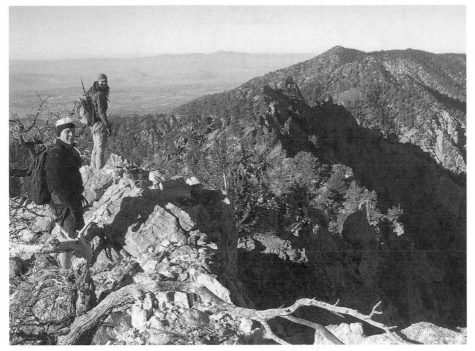

Little San Gorgonio Peak and the eastern Yucaipa Ridge

ribs separating upper forks of the canyon make the traverse very tedious. The ridge has been partially logged at about 6600 feet. The trip ends behind the houses on Prospect Dr., where your getaway vehicle awaits.

VARIATIONS

There are several alternatives for this trip. Local hikers have discovered a number of steep and devious routes from Forest Falls to the Yucaipa Ridge. It is possible to climb to a point 0.5 mile west of Little San Gorgonio Peak from the Vivian Creek Trailhead by way of Camp Creek (see Trip 5.2). From here, you can make a shorter loop east to Galena Peak or west to Birch Mtn. Another option is to continue west from Birch Mtn. along the Oak Glen Divide Trail to the Yucaipa Ridge fire road, which was once a popular point of entry. Access to this road from both the south and north is now cut off by landowners.

San Gorgonio
Wilderness

chapter 6

High Desert

The High Desert encompasses the Mojave Desert in San Bernardino County. It generally sits at elevations of 2000–4000 feet, in contrast to the Low Desert around the Coachella Valley, which is near or below sea level. The High Desert is thus cooler and moister than its lower counterpart. Creosote bush and Joshua tree are two of the characteristic plants. This chapter covers hikes in the vicinity of Victorville and Barstow, the High Desert's major communities. Chapters 15 and 16 cover other regions of the Mojave Desert.

The High Desert is a gigantic plateau that began pushing up about 140 million years ago as the Pacific and North American plates crashed together. More recently, the same forces pushed up some of the minor desert mountain ranges and volcanoes. Until recently, geologically speaking, the region received regular rainfall and was the site of enormous lakes. Large land animals once roamed the area. About 10,000 years ago, at the end of the last Ice Age, the Mojave fell into the rain shadow of the rising Transverse and Peninsular Mountain Ranges (the San Gabriels, San Bernardinos, and San Jacintos), which were pushed up by the infamous San Andreas Fault. Moisture from the ocean seldom crosses these formidable barriers, so the lakes dried up and the land changed dramatically.

The Mojave River is one of the few major water sources in this desert. Its waters flow briskly off the north slopes of the San Bernardino Mountains, but soon sink into the sands near Hesperia. The river mostly flows underground, but occasionally emerges to the surface at bottlenecks such as Afton Canyon, or when intense thunderstorms send flash floods down the riverbed. Flash floods can radically change the terrain in canyons and washes, so be prepared for conditions to differ from these route descriptions.

Although many people think of the desert as lifeless, a wide variety of animals scratch out a living in these harsh conditions. Dawn and dusk are great times to watch for wildlife, but observant hikers will see tracks and scat any time of day.

The best time to visit the High Desert is between late fall and early spring. Summer temperatures routinely exceed 100°F in the shade. However, subfreezing temperatures are not uncommon in the winter. The desert is especially beautiful after the occasional snowstorm. Temperatures can fluctuate dramatically between day and night time, so come prepared.

Owl Canyon

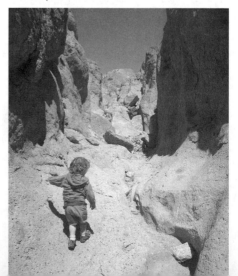

trip 6.1 Mormon Rocks Nature Loop

Distance	1 mile (loop)
Hiking Time	30 minutes
Elevation Gain	200'
Difficulty	Easy
Trail Use	Dogs, good for children
Best Times	October–April
Agency	Angeles National Forest (Cajon Ranger Station)
Optional Map	*Telegraph Peak, Cajon* 7.5'

DIRECTIONS From Interstate 15 south of Cajon Pass, exit west on Highway 138. Proceed 1.6 miles and turn left into the Mormon Rocks Forest Service Fire Station.

At the junction of Interstate 15 and Route 138, oddly tilted sedimentary rock formations stand sentinel below Cajon Pass. Officially named Rock Candy Mountains, but locally known as the Mormon Rocks, the formations have been riddled with holes by strong winds and weather. Lizards, owls, and pack rats make their homes in these small caves. The wild contortions of the San Andreas Fault have thrust these cemented sandstone beds upward toward the sky. Although the Mormon Rocks appear to be weather-worn and crumbly, they remain standing because they erode more slowly than the sand and silt of the alluvial flats of the Cajon Canyon Wash.

Behind the pine-shaded Mormon Rocks Fire Station and across a picturesque footbridge is a well-marked 1-mile nature trail. The trail was built by the Forest Service in 1975 to provide hikers with panoramic views of the Mormon Rocks and the Cajon Pass. The trail's numbered interpretive markers provide history and geological information about the surrounding area. Be sure to pick up the informative brochure at the beginning of the trail.

The trail switchbacks through areas of creosote and sage bushes, manzanitas, and yuccas. Note that this trail does not weave its way through the rocks themselves, but is across the highway, and provides expansive views of the formations. To explore the rock formations more closely, simply cross Highway 138 and wander to your heart's content.

Mormon Rocks

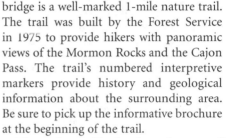

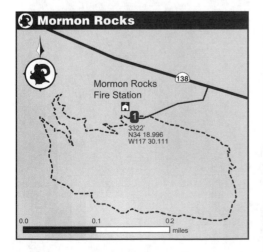

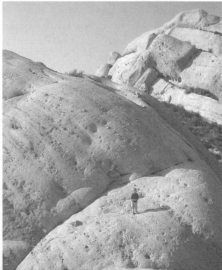

trip 6.2 East Ord Mtn.

Distance	2.5 miles (out-and-back or semi-loop)
Hiking Time	3–4 hours
Elevation Gain	2000'
Difficulty	Moderate
Trail Use	Dogs
Best Times	October–April
Agency	BLM Barstow Field Office
Required Map	*Fry Mountains, Camp Rock Mine, Ord Mountain* 7.5'

see map on p. 143

DIRECTIONS A high clearance vehicle is useful to reach the trailhead. From Interstate 15 in Victorville, turn east on Highway 18 and proceed 25 miles to Lucerne Valley. At a stop sign, continue straight (east) to join Highway 247 and go 5.1 miles. At an intersection 0.4 mile east of mile marker 247 SBD 40.00, turn left (north) on Camp Rock Rd. In 4.0 miles, stay right to remain on Camp Rock Rd. In another 2.3 miles, the road turns to excellent dirt. Continue 7.6 miles to a junction beneath the huge transmission lines; turn left on the fair dirt BLM Road 6657. A high clearance vehicle may be helpful if this road hasn't been maintained recently. Go 0.9 mile to a junction, then turn right and continue 0.7 mile up a rocky dirt road to a turnout beside the ruins of a corrugated metal water tank. If you have 4WD and plenty of clearance, you can continue 0.3 mile farther up the road to park at a second turnout where the road passes near the wash to the north.

E ast Ord Mtn. is a volcanic desert peak overlooking the Lucerne Valley between Victorville and Joshua Tree. It is slightly shorter than its neighbor, Ord Mtn., but is nevertheless the most prominent mountain in the range. The Ord Mountains were named for Major General E. O. C. Ord who led the first official survey of Los Angeles. Finding the remote trailhead is half the fun of this short but steep cross-country jaunt. Despite its short length, the trip is not recommended for inexperienced desert travelers. The summit offers outstanding 360° views of snowcapped ranges and desert basins on a clear winter day, from San Gorgonio in the south to the Panamint Mountains to the north. The mountain overlooks the Johnson Valley Off-Highway Vehicle Recreation Area; the incessant whine of dirt bikes and ATVs can detract from the wilderness experience.

From the lower parking area, hike west up the rough and rocky mining road for 0.3 mile. After passing around a ridge coming down from the north, the road runs adjacent to a boulder-strewn dry wash before climbing steeply up a hill. 4WD vehicles can park here, just before the hill and a white

cable fence. From this upper parking area, study the view of the peak to the north-northwest and pick out your route. The summit is identifiable by the brown line of cliffs underneath and the dirt saddle immediately to the left (west). This trip climbs the mountain by way of the saddle.

Leave the road at the 4WD parking area and hike up the wash for 0.2 mile to the

East Ord Mountain

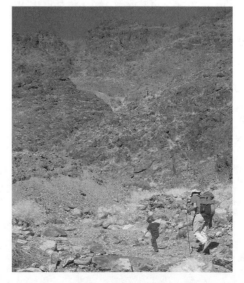

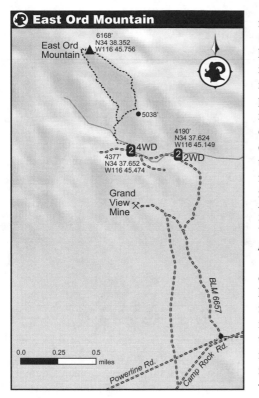

East Ord Mountain

6168'
N34 38.352
W116 45.756

East Ord
Mountain

● 5038'

4190'
N34 37.624
W116 45.149

4WD

2WD

4377'
N34 37.652
W116 45.474

Grand
View
Mine

BLM 6657

0.0   0.25   0.5
miles

Powerline Rd.

Camp Rock Rd.

first place you can easily exit on the right (north). Follow a smaller gully system that leads up to the saddle left of the peak. This is steep hiking, climbing 1500 feet in 1 mile and involves plenty of boulder hopping, but no difficult climbing. The region is home to creosote bushes and hedgehog cacti, yielding to barrel and Mojave mound cacti at higher elevations. Upon reaching the saddle, turn right (east) and climb 150 feet more to the summit. If you pick a careful path that loops around the north side, you can avoid scrambling up large rocks. Descend the way you came.

ALTERNATIVE FINISH

Alternatively, it is possible to climb or descend the southeast ridge, making a semi-loop trip. The ridge is most easily accessed from a saddle next to Point 5038'. The ridge route is of comparable difficulty to the gully route, involving mostly straightforward walking with one band of rock to navigate through.

trip 6.3 Owl Canyon

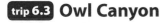

Distance	4 miles (out-and-back)
Hiking Time	3 hours
Elevation Gain	1000'
Difficulty	Moderate
Trail Use	Dogs, good for children
Best Times	October–April
Agency	BLM Barstow Field Office
Recommended Map	*Mud Hills 7.5'*

see map on p. 144

DIRECTIONS From Interstate 15 in Barstow, exit north on Barstow Rd. Go 1 mile to a T-junction at Main St. and turn left (west). In 0.2 mile, turn right (north) on 1st Ave., which crosses the rail yard and Mojave River. In 0.9 mile, turn left on Irwin Rd. In another 6.1 miles, turn left onto the excellent dirt Fossil Bed Rd. In 2.9 miles, turn right (north) at a signed turnoff for Rainbow Basin Scenic Dr. and Owl Canyon Campground. In 0.4 mile, come to a signed junction with a road leading right to Owl Canyon Campground.

The trailhead starts at the Owl Canyon Campground. However, before you go there, it is worth taking a driving tour through Rainbow Basin. Continue straight (north) on the 3.7-mile, one-way loop through the spectacular multi-hued canyon, which is too narrow for motor homes or cars pulling trailers. Watch for the famous bent rock bands of the Barstow Syncline.

When you get back to the main Fossil Bed Road, turn left and return 0.7 mile to the junction you had originally reached leading to Rainbow Basin and Owl Canyon. Drive 0.4 mile to the Owl Canyon turnoff, then 1.4 miles to the campground. Park at the far north end at the signed Owl Canyon Hiking Trail.

High Desert

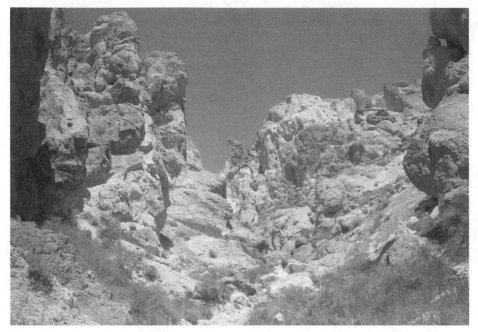

Upper Owl Canyon

During the Barstovian Land Mammal age 12–16 million years ago, the Mojave Desert received much more rainfall and resembled the savannas of Africa. Large animals, including mastodons, camels, and dog-bears roamed the grasslands. Their fossils can be found today in the green, brown, and white sedimentary rock around Rainbow Basin. The basin also contains a complex mix of older granite rock and recent volcanic rock, all of which has been bent and twisted by fault action into an exotic badland. Because of its unique paleontological and geological value, the area has been designated a National Natural Landmark and an Area of Critical Environmental Concern. Collecting fossils without a permit is illegal. Bring a flashlight to explore an unusual natural tunnel along the way.

Owl Canyon is one of the best places to see the geological splendors of this area for yourself. As interesting as the Rainbow Basin drive may be, navigating the rock formations close up as you hike and scramble through the narrows is far better. At the time of this writing, Owl Canyon Campground offered picnic tables and outhouses but no running water, and cost $6/night for camping.

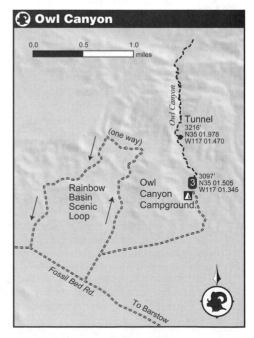

The signed "trail" leads down from the parking area into the wash and promptly vanishes. Follow the wash north; the majority of the hike is easy walking, but there is some rock-hopping and an occasional 6-foot dry waterfall to scramble up, so young children will need a boost. The geologic formations at the start are interesting and become even more dramatic as you ascend.

In 0.7 mile, reach a remarkable tunnel on the right side of the canyon. This rare feature penetrates about 100 feet through the sedimentary wall to reach the mouth of a tributary wash. The middle portion is completely dark. After exploring, return to the main canyon.

In another 0.1 mile, enter a section of spectacular narrows. In another 0.4 mile, the canyon opens up into an amphitheater splashed with swathes of green, orange, purple, and gray rock. At the north end, pass through a final section of narrows before emerging in a valley below some hills.

The wash divides. Take the right fork, which soon becomes a trail leading toward a huge purple rock formation. The hills here are chopped up with a maze of ATV trails. Climb a quarter mile for good views back over the valley before returning the way you came.

trip 6.4 Afton Canyon

Distance	4 miles (out-and-back)
Hiking Time	2.5 hours
Elevation Gain	200'
Difficulty	Easy
Trail Use	Dogs, equestrians, good for children
Best Times	October–April
Agency	BLM Barstow Field Office
Recommended Map	*Dunn, Cave Mountain 7.5'*

DIRECTIONS From Interstate 15, take the Afton Rd. exit south. It is located 36 miles east of Barstow, at mile marker 15 SBD 111. Follow the good dirt road. Stay left at a junction with the old Mojave Rd., then left again to pass the Afton Canyon Group Camping Area. In 3.5 miles from the freeway, arrive at the Afton Canyon Campground.

This hike follows the Mojave River through the colorful Afton Canyon to a pair of shallow caves. The Mojave River normally flows underground, but impermeable rocks keep the waters on the surface in this region. During the wet season, the river is a dependable source of water here and it was an important resource to the Native Americans who lived in the region. In the past two centuries, the river has supported explorers, prospectors, and settlers following the Mojave Trail across the vast parched desert. In 1905, railroad tracks were built through the river canyon to link Utah to Los Angeles. The Union Pacific Railroad now operates these tracks. You are likely to get your feet wet, so sandals are recommended. At rare times of heavy flow in the Mojave River, this hike is not advisable.

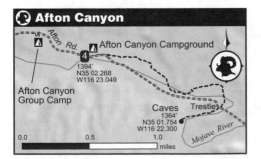

High Desert

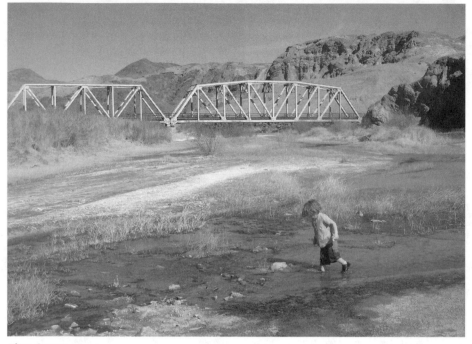

Afton Canyon

Afton Canyon was cut during the Ice Age about 19,000 years ago. When the climate was much wetter, a chain of large lakes filled the basins between Barstow and Death Valley. Lake Manix burst its basin and cut the deep canyon that the Mojave River now follows.

Park in the large clearing at the entrance to the Afton Canyon Campground, taking care not to block any campsites. If you wish to camp here, the fee is presently $6/night. There is an outhouse, but do not rely on water being available here.

From the campground, continue east on foot along the main dirt road that you had been driving. In 0.2 mile, the road turns right (south) and crosses the Mojave River. At this point, leave the road and begin following the river. The best route varies from season to season and year to year, so use your judgment. You may find sporadic traces of trail along the north bank. Depending on the water levels and vegetation, it may be easier to walk on the salt-encrusted sandy riverbed. If neither of these options looks good, you can ford the river and follow the road along the south side.

The walls of the canyon begin to rise. Some are carved from spectacular sedimentary rock tinted red, brown, tan, green, and black. In 1.5 miles, follow the riverbed as it turns right (south) and crosses under a large railroad trestle and recrosses the road. In another 0.4 mile, look for a shallow cave in the mountainside where the river bends back to the left. A second cave can be found just to the east.

Return the way you came. When you reach the trestle, you can follow the road back; this is easier walking and a slightly shorter route, but receives heavy ATV traffic. Or if you want a longer hike, Afton Canyon continues another 6 miles. Many of the tributary canyons are also interesting, and the unusual geology draws rock hounds seeking specimens.

chapter 7

Urban Parks

This chapter covers a potpourri of trails scattered through urban areas in the Inland Empire. It would take a much larger book to describe every trail in every city, so these trips were selected because they are popular, noteworthy, and close to large numbers of people. Few people travel long distances to visit these parks. But, for those who live nearby, it is a great pleasure to take a stroll or jog in these hills at the start or end of a busy day. By watching the seasons pass and the plants and birds going through their cycles of life, you strengthen your connection to the land and enrich your own life.

Three of these trips are in Box Springs Regional Park, which encompasses 1155 acres overlooking UC Riverside. The boulder-studded hills are laced with numerous trails popular among hikers, equestrians, and mountain bikers. The park is located in a transitional zone between coastal sage scrub and chamise chaparral. The park provides habitat for many species of reptiles, mammals, and birds that are under pressure because of the unrelenting urban growth in the Inland Empire. The park is open daily from 8 A.M. to sunset.

Box Springs Skyline Trail

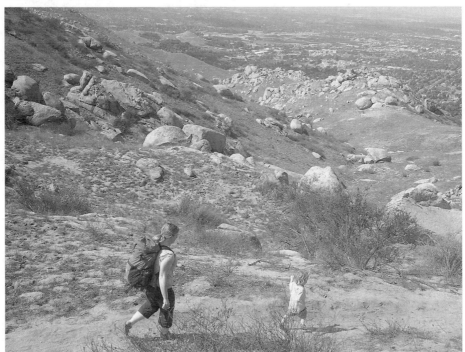

trip 7.1 Walnut Creek

Distance	up to 5.5 miles (out-and-back)
Hiking Time	2-3 hours
Elevation Gain	400′
Difficulty	Easy
Trail Use	Dogs, equestrians, good for children
Best Times	All year, sunrise to sunset
Agency	Los Angeles Department of Parks and Recreation
Optional Map	*San Dimas* 7.5′

DIRECTIONS In San Dimas exit the 57 Freeway at Via Verde (one exit north of Interstate 10), go west for 0.1 mile, then turn right on San Dimas Ave. Proceed north for 1.0 mile to a signed parking area for the Michael D. Antonovich Trail on the west side of the road. The trailhead is located just south of the 57 overpass. Alternatively, exit the 210 Freeway on San Dimas Ave. and take it 2.4 miles south to the same point.

It is also possible to access Walnut Creek from the bottom (west) end. From the 57 Freeway, take Via Verde 0.8 mile west, then turn right on Puente St. Continue 1.5 miles northwest where the street becomes Reeder Ave. Park at a small turnout on the left (south) side just before the road turns right. The signed Michael D. Antonovich Trail begins on the north side of the road.

Tucked away in a narrow canyon scarcely a stone's throw from expensive, sprawling homes, Walnut Creek remarkably offers the feeling of being alone in the wilderness. The Antonovich Trail criss-crosses the creek innumerable times and through much of the year there is no choice but to wade through the knee-deep waters. The shady canyon and frequent stream crossings make this an enticing option for a warm spring afternoon or summer morning. The length of the hike is up to you; for a shorter excursion, it is easy to turn back part way along the trail. Sandals are recommended because of the many stream crossings.

This hike starts inauspiciously at a turnout littered with broken glass. Overhead, a cacophonous din rains down as trucks thunder along the freeway. Almost immediately, the trail drops steeply into the cool, mysterious depths of the canyon. Sycamores, oaks, willows, palms, eucalyptus, and even the occasional walnut tree cover the canyon bottom with a dense canopy. In 0.3 mile, reach the first of many creek crossings. There are various forks along the way; follow the main trail along the bottom of the canyon westward. Cross a bridge in 0.3 mile, then a paved road in 0.2 mile, then

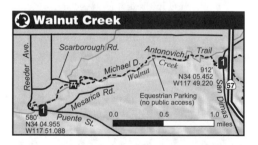

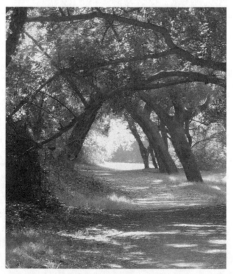

Michael D. Antonovich Trail

Urban Parks

come to a dirt equestrian parking area 0.1 mile beyond. Shortly after leaving the lot, the trail forks again. Take the right fork up a small hill and back down to the canyon bottom. (The left fork leads to a clearing with a rope swing over the creek; check the condition of the rope before trusting it!)

Continue west, passing behind mansions in 0.6 mile, and then in another 0.4 mile reach a dirt parking lot with picnic benches. This parking area can be reached from Scarborough Rd. off Renshaw in San Dimas. Beyond, the trail crosses the creek several more times and forks to reach paved roads at several places near the junction of Puente St. and Reeder Ave. in San Dimas, 2.8 miles from the start.

Unless you have left a bicycle or car at this end, return the way you came. The final 200 feet back out of the canyon to San Dimas Rd. are especially steep.

trip 7.2 Bonelli Park

Distance	6 miles (loop)
Hiking Time	3 hours
Elevation Gain	400'
Difficulty	Moderate
Trail Use	Dogs, equestrians, cyclists
Best Times	All year
Agency	Los Angeles County Department of Parks and Recreation
Optional Map	Ask at park entrance or *San Dimas* 7.5'

see map on p. 150

DIRECTIONS In San Dimas exit the 57 Freeway at Via Verde (one exit north of Interstate 10). You can pay the vehicle entry fee ($8 at the time this was written) and park at the picnic area. To reach the picnic area, drive east to the entrance station, then make an immediate left on Eucalyptus into the parking area. Alternatively leave your car at a Park and Ride lot and walk or cycle into the park. The Park and Ride is located immediately west of the freeway on the north side of Via Verde. There is normally plenty of room on the weekends, but it can fill up on weekdays. If you park here, walk 0.25 mile east on Via Verde across the 57 overpass to reach the Bonelli Park entrance station.

Frank G. Bonelli Regional Park covers nearly 2000 acres in the hills at the western end of the Inland Empire. It features 250-acre Puddingstone Reservoir and countless amenities such as boat rentals, picnic areas, playgrounds, golfing, hot tubs, the Raging Waters theme park, and even a wedding chapel! Hikers will find a paved trail around the lake (described in this trip) and a network of trails in the hills (shown on the map). The Park is open sunrise–7 P.M. from Nov. to Feb., and sunrise–10 P.M. from March to October.

The general principle of this hike is to make a counterclockwise loop around the lake. There are too many variations to describe, so just keep the lake on your left and pick a path that looks good. Start walking on a paved path leading east. In many stretches, a dirt trail runs alongside the paved path closer to the lake and may be more enjoyable. Near the northeast corner of the lake, pass a gate into an RV campground and continue through until you reach the end of McKinley Ave. at the west end of Brackett Airfield. If you follow McKinley east for a half mile, you will reach the general aviation terminal, where Norm's Hanger Cafe serves up delicious pancakes and burgers. The Café closes at 2 P.M., so if you plan to stop and eat, plan your hike accordingly.

Otherwise, turn left on a dirt track that follows the fenceline along the west end of Brackett Airfield; you can usually watch small aircraft taking off directly overhead. At

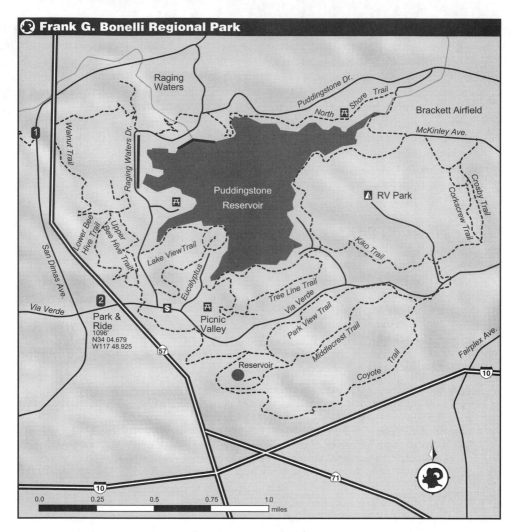

Frank G. Bonelli Regional Park

Raging Waters

Puddingstone Dr.

North Shore Trail

Brackett Airfield

McKinley Ave.

Walnut Trail

Raging Waters Dr.

1

Puddingstone Reservoir

RV Park

Crosby Trail

Corkscrew Trail

Lower Bee Hive Trail

Upper Bee Hive Trail

Lake View Trail

Eucalyptus

Kiko Trail

San Dimas Ave.

Via Verde

2

Park & Ride
1096'
N34 04.679
W117 48.925

S

57

Picnic Valley

Tree Line Trail

Via Verde

Park View Trail

Middlecrest Trail

Coyote Trail

Fairplex Ave.

Reservoir

10

10

0.0   0.25   0.5   0.75   1.0

miles

71

Puddingstone Reservoir

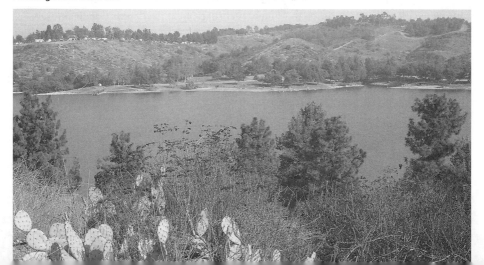

a T-junction with another dirt road, turn left and follow the north shore of the lake past a vast picnic complex and enormous parking lot, then past a sandy swimming beach. Take another dirt road west past the spillway until you reach the paved Raging Waters Dr. Turn left and cross the dam above the water park.

Continue on the road, passing the angler's picnic area and the next dam. Finally, either follow the paved road back to the entrance station or follow a dirt track down to the lake. The dirt track provides an opportunity to climb a hill with panoramic views of the San Gabriel Mountains.

trip 7.3 Prado Lake

Distance	2.5 miles (loop)
Hiking Time	2 hours
Elevation Gain	50'
Difficulty	Easy
Trail Use	Dogs, cyclists, equestrians, good for children
Best Times	September–June
Agency	San Bernardino County Regional Parks District
Optional Map	*Prado Regional Park* (available at entrance station)

DIRECTIONS From the 60 or 10 freeways in Ontario, exit south on Euclid. After passing Chino Airport and Pine Ave., turn left on McCombs, the entrance road. Pay the hefty entry fee at the gate and pick up a copy of the park map. Make a right at the first intersection and follow a short road to the #1 parking area.

Prado Regional Park is a popular destination for families and anglers. Located on 2200 acres leased by San Bernardino County from the Army Corps of Engineers, it features a 60-acre lake, sports fields, an enormous playground, camping, picnicking, and, of course, a walking trail. It is located close to Chino Airport, which is home to excellent aircraft museums; you may see vintage bombers and fighter planes circling overhead. The Prado Flood Control Basin to the south attracts copious wildlife because it is one of the few remaining undeveloped areas in the region. The park is open year-round, though it can be very hot during summer days. For current hours and information, contact the park at (909) 697-4260.

From the parking lot, a 2.5-mile trail leads around the many tentacles of this oddly-shaped lake. Start walking west, then south around the small dam at the west end of the lake, and follow a series of trails counterclockwise around the lake. Native vegetation and plentiful wildlife are found on the south side of the lake, while the north side has grass, picnic areas, and playgrounds. In 0.8 mile, pass the outlet on the south end of the lake. Pass the campground and picnic area at the east end of the lake, then come to a huge playground and water play park. Rowboats and pedal boats can be rented at the nearby ramp. Continue north around the last tentacle of the lake past athletic fields and return to your vehicle.

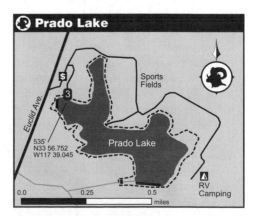

trip 7.4 Mt. Rubidoux

Distance	3.3 miles (loop)
Hiking Time	1.5 hours
Elevation Gain	450 feet
Difficulty	Easy
Trail Use	Cyclists, dogs
Best Time	All year but hot in summer
Agency	City of Riverside Parks & Recreation Department
Optional Map	*Riverside West 7.5´*

DIRECTIONS From Riverside on the 60 Freeway exit south on Rubidoux Blvd. In 0.3 mile, turn left on Mission Blvd. Follow it 1.5 miles across the Santa Ana River to where the name changes to Mission Inn Ave., then turn right on Redwood Dr. Go 0.2 mile to 9th St., then turn right again and park along the street in one block near the corner of Mt. Rubidoux Dr. The trailhead is located in a residential neighborhood with strict parking enforcement. Take care to observe the signed parking restrictions.

Mt. Rubidoux is a prominent granite hill located west of downtown Riverside and south of the Santa Ana River. The mountain is named for Louis Rubidoux, who settled the area in the mid-1800s, but it was Frank Miller, one of Riverside's early promoters and the builder of the historic Mission Inn, who transformed Mt. Rubidoux from an anonymous bump to a much-loved and inspirational park. Miller originally intended to develop the mountain for expensive homes, but his plans failed. Instead, Miller graded a road circling up the mountain; it is this road that hikers, cyclists, joggers, and strollers enjoy today.

Miller's estate donated Mt. Rubidoux to the people of Riverside in 1955, and it is now a favorite city park. The long list of restrictions at the entrance gate forbids alcohol, smoking, fires, gambling, weapons, unleashed dogs, off-trail travel, skateboards, horses, camping, motorized vehicles, fireworks, cutting plants, and, last but not least, soliciting. The park is open year-round from one-half hour before sunrise to one-half hour after sunset.

There are two paved trails that wind up the mountain like intertwined corkscrews. The gentle route is 2 miles long and loops the mountain twice, while the steeper route is 1 mile and loops the mountain only once. The two trails intersect twice.

This trip begins at the Mt. Rubidoux Dr. Trailhead and winds along the bottom of the mountain. Gnarly prickly pear cactus intermingle with coastal sage scrub and drift downward into the backyard gardens of homes at the base of the mountain. The yuccas, aloes, agaves, and cacti were planted by Miller. In 0.5 mile, reach a signed four-way junction and make a hairpin right turn to take the longer trail. As you climb there are views of downtown Riverside, Evergreen Memorial Cemetery, the Santa Ana River, and Flabob Airport. Flabob is one of the older airports in America and is a famous base for antique and home-built aircraft. Keep your eyes out for unusual planes on approach into the field.

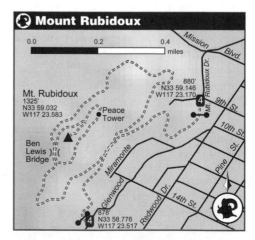

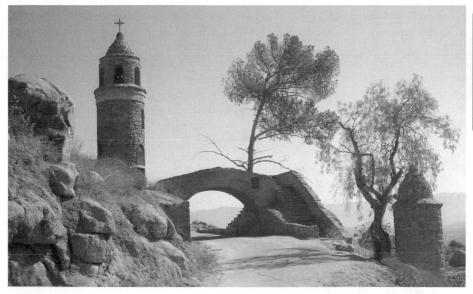

Peace Tower

Pass the short trail a second time as you cross under the Ben Lewis Bridge, then reach the Peace Tower, built by "friends of Frank Augustus Miller in recognition of his constant labor in the promotion of civic beauty, community righteousness, and world peace." Once you reach the top of the mountain, explore the amphitheater, the plaque honoring Father Junipero Serra, the flagpole, and the large cross. On a clear day there are spectacular views south over Riverside.

Return via the steeper trail, which leads west along the north side of the mountain and over the Ben Lewis Bridge. When you reach the signed junction on the south side, continue east along your original route back to the trailhead.

trip 7.5 California Citrus State Historic Park

Distance	1.25 miles (out-and-back)
Hiking Time	1 hour
Elevation Gain	80'
Difficulty	Easy
Best Time	Year round, but can be hot in the summer and early fall
Agency	California Citrus State Historic Park
Optional Map:	none

DIRECTIONS From the 91 Freeway, exit southeast on Arlington Blvd. and go 2 miles. Turn left on Dufferin, then make an immediate right into the park and then a left into the first parking lot. A brightly colored replica of a vintage orange juice stand on the corner of Van Buren Blvd. and Dufferin Ave. marks the entrance to the California Citrus State Historic Park. There is a $4/day parking fee.

The California Citrus State Historic Park opened in 1993 as a living history museum dedicated to preserving a rapidly fading facet of Southern California's history. It is often hard to imagine the tract homes and strip malls that make up sprawling

Southern California are on land that once held vast expanses of lush, sweet-smelling citrus groves.

In 1873, Eliza Tibbets obtained two experimental navel orange trees from the United States Department of Agriculture. The two trees thrived in Southern California's Mediterranean climate, growing to produce oranges that were intensely sweet and flavorful, seedless, and easy to peel. The fruit quickly became highly coveted by both growers and consumers and by 1887 the navel orange had become the dominant fruit crop in Riverside. By 1895, Riverside had become California's richest city per capita. The "second gold rush" was in full swing and would continue well into the 20th Century. As water and land prices soared, growing citrus became less lucrative. Today, less than 20 percent of Southern California's citrus groves remain. The California Citrus State Historic Park preserves roughly 200 acres of those groves.

The interpretive trail starts at the gazebo near the Sunkist center. Trail guide pamphlets can usually be found at the gazebo. This leisurely trail wanders through the park's Varietal Collection featuring more than one hundred types of citrus trees. In addition to the common orange and lemon, more exotic citrus varieties are represented. Of particular interest are the Ponderosa Lemon, weighing in at 5 pounds or more, and the fingered citron (also known as Buddha's Hand), an oddly shaped variety resembling a bunch of green fingers languidly hanging from the tree. The fruit is incredibly sour and is most often used as flavoring in candies in fruitcakes.

As the trail gently climbs, old smudge pots and rusting farm machinery peek out from among the trees. Signs on the trail explain how citrus farmers used such equipment. From the top of the knoll, take in the view of the surrounding groves. Many citrus farmers built their homes on hillsides to have an all-encompassing view of their groves. San Gorgonio Mtn. and Mt. Baldy can be seen on a clear day.

The trail follows the Gage Canal downhill. Built by Matthew Gage between 1885 and 1889, the 12-mile-long canal diverted water from the Santa Ana River to citrus groves in Riverside and San Bernardino. This engineering accomplishment doubled the citrus producing area in Riverside and ensured a regular supply of water for the groves in drought-prone Southern California. The canal still provides water for the groves in the park.

The trail ends at the Visitor's Center. Make sure to stop in and learn more about the history of citrus in Southern California. On the way back to the start of the interpretive trail, take some time to enjoy the park within a park. The rolling green expanses of grass and picnic areas evoke an early 20th Century park and entice harried urbanites to relax and restore their spirits in quiet peace.

The California Citrus State Historic Park is still under development and future plans for the park include an operating packinghouse, a replica of a period worker's camp, and a restaurant housed in a turn-of-the-century grower's mansion. Construction is currently underway on the grower's mansion. The park is open from 8 A.M.–5 P.M. October through March, and from 8 A.M.-7 P.M. April through September. The Visitors Center is open every Wednesday, Saturday, and Sunday from 10 A.M.–4 P.M. There is also a summer concert series.

trip 7.6 Box Springs: Two Trees Trail

Distance	3 miles (out-and-back)
Hiking Time	2 hours
Elevation Gain	1000'
Difficulty	Moderate
Trail Use	Dogs, cyclists, equestrians
Best Times	September–June
Agency	Riverside County Regional Park and Open-Space District
Optional Map	*Riverside East, San Bernardino South 7.5'*

DIRECTIONS From the 215 Freeway in Riverside, exit on Blaine St. and drive east 2 miles to where the road turns to dirt. Park at a turnout on the right. The trail starts in a residential development nearby, but this is the closest hiker parking.

The Two Trees Trail offers a short and steep workout with convenient access from Riverside. It follows a canyon from the edge of town to the trailhead on the ridge. From there, you can make a longer hike by linking up with the Skyline or Towers loops (see Trips 7.7 and 7.8).

From the parking area, walk east on the dirt road to a four-way junction. A private driveway continues east; you turn left (north) and follow another dirt road beside some houses for 0.2 mile to Two Trees Rd. Turn right on the road and soon reach the signed Two Trees Trailhead next to a gate.

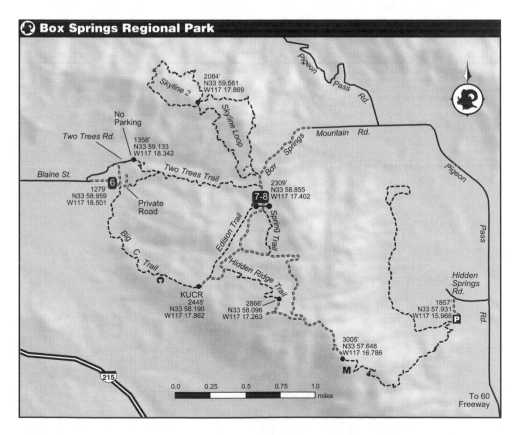

Box Springs Regional Park

Pigeon Pass Rd.

Skyline 2
2064'
N33 59.561
W117 17.869

No Parking

Skyline Loop

Mountain   Rd.

Two Trees Rd.
1358'
N33 59.133
W117 18.342

Box   Springs

Pigeon

Blaine St.

Two Trees Trail

6
1279'
N33 58.959
W117 18.501

Private Road

2309'
N33 58.855
W117 17.402

7-8

Pass

Spring Trail

Edison Trail

Big   C   Trail

Hidden Ridge Trail

Hidden Springs Rd.

KUCR
2448'
N33 58.190
W117 17.862

2866'
N33 58.096
W117 17.263

1857'
N33 57.931
W117 15.968

P

Rd.

3005'
N33 57.648
W117 16.786

M

215

0.0   0.25   0.5   0.75   1.0
miles

To 60 Freeway

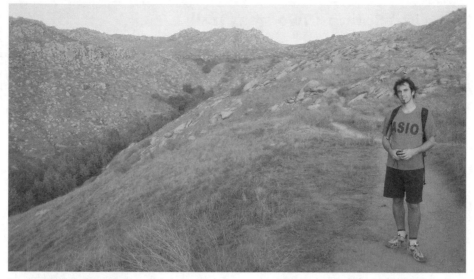

Box Springs Two Trees Trail

There is no parking here. Cross a small bridge and pass a sycamore-filled canyon, then hike up to a ridge where you may see another equestrian trail coming up from the houses at the end of Blaine. Continue east up to the trail's end on Box Springs Mountain Rd., 1.3 miles from the start. The upper trailhead parking area is located to the right (south) beyond a private residence. Please respect the homeowner's privacy.

trip 7.7 Box Springs: Skyline Trail

Distance	3 or 4.5 miles (loop)
Hiking Time	2 hours
Elevation Gain	600' or 1300'
Difficulty	Moderate
Trail Use	Dogs, cyclists, equestrians
Best Times	September–June
Agency	Riverside County Regional Park and Open-Space District
Optional Map	*Riverside East, San Bernardino South 7.5'*

see map on p. 155

DIRECTIONS From the 60 Freeway in Moreno Valley, exit on Pigeon Pass Rd. and drive north and then west 4 miles to where the road turns right in the pass. Stay straight on Box Springs Mountain Rd., which soon turns to dirt. In 1.2 miles, reach the trailhead parking area on the right beside a gate and a private residence.

The Skyline Trail makes a loop on the northern end of the Box Springs Mtn. ridge. On a clear day, it has terrific views of the Inland Empire's major peaks towering over the endless suburban sprawl.

From the parking area, walk north back down Box Springs Mountain Rd. for 0.2 mile, passing the top of the Two Trees Trail. Look on the left side of the road for the post marking the start of the Skyline Trail at the foot of a small hill. The Skyline Trail promptly forks. It makes a 2.5-mile loop around the ridge, with fine views along the way. Consider scrambling up one of the

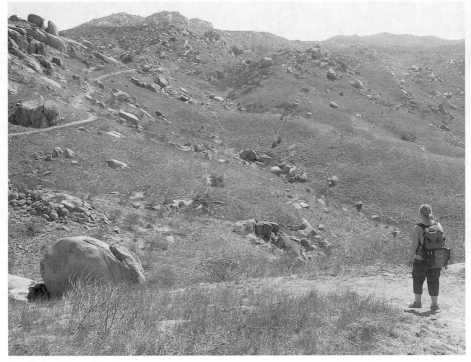

Box Springs Skyline Trail

hills near the start of the trail for even better vistas.

VARIATION

At the northwest end where the Skyline Trail crosses a saddle on the ridge, the less-maintained Skyline 2 trail continues northwest around the next part of the ridge. If you choose to take the second loop, you can add 1.5 miles and 700 feet of elevation gain and loss on numerous steep ups and downs. A new map at the trailhead shows yet a third loop around Sugarloaf Mountain connecting to the west end of Skyline 2, but the authors have not surveyed the Sugarloaf Trail on foot.

trip 7.8 Box Springs: Towers Loop

Distance	3.5 miles (loop, with many possible variations)
Hiking Time	2 hours
Elevation Gain	800'
Difficulty	Moderate
Trail Use	Dogs, cyclists, equestrians
Best Times	September–June
Agency	Riverside County Regional Park and Open-Space District
Optional Map	*Riverside East, San Bernardino South 7.5'*

see map on p. 155

DIRECTIONS From the 60 Freeway in Moreno Valley, exit on Pigeon Pass Rd. and drive north 4 miles to where the road turns right in the pass. Stay straight on Box Springs Mountain Rd., which soon turns to dirt. In 1.2 miles, reach the trailhead parking area on the right beside a gate and a private residence.

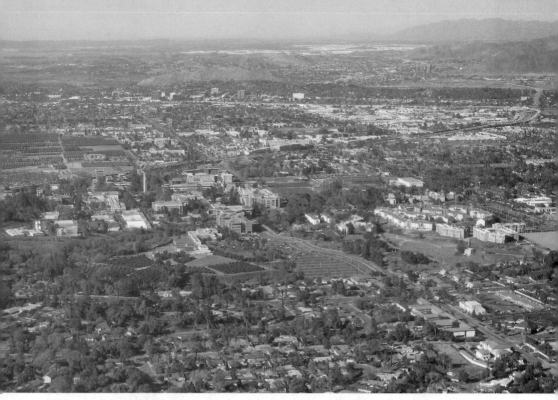

UC Riverside from Box Springs Mountain

The Towers Loop climbs to the antennas on the tallest hills of Box Springs Mtn. On a clear winter day, it offers stunning views over Riverside and Moreno Valley. You can choose your route, staying mostly on dirt service roads or exploring the trails that parallel the road.

The Towers Loop begins at the service road leading south past the gate from the parking area. In 0.1 mile, it reaches the signed Spring Trail warning: DANGER: NO HORSES. You can follow this past Cassina Spring for 0.4 mile to where it rejoins the service road. Alternatively, continue on the service road for 0.6 mile, staying left at a fork, to where it meets the southern terminus of the Spring Trail.

The service road climbs the hill toward the antenna farm. In 1.0 mile, it branches again at a cluster of antennas. The left fork leads down to an overlook above Moreno Valley's Big M sign, while the right fork continues past more antennas on the ridge. Take the right fork, then stay right again at a second junction, and reach the road's end in 0.4 mile at a rectangular tower with white horns.

From this tower, the enjoyable Hidden Ridge Trail descends 0.7 mile northwest toward the lone KUCR antenna. The trail ends at another service road. Turn right at the service road junction and go 0.3 mile back to the main service road, which leads north back to the trailhead.

ALTERNATIVE FINISHES

From the bottom of Hidden Ridge Trail, you can turn left and follow the service road southwest. In 0.2 mile, reach the Edison Trail, which leads north-northeast 0.8 mile under the power lines to the trailhead.

Yet another option is to continue 0.1 mile farther on the service road to the solitary antenna. From here, you can descend to UC Riverside's Big C sign; a steep and loose trail continues down from the C to the railroad tracks, then turns north toward Blaine St., where you could loop back on the Two Trees Trail (see Trip 7.6).

trip 7.9 Terri Peak

Distance	4 miles (out-and-back)
Hiking Time	2 hours
Elevation Gain	800'
Difficulty	Moderate
Trail Use	Dogs, equestrians, cyclists
Best Times	October–May
Agency	Lake Perris State Recreation Area
Optional Map	*Perris, Sunnymead* 7.5'

DIRECTIONS From the 60 Freeway in Moreno Valley, 6 miles east of Highway 215, exit south on Moreno Beach Dr. Follow Moreno Beach Dr. for 3.4 miles, then turn left on Via Del Lago.

This hike can begin inside or outside of the Lake Perris State Recreation Area. To begin outside, pull off the right side of Via Del Lago in 0.4 mile at the south end of a gated development near the beginning of a white-fenced walking trail. To begin inside, continue another 0.8 mile to the entry station and pay your admission fee ($8 at the time of this writing). Turn right on a paved road 0.1 mile beyond the entry station. Go 0.4 mile, then immediately beyond the Campfire Center, turn right on a good dirt road to the Horse Group Camp. Follow it 0.4 mile, staying left at a junction with a service road, and park near a corral, taking care not to block anyone camping there.

Lake Perris was built in 1973 as a reservoir at the southern end of the 444-mile California Aqueduct. Each year nearly 100 billion gallons of water flow through the lake and on to Riverside and San Diego Counties. The land around Lake Perris has been set aside as a California State Recreation Area. It primarily draws boaters, picnickers, and anglers, but the hills surrounding the lake are of interest to hikers and rock climbers. Terri Peak overlooks the facilities on the northwest side of the lake and offers a moderate climb with fine views of the lake and nearby communities. It is especially worth visiting in March and April when the wildflowers are in bloom.

The hike can begin inside or outside of the State Recreation Area and can involve a simple jaunt to the peak and back or a longer loop. Starting inside involves a paying substantial admission fee and the trailheads lack good parking and signage, so the outside start is recommended unless you want to visit the Indian Museum and picnic by the lake.

If you start on the north side outside the park, follow the fenced walking path along the southeast boundary of the gated community. Young children may be frightened by aggressively barking dogs roaming the backyards. In 0.4 mile, reach a water tank and flood control basin. Turn left, pass a gate, and follow a paved road up toward another water tank. In 0.1 mile, just before reaching the second tank, turn left again, pass another gate, and hike up a dirt road that is now closed to vehicles. The road leads past brittlebushes and other coastal sage scrub for 0.6 mile to a T-junction with the trail from Horse Group Camp. Turn right and continue 0.9 mile to the summit.

If you start at the Horse Group Camp, walk back up the road 0.1 mile, then turn

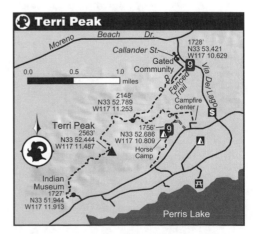

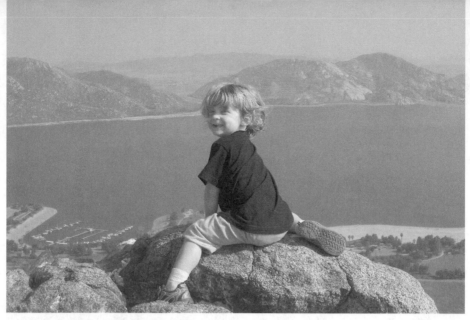
Lake Perris from Terri Peak

left onto a trail marked with a wooden post and horseshoe. The trail is a shortcut to the service road that you passed on the way in. Follow the road up for another 0.1 mile to a water tank in a grove of trees. On the north side of the road, look for two trails. One leads east down to the campfire circle, but our trail goes northwest up the mountain. It gradually climbs for 0.7 mile to reach the junction with the trail from the north side of the mountain. Continue up another 0.9 mile to the summit. Retrace your steps to your vehicle.

ALTERNATIVE FINISH

If you started in the park, consider making a longer loop down to the Indian Museum and back along the lakeshore. A faint 1.2-mile trail continues west from Terri Peak and descends the southwest ridge before turning south and arriving at a marker at the west end of the Ya'i Heki' Regional Indian Museum parking area. Unfortunately, the path is rarely maintained and can be overgrown with scratchy brush, which detracts from this otherwise appealing route. Long pants are strongly recommended. At the time of this writing, the museum was open 10 A.M.–4 P.M. on weekends and 10 A.M.–2 P.M. on Wednesdays. Then pick a path through the intricate network of roads, sidewalks, and beaches back along Lake Perris before returning to your starting point.

chapter 8

Santa Rosa Plateau Ecological Reserve

If you ever wondered what Southern California looked like before the arrival of European settlers, you can find out by visiting the Santa Rosa Plateau Ecological Reserve (not to be confused with the Santa Rosa Mountains covered in Chapter 12). The reserve is located at the southern end of the Santa Ana Mountains and is home to some of the finest remaining bunchgrass prairie in the state, along with endangered Engelmann oak woodlands, vernal pools, and chaparral. The best time to visit is in March or April after a wet winter, when the vegetation is lush, the pools and creeks are full, snow-capped mountains stand sentry above the horizon, and the wildflowers are in bloom. Birdsong carries playfully through the trees and on the breeze; you are likely to see raptors, coyotes, and smaller animals if you are quiet and watchful.

The 7000-acre Santa Rosa Plateau Ecological Reserve is jointly managed by a public-private partnership involving the Nature Conservancy, the Riverside County Regional Park District, the California Department of Fish and Game, the US Fish and Wildlife Service, and the Metropolitan Water District. The Nature Conservancy purchased half of the land in 1984 from a housing development company. The rest was intended for houses, shopping centers, and golf courses before it was purchased with government assistance in 1991–1995. From vantage points where you can compare the

Aerial view of the Santa Rosa Plateau and Vernal Pool

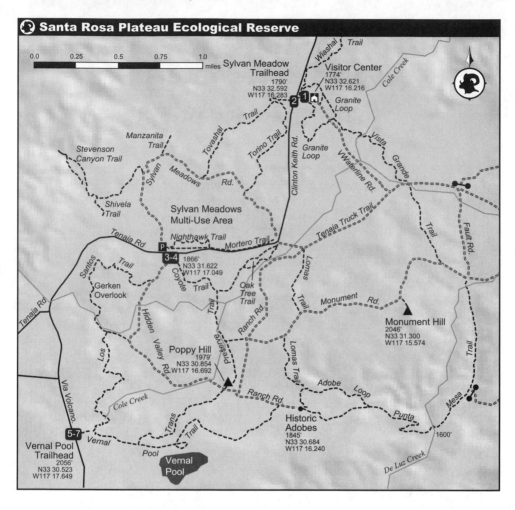

Santa Rosa Plateau Ecological Reserve

pristine reserve to the nearby hills scarred by ostentatious development, it is easy to appreciate some of the reasons why it was so important to set this land aside. Careful study of the unique and endangered ecology reveals many more reasons to treasure the reserve.

The geology of the plateau contributes to its unique environment. Seven million years ago, this part of Southern California consisted of gently rolling hills. Volcanic eruptions filled the valleys with lava. You can see the eroded remnants of the lava flows in the mesas at the eastern edge of the park and in the basalt rocks around the vernal pools and tenajas (natural catch-basins). The pool floors are made of decomposed

volcanic rock clay, which is nearly impermeable to water. Winter rains collect in the ponds and remain until they evaporate.

The reserve is open to the public daily from sunrise to sunset. Fees are $2 for adults and $1 for children and can be paid at the visitor center or at the trailheads. Park maps are also available at these locations. The visitor center is open 9 A.M.–5 P.M. on weekends and 10 A.M.–4 P.M. on Thursdays and Fridays. Do not disturb the plants, animals, and rocks within the reserve. Horseback and bicycle riding and dogs are allowed in the Sylvan Meadows multi-use area only. Trail runners enjoy all of the paths, which are relatively level and well-marked. Visitors must remain on marked trails.

trip 8.1 Granite Loop

Distance	1.2–1.6 miles (loop)
Hiking Time	45 minutes
Elevation Gain	100'
Difficulty	Easy
Trail Use	Good for children
Best Times	October–May
Agency	Santa Rosa Plateau Ecological Reserve
Optional Map	*Santa Rosa Ecological Reserve* or *Wildomar* 7.5'

see map on p. 162

DIRECTIONS From Interstate 15 in Murrieta, exit southwest on Clinton Keith Rd. Drive 4.1 miles to the visitor center on the left. The dirt entrance road is easy to miss.

The Granite Loop is an easy introduction to the pleasures of the Santa Rosa Ecological Reserve. It tours three of the major ecosystems: oak woodlands, chaparral, and riparian zones. Benches along the way welcome you for a picnic, bird watching, or quiet contemplation. This trip describes the loop in the clockwise direction.

The signed Granite Loop Trail begins at the north end of the parking area at the visitor center. It leads through chaparral for 0.1 mile to an oak-shaded picnic area by the creek. If you have children along, be sure they stay in the clearing; the brush is infested with poison oak.

In another 0.2 mile, stay left at a signed junction; the unmarked path on the right cuts back to the visitor center. The trail leads through more chaparral encrusted in thick green lichen. In 0.2 mile, pass the Vista Grande Trail. Consider making a short detour to the left (east) on this trail to the Tenajas Overlook where during wet years you can admire a pool in Cole Creek. Then return to the Granite Loop.

Immediately beyond the Vista Grande Trail, cross the dirt Waterline Rd., then reach benches beneath a coast live oak patriarch. Beyond, pass piles of granite boulders and cross a branch of Cole Creek. Climb a small hill overlooking the visitor center, where you can see the contrast between the pristine reserve and the nearby hills scarred by development. Soon the loop ends at the south end of the visitor center parking lot.

Granite Loop signpost

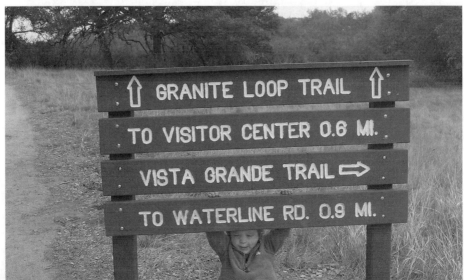

trip 8.2 Sylvan Meadows

Distance	4.5 miles (loop)
Hiking Time	2.5 hours
Elevation Gain	300'
Difficulty	Easy
Trail Use	Equestrians, cyclists, dogs
Best Times	October–May, especially March–April
Agency	Santa Rosa Plateau Ecological Reserve
Recommended Map	*Santa Rosa Ecological Reserve* or *Wildomar* 7.5'

see map on p. 162

DIRECTIONS From Interstate 15 in Murrieta, exit southwest on Clinton Keith Rd. Drive 4.1 miles and park on the right (west) side of the road opposite the visitor center entrance.

Sylvan Meadows is one of California's finest remaining native bunchgrass prairies. The meadow is dotted with magnificent oaks. The dirt Sylvan Meadows Rd. encircles the meadow. It is a designated multi-use trail, popular with equestrians and mountain bikers as well as hikers and joggers. The best time to visit is the spring, when the meadow is lush and the wildflowers are in bloom. This is also a good area for bird watching. Ask at the visitor center for more information about birding.

From the trailhead parking, follow the Tovashal Trail west. In 0.2 mile, cross a bridge and come to a junction with the Torino Trail. Stay right on the Tovashal Trail. In 0.8 mile, reach a T-junction with Sylvan Meadows Rd. Turn right and follow it around the meadow. In 0.3 mile, pass a signed turnoff for Manzanita Trail, which leads to the subdivision outside the reserve. Stay on the road and in another 0.2 mile, reach the Shivela Trail on the right.

VARIATION

If you have time, a scenic detour into a lovely canyon is recommended here. Follow the Shivela Trail southwest for 0.4 mile, then turn right on a trail leading into the mouth of Stevenson Canyon. In 0.1 mile, the trail forks. Follow either side 0.3 mile up along a creek through the oak-shaded canyon where the forks rejoin, then return by the other fork, and retrace your steps to Sylvan Meadows Rd. This variation adds 1.6 miles round trip.

Continue along Sylvan Meadows Rd. past mistletoe-laden sycamores for 0.5 mile to the Hidden Valley Trailhead. The Nighthawk and Mortero Trails lead east, parallel to Tenaja Rd. Follow the Nighthawk Trail (which is set farther back from the road) for 0.4 mile until it rejoins the Mortero, then continue another 0.4 mile east alongside the road to a junction.

Turn left onto Sylvan Meadows Rd. and go 0.5 mile to a junction with the Torino Trail. Turn right and follow it 0.8 mile back to the Tovashal Trail near the bridge. Then turn right again and return to the trailhead.

Sylvan Meadows and Mesa sin Nombre

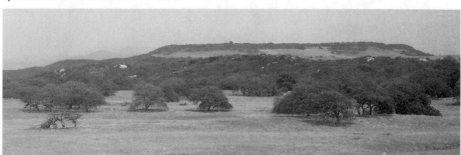

trip 8.3 Oak Tree Trail

Distance	2 miles (semi-loop)
Hiking Time	1 hour
Elevation Gain	100'
Difficulty	Easy
Trail Use	Good for children
Best Times	October–May, especially March–April
Agency	Santa Rosa Plateau Ecological Reserve
Recommended Map	*Santa Rosa Ecological Reserve* or *Wildomar 7.5'*

see map on p. 162

DIRECTIONS From Interstate 15 in Murrieta, exit southwest on Clinton Keith Rd. Drive 5.8 miles to the Hidden Valley Trailhead on the left side of the road. The trailhead is located shortly beyond where the road makes a sharp left turn and changes name to Tenaja.

The Santa Rosa Plateau is home to some of the last remaining Engelmann oaks. The majestic trees can live up to 300 years, and their many twisting limbs and gray-green leaves distinguish them from the more common coast live oaks. These spectacular oaks prefer to grow on mesas and foothills at least 20 miles inland from the ocean. Construction of subdivisions has led to the destruction of most of the native Engelmann oak woodlands, especially in the hills above Pasadena and Pomona. The Oak Tree Trail makes a short loop through a fine stand of Engelmann oaks along Cole Creek.

Look for two paths leading south from the Hidden Valley Trailhead. The Coyote Trail immediately branches left off Hidden Valley Rd. Here observant hikers may see coyotes and their prey intently engaged in the game of life.

Follow it for 0.5 mile through undulating grasslands to a junction. Turn left and follow the Trans Preserve Trail 0.3 mile to the beginning of the Oak Tree Loop. You can then tour the 0.6-mile loop either clockwise or counterclockwise. When you are done, return the way you came.

trip 8.4 Los Santos Loop

Distance	5 miles (loop)
Hiking Time	2.5 hours
Elevation Gain	500'
Difficulty	Easy
Best Times	October–May, especially March–April
Agency	Santa Rosa Plateau Ecological Reserve
Recommended Map	*Santa Rosa Ecological Reserve* or *Wildomar 7.5'*

see map on p. 162

DIRECTIONS From Interstate 15 in Murrieta, exit southwest on Clinton Keith Rd. Drive 5.8 miles to the Hidden Valley Trailhead on the left side of the road. The trailhead is located shortly beyond where the road makes a sharp left turn and changes name to Tenaja.

The hills and meadows in the southwestern corner of the Santa Rosa Plateau are dotted with some of the stateliest Engelmann oaks in the reserve. This counterclockwise loop offers a scenic tour of

the area along the Los Santos and Trans Preserve Trails. Other highlights include the basalt Mesa de Colorado, Poppy Hill, and an optional short detour to the fascinating seasonal vernal pool. Quiet and observant

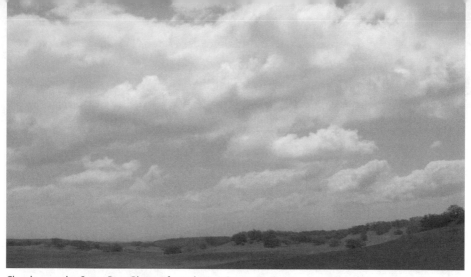

Clouds over the Santa Rosa Plateau from the Los Santos Trail

hikers often see the coyotes and raptors that hunt in these hills.

Two paths lead south from the trailhead. Take the right fork, Hidden Valley Rd. You will return by the Coyote Trail later. The dirt road leads through a meadow. In 0.2 mile turn right onto the narrow Los Santos Trail, which winds around and climbs a low ridge. In another 0.8 mile, reach a bench with terrific views at the Walter B. Gerken overlook, named for the former chairman of the Nature Conservancy. In 0.4 mile, the trail descends to another junction, where a connector path to the left leads back to Hidden Valley Rd. Stay right and climb onto the Mesa de Colorado. As the soil becomes more volcanic in composition,

the vegetation becomes noticeably different and varied. The prickly pear cacti produce spectacular flowers in late spring, but watch for poison oak if you stray from the trail.

In 1.1 miles, reach the Vernal Pool Trail, marking the halfway point of your hike. Turn left and go 0.3 mile to a junction with the Trans Preserve Trail. In the spring, it is well worth taking a 0.2-mile detour onward to the big pool (see Trip 8.5) before returning via the Trans Preserve Trail. In 0.8 mile, cross Hidden Valley Rd. and pass Poppy Hill, which ignites with California poppies in the spring. In another 0.8 mile, turn left on the Coyote Trail and follow it the last half mile back to the Hidden Valley Trailhead.

Cactus blooming along the Los Santos Trail

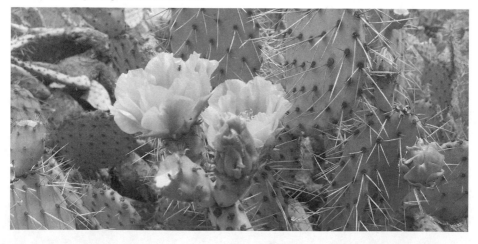

trip 8.5 Vernal Pool

Distance	1.5 miles (out-and-back)
Hiking Time	45 minutes
Elevation Gain	100′
Difficulty	Moderate
Trail Use	Good for children
Best Times	March–April
Agency	Santa Rosa Plateau Ecological Reserve
Optional Map	*Santa Rosa Ecological Reserve* or *Wildomar 7.5′*

see map on p. 162

DIRECTIONS From Interstate 15 in Murrieta, exit southwest on Clinton Keith Rd. Drive 6.9 miles. Clinton Keith changes names to Tenaja Rd. At a stop sign, stay left onto Via Volcano. In another 0.8 mile, park along the side of the road at the Vernal Pool Trailhead.

In the southwest corner of the reserve is a shallow basalt basin that fills with water during the winter rains. Such vernal pools, so named because they usually hold an abundance of water in the spring, were once common in California, but over 90 percent have been destroyed by development or agriculture. Vernal pools nourish a variety of endangered species. The Santa Rosa Plateau has some of the last remaining vernal pools. This one, the largest pool in the reserve, supports fairy shrimp, frogs, and water birds. Wildflowers encircle the pool and creep toward the center as the water evaporates in May. A short well-marked trail leads to a boardwalk over the pool so that you can enjoy its wonders without trampling the fragile environment.

From the trailhead, hike east for 0.1 mile to a junction. The Los Santos Trail forks off to the left (see Trip 8.4), but the Vernal Pool Trail continues straight. Hike through a meadow dotted with oaks; keep your eyes out for the occasional small pool. In 0.3 mile, reach a second junction with the Trans Preserve Trail, which also forks to the left. Continue straight 0.2 mile to the large vernal pool. Look for the boardwalk that leads over the pool. Interpretive signs explain some features of the site. Stay on the trail so that you do not disturb the sensitive wildlife.

Return the way you came. Or for a longer walk, continue along the trail to the historic adobes (see Trip 8.6) or take a loop to the north toward Poppy Hill.

Vernal Pool boardwalk

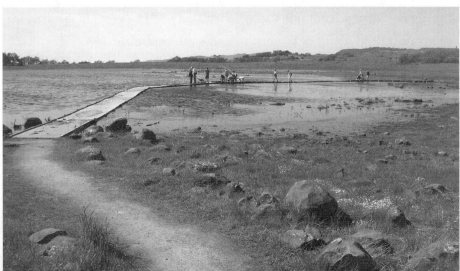

trip 8.6 Historic Adobes

Distance	3.5 miles (out-and-back)
Hiking Time	2.5 hours
Elevation Gain	300'
Difficulty	Easy
Best Times	October–May, especially March–April
Agency	Santa Rosa Plateau Ecological Reserve
Recommended Map	*Santa Rosa Ecological Reserve* or *Wildomar* 7.5'

see map on p. 162

DIRECTIONS From Interstate 15 in Murrieta, exit southwest on Clinton Keith Rd. Drive 6.9 miles. Clinton Keith changes names to Tenaja. At a stop sign, stay left onto Via Volcano. In another 0.8 mile, park along the side of the road at the Vernal Pool Trailhead.

In 1846, Pio Pico, governor of California, granted the 48,000-acre Santa Rosa Rancho to Juan Moreno. Moreno built a ranch where he and his family grazed cattle. The small Moreno adobe is the oldest building in Riverside County, and the large Machado adobe, built later around 1855, is the second oldest. This hike visits the restored ranch, passing by way of the vernal pool and a shady creek. It is ideal in the spring, when the pool is full and the wildflowers are in bloom.

Follow the trail east for 0.6 mile through meadows dotted with oaks to the large vernal pool (see Trip 8.5), staying right at junctions with the Los Santos and Trans Preserve Trails along the way. This site is worth exploring, but stay on the marked trail and boardwalk to protect the endangered species living near the pool.

Continue along the trail for 0.9 mile, dropping down through a band of chap-

arral to Ranch Rd. Turn right and follow the road 0.1 mile to the historic ranch. Interpretive signs and a botanical garden walk explain the history and environment of the ranch.

VARIATION

For a scenic detour, continue east from the ranch toward the Punta Mesa Trail. In 0.5 mile, turn left at a sign for the Adobe Loop Trail. This trail leads back west along bubbling Adobe Creek beneath the oak canopy. Beware of the poison oak, which grows thick alongside the trail. Keep your eyes out for a tenaja, a pool formed by erosion along the stream. In another 0.5 mile, reach a T-junction with the Lomas Trail. Turn left and hike 0.1 mile back to the ranch.

Return the way you came, or explore an alternate route along the rich network of trails in this corner of the former Rancho.

Santa Rosa Ranch

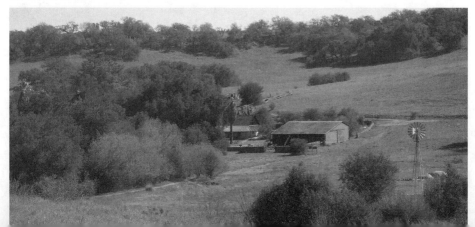

trip 8.7 Santa Rosa Plateau Loop

Distance	11 miles (loop)
Hiking Time	6 hours
Elevation Gain	700'
Difficulty	Strenuous
Best Times	October–May, especially March–April
Agency	Santa Rosa Plateau Ecological Reserve
Recommended Map	*Santa Rosa Ecological Reserve* or *Wildomar 7.5'*

see map on p. 162

DIRECTIONS From Interstate 15 in Murrieta, exit southwest on Clinton Keith Rd. Drive 6.9 miles. Clinton Keith changes names to Tenaja. At a stop sign, stay left onto Via Volcano. In another 0.8 mile, park along the side of the road at the Vernal Pool Trailhead.

This trip offers a grand tour of the Santa Rosa Plateau including the vernal ponds, the historic adobes, and the volcanic mesas, culminating with a panoramic view from Monument Hill. If you have a full day to hike, this is a great way to see many of the diverse features in the reserve. The trail also features fine views of San Jacinto Peak, San Gorgonio Mtn., and Mt. Baldy, the three tallest peaks ringing the Los Angeles Basin. There are many variations possible, so you can shorten or lengthen the trip as you prefer. For example, you could start or end at the visitor center, and could extend the hike to include the Los Santos Trail (see Trip 8.4) and/or the Sylvan Meadows Loop (see Trip 8.2).

From the Vernal Pool Trailhead, hike 0.6 mile east through a meadow dotted with oaks, passing the Los Santos and Trans Preserve Trails, to the big pool, which is full of water after winter's rains. After visiting the boardwalk along the pool, continue 0.9 mile to Ranch Rd. Turn right (east) and hike 0.1 mile to the historic Santa Rosa Ranch, which is a good place to stop for a break.

Next, follow the Lomas Trail north along the west side of the ranch for 0.1 mile to a gate marking the entrance to the Adobe Loop Trail. Turn right and follow the creek under the shady oaks for 0.5 mile to a T-junction with the Punta Mesa Trail. Turn left (east) and follow the Punta Mesa Trail down through the chaparral to a small creek crossing, then continue up and north. Pass an intersection in 1.9 miles with Monument Rd. and continue another 0.7 mile across a wide meadow to a junction with the Tenaja Truck Trail. The construction scars on the hills to the northwest show how fortunate it was that this pristine plateau was saved from development.

Hikers at Monument Hill

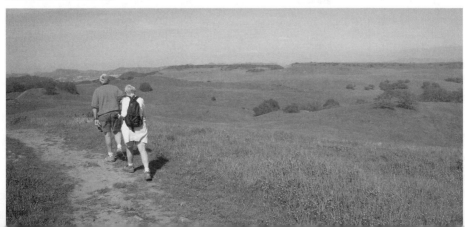

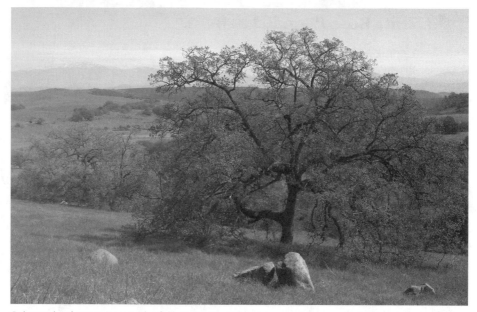

Oak grassland comprises much of the Santa Rosa Plateau

Turn left (west) and follow the dirt road for 0.5 mile, then turn right and follow Waterline Rd. for 0.7 mile toward the visitor center passing oaks and granite boulders in the meadow. Shortly before reaching the visitor center, turn right on the Granite Loop Trail and go less than 0.1 mile, then turn right again on the Vista Grande Trail. The trail forks but both branches rejoin shortly near a bridge over Cole Creek and a bench overlooking the tenajas. In 0.9 mile, cross the Tenaja Truck Trail again and continue 0.7 mile to a T-junction with Monument Hill Rd. Turn right (west) and climb 0.4 mile to a spur trail that leads 0.1 mile to the summit of Monument Hill (2046′), where you can take in views of the entire eastern half of the reserve that you have just explored.

Continue west along Monument Rd., passing two junctions with the Lomas Trail, to reach Ranch Rd. in 1 mile. Turn left (south) and go 0.4 mile. At a junction near Poppy Hill, turn right (west) and hike 0.1 toward the hill, then turn left (southwest) on the Trans Preserve Trail. Follow it 0.8 mile to a T-junction with the Vernal Pool Trail on Mesa de Colorado. Turn right (west) and retrace your steps 0.4 mile to where you began this big loop.

chapter 9

San Jacinto Mountains National Monument

The San Jacinto Mountains are the northernmost crest of the Peninsular Ranges, a spiny backbone that stretches roughly 900 miles from Southern California to the southern tip of the Baja California Peninsula. During the Cretaceous period, about 100 million years ago, magma welled up beneath the earth's surface and slowly cooled, forming a vast expanse of granite called a batholith. The region was subsequently thrust upward by seismic activity along the San Andreas Fault. Millions of years of erosion have stripped off the overlaying rock, cutting deep canyons and revealing the spectacular granite of the San Jacintos.

Extending 30 miles from Interstate 10 to the Santa Rosa Mountains, the San Jacinto Mountains form the eastern wall of the greater Los Angeles Basin. Palm Springs nestles against the eastern side of the range; beyond lies the Coachella Valley and endless miles of the Colorado Desert. The mountain town of Idyllwild is perched on the western slope beneath Tahquitz Peak. San Gorgonio Pass, also known as Banning Pass, separates the range from the San Bernardino Mountains in the north. The range is also home to Southern California's second tallest peak: San Jacinto's (10,834´) summit towers nearly 2 vertical miles above Banning Pass.

The earliest known inhabitants of the San Jacinto Mountains and the surrounding deserts were the Cahuilla Indians. The Cahuilla routinely traveled into the

The San Jacinto Mountains from the Coachella Valley

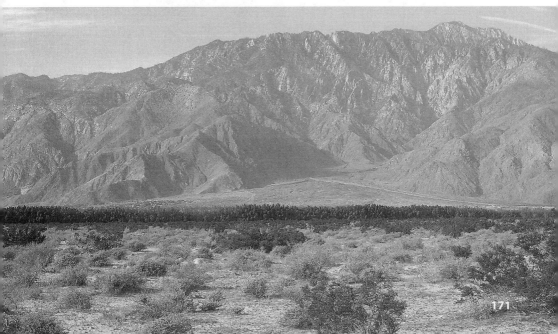

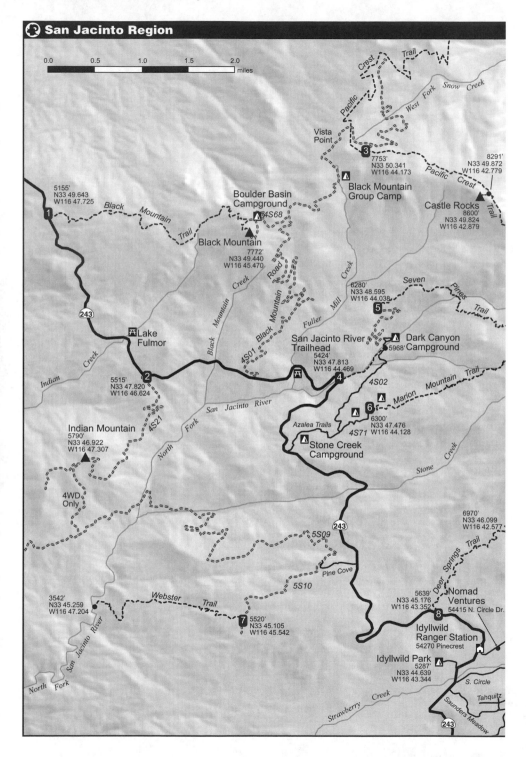

San Jacinto Region

0.0   0.5   1.0   1.5   2.0
miles

1
5155'
N33 49.643
W116 47.725

Black   Mountain   Trail

Boulder Basin
Campground
4S68

Black Mountain
7772'
N33 49.440
W116 45.470

Vista
Point

Pacific   Crest   Trail

3
7753'
N33 50.341
W116 44.173

Black Mountain
Group Camp

West Fork   Snow Creek

8291'
N33 49.872
W116 42.779

Pacific   Crest

Castle Rocks
8600'
N33 49.824
W116 42.879

243

Lake
Fulmor

Black   Mountain   Creek

Black   Mountain   Road

Fuller   Mill   Creek

Seven   Pines   Trail

6280'
N33 48.595
W116 44.038

5

San Jacinto River
Trailhead
5424'
N33 47.813
W116 44.469

Dark Canyon
Campground
5968'

4   4S02

Marion   Mountain   Trail

2
5515'
N33 47.820
W116 46.624

4S01

Indian   Creek

San Jacinto River

North   Fork

Indian Mountain
5790'
N33 46.922
W116 47.307

4S21

Azalea Trails

6
6300'
N33 47.476
W116 44.128
4S71

Stone Creek
Campground

Stone   Creek

4WD
Only

5S09

243

6970'
N33 46.099
W116 42.577

Pine Cove

5S10

Deer   Springs   Trail

3542'
N33 45.259
W116 47.204

Webster   Trail

7   5520'
N33 45.105
W116 45.542

San Jacinto River

North   Fork

5639'
N33 45.176
W116 43.352

Nomad
Ventures
54415 N. Circle Dr.

8

Idyllwild
Ranger Station
54270 Pinecrest

Idyllwild Park
5287'
N33 44.639
W116 43.344

S. Circle

Tahquitz

Strawberry   Creek

Saunders   Meadow

243

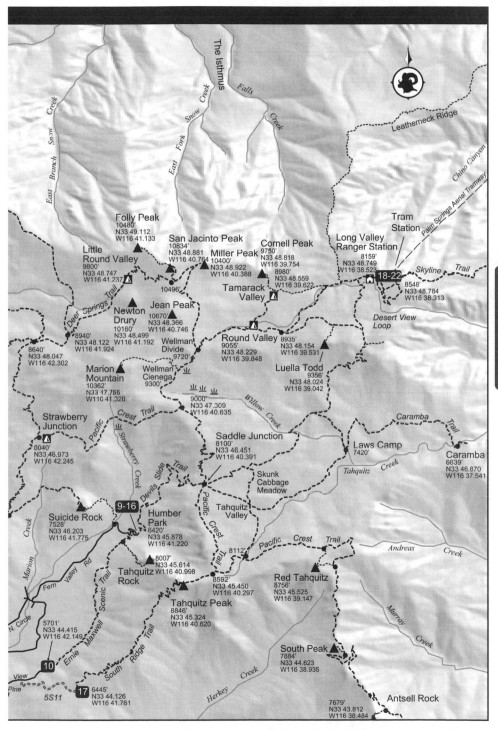

The Isthmus

Falls

East Fork Snow Creek

Snow Creek

Creek

East Branch Snow Creek

Leatherneck Ridge

Chino Canyon

Palm Springs Aerial Tramway

Folly Peak
10480'
N33 49.112
W116 41.133

Little
Round Valley
9800'
N33 48.747
W116 41.237

San Jacinto Peak
10834'
N33 48.881
W116 40.764

Miller Peak
10400'
N33 48.922
W116 40.388

Cornell Peak
9750'
N33 48.818
W116 39.754

8980'
N33 48.559
W116 39.622

Tram
Station

Long Valley
Ranger Station
8159'
N33 48.749
W116 38.523

18-22

Skyline   Trail

8548'
N33 48.784
W116 38.313

10496'

Deer Springs Trail

Tamarack
Valley

Jean Peak
10670'
N33 48.366
W116 40.746

Newton
Drury
10160'
N33 48.499
W116 41.192

Wellman
Divide
9720'

Round Valley
9055'
N33 48.229
W116 39.848

8935'
N33 48.154
W116 39.531

Desert View
Loop

8940'
N33 48.122
W116 41.924

8640'
N33 48.047
W116 42.302

Marion
Mountain
10362'
N33 17.766
W116 41.328

Wellman
Cienega
9300

Luella Todd
9356'
N33 48.024
W116 39.042

9000'
N33 47.309
W116 40.635

Willow Creek

Strawberry
Junction
0040'
N33 46.973
W116 42.245

Crest Trail

Pacific

Strawberry Creek

Caramba   Trail

Saddle Junction
8100'
N33 46.451
W116 40.391

Laws Camp
7420'

Tahquitz Creek

Caramba
6639'
N33 46.870
W116 37.541

Devils Slide Trail

Skunk
Cabbage
Meadow

9-16

Suicide Rock
7528'
N33 46.203
W116 41.775

Humber
Park
6420'
N33 45.878
W116 41.220

Tahquitz
Valley

Pacific Crest

Pacific   Crest   Trail

Andreas   Creek

Marion Creek

8007'
N33 45.614
W116 40.998

Tahquitz
Rock

8112'

Trail

8592'
N33 45.450
W116 40.297

Red Tahquitz
8756'
N33 45.525
W116 39.147

Fern Valley Rd

Scenic

Maxwell

Tahquitz Peak
8846'
N33 45.324
W116 40.620

Murray   Creek

Ernie

5701'
N33 44.415
W116 42.149

N. Circle

South Ridge Trail

South Peak
7884'
N33 44.623
W116 38.935

10

View

17   6445'
N33 44.126
W116 41.761

Pine

5S11

Herkey   Creek

7679'
N33 43.812
W116 38.484

Antsell Rock

mountains to hunt and to escape the summer heat. They first came in contact with the Spanish in 1774 when Juan Bautisa de Anza was looking for an overland route between Monterey, California and Sonora, Mexico. With the aid of Sebastian Tarabal, an Indian from the San Gabriel Mission who spoke Spanish and a number of native languages, Anza "discovered" the San Jacinto Valley, with the imposing snow-capped San Jacinto Mountains standing sentinel over the surrounding valleys and deserts. Under the aegis of the San Luis Rey Mission, cattle ranching was soon established in the San Jacinto Valley. Cattle ranching and sheep herding would come to dominate the San Jacinto landscape for the next 150 years.

Much like the Cahuilla before them, today's hikers escape the summer heat of the Coachella Valley by retreating to the mountains of San Jacinto. Where the Cahuilla had to negotiate the tricky granite mountainsides by foot to reach the cooler elevations, today's hikers only have to hop onto the Palm Springs Aerial Tramway and in minutes they are whisked up where the cool breezes and whispering pines are found. The tram offers a breathtaking ride in a rotating car up the rocky and steep Chino Canyon with awe-inspiring views of the Coachella Valley. The tram opened in 1963 after 17 years of bitter dispute between developers and conservationists. Even now, there are still serious concerns about the impact hundreds of thousands of annual tram riders have on the wilderness; however, the tram station is undoubtedly the most popular trailhead for San Jacinto Peak.

The Palm Springs Aerial Tramway is not the only attraction that lures people to the San Jacinto Mountains. Tahquitz Rock was the birthplace of technical rock climbing in Southern California and remains a mecca for rock climbers. The modern system of rating climbs within the fifth class, now called the Yosemite Decimal System, was developed at Tahquitz.

The San Jacinto Mountains are part of a national monument and include both a state park and a federal wilderness area within the monument boundaries. Mt. San Jacinto State Park and Wilderness encompasses the peak, the tram, and much of the high country. San Jacinto Wilderness, administered by the Forest Service, extends north and south from the state park and includes Tahquitz and the Desert Divide as far south as Spitler Peak. The 272,000-acre Santa Rosa and San Jacinto Mountains National Monument was established by Congress in 2000 "in order to preserve the nationally significant biological, cultural, recreational, geological, educational, and scientific values found in the Santa Rosa and San Jacinto Mountains and to secure now and for future generations the opportunity to experience and enjoy the magnificent vistas, wildlife, land forms, and natural and cultural resources in these mountains and to recreate therein." Congresswoman Mary Bono Mack, who represents the 45th district spanning central and eastern Riverside County including the Coachella Valley, championed the monument designation bill.

A free wilderness permit is necessary for hiking anywhere within the state park or wilderness. The wilderness permit can be obtained from either the State Park or Forest Service depending on your entry location. At the time of this writing, the quota for permits entering via the Devils Slide Trail from Idyllwild fills up in advance on summer weekends. Leashed dogs are allowed in the federal wilderness, but not in the state park. Groups are limited to 12 in San Jacinto Wilderness and 15 in the State Park.

A camping permit is required to stay overnight in either the state park or wilderness. The campgrounds are divided into zones, each with a separate quota. The zones include Round Valley, Tamarack Valley, Little Round Valley, and Strawberry Junction within the State Park and Skunk Cabbage,

Tahquitz, Chinquapin, North Rim, Lower Basin, and Desert View within the federal Wilderness. The camping permits must be obtained directly from the State Park or the Forest Service depending on where you plan to stay. A backpacking trip with nights in both zones requires separate camping permits. Many of these zones fill a month in advance during the summer, so plan ahead. Campfires are not permitted in any zone.

Camping permits for the State Park can be obtained in person or by mail up to 56 days in advance from the Mt. San Jacinto State Park headquarters in Idyllwild, or in person from the Long Valley Ranger Station

located west of the tram station. Hiking and camping permits for the federal Wilderness can be obtained in person, by mail, or by fax from the Idyllwild Ranger Station up to 90 days in advance. (See Appendix B.)

The elevation of San Jacinto Peak has been a subject of some discussion. The 1996 edition of the USGS *San Jacinto Peak* 7.5′ topographic map erroneously lists the elevation at 10,804 feet. More recently, the elevation has been corrected to 10,834 feet. Some mountaineers argue that the survey benchmark sits 8 feet below the natural summit, so the true elevation of the peak should be 10,842 feet.

trip 9.1 Black Mtn.

Distance	7 miles (out-and-back)
Hiking Time	4 hours
Elevation Gain	2700′
Difficulty	Strenuous
Trail Use	Dogs, suitable for backpacking
Best Times	May–October
Agency	San Bernardino National Forest (Idyllwild Ranger Station)
Recommended Map	Tom Harrison *San Jacinto Wilderness* or *Lake Fulmor* 7.5′

see map on p. 172

DIRECTIONS From Banning drive southeast on State Highway 243, to the beginning of the Black Mtn. Trail (2E35), at mile marker 243 RIV 16.75, 1.0 mile beyond Vista Grande Ranger Station. Turn left and drive 100 yards up a dirt road to the parking area.

Black Mtn. (7772′) stands back from the bulk of San Jacinto on the northwest side. Not surprisingly, it offers fantastic views of the surrounding mountains and chaparral. The Forest Service takes advantage of these views with a fire lookout on the summit, staffed by volunteers. It is open to visitors 9 A.M.–5 P.M. when the access road is open (typically Memorial Day through Labor Day). The volunteers are happy to share their mountain knowledge with hikers. The vigorous hike to the lookout makes for an enjoyable excursion through the forest and granite boulders typical in this mountain range.

Hike up the trail through bands of pine and oak forest and chaparral. Initially the

climbing is steep, but soon becomes more gradual on the boulder-strewn ridge. Cross a low divide into Hall Canyon, then contour across the head of the fern-filled canyon,

Boulders and pines from the Black Mtn. Trail

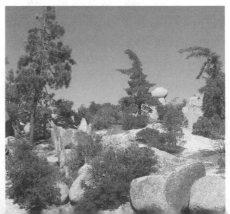

San Jacinto Mountains National Monument

where Indian Creek flows in the spring. Then climb steeply again to reach a spur of the Black Mtn. lookout road just north of the summit.

Turn right and walk past a water tank, then follow a steep faint use trail up to the lookout tower on the top. If you lose your way, just choose your own route, avoiding the jumbo boulders along the way. Alternatively, descend the spur road east to the Boulder Basin Public Campground, turn right, and hike 0.5 mile up the gated dirt road to the lookout.

Return the way you came.

ALTERNATIVE FINISH

Another option is to make a one-way hike by arranging a car or bicycle shuttle at the Boulder Basin Public Campground. To reach the campground from Highway 243, go 4.2 miles southeast from the Black Mtn. Trailhead. Turn left (north) on Black Mtn. Rd.(4S01). Drive 4.8 miles up the good dirt road, then turn left on 4S68 and proceed 0.4 mile to the campground.

trip 9.2 Indian Mtn.

Distance	5.5 miles (out-and-back)
Hiking Time	3 hours
Elevation Gain	1300′
Difficulty	Moderate
Trail Use	Dogs
Best Times	October–June
Agency	San Bernardino National Forest (Idyllwild Ranger Station)
Recommended Map	Tom Harrison *San Jacinto Wilderness* or *Lake Fulmor* 7.5′

see map on p. 172

DIRECTIONS From Banning, drive southeast on State Highway 243 to the Indian Vista overlook parking area 0.6 mile past the Lake Fulmer picnic area and just past mile marker 243 RIV 14.00. The Indian Mtn. Fire Rd. (4S21) begins just northwest of the overlook parking area.

Indian Mtn. is perched amidst the chaparral on the western slopes of the San Jacinto Mountains. It is named for the nearby Indian Creek, which runs through the Soboba reservation. The approach along a fire road is unpleasantly hot in the summer, but on a crisp winter day, it offers a fine walk and an unforgettable view of snow-clad San Jacinto Peak towering above. Even if the fire road is blanketed by recent snowfall, the hike is straightforward so long as you have adequate footwear.

Follow the Indian Mtn. Fire Rd.(4S21) down to a saddle, then up the east and south side of Indian Mtn. When the road reaches its highest point immediately south of the summit, turn right and follow the partly overgrown trail to the summit boulders. Return the way you came.

Snowy San Jacinto from Indian Mtn.

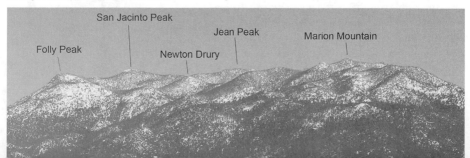

Folly Peak · San Jacinto Peak · Newton Drury · Jean Peak · Marion Mountain

trip 9.3 San Jacinto Peak via Fuller Ridge

Distance	15 miles (out-and-back)
Hiking Time	8 hours
Elevation Gain	4100′
Difficulty	Strenuous
Trail Use	Suitable for backpacking
Best Times	June–October
Agency	San Bernardino National Forest (Idyllwild Ranger Station) and Mt. San Jacinto State Park
Recommended Map	Tom Harrison *San Jacinto Wilderness, Santa Rosa and San Jacinto Mountains National Monument* or *Lake Fulmor, San Jacinto Peak 7.5′*
Permit	San Jacinto Wilderness Permit Required

see map on p. 172

DIRECTIONS From State Highway 243, 0.5 mile past mile marker 243 RIV 13.00, turn northeast up the good dirt Black Mtn. Rd. (4S01). After 4.8 miles, pass a side road on your left to Black Mtn. Campground and fire lookout. Your road winds to the right through spectacular open forest dotted with giant granite boulders. It passes the entrance of the Black Mtn. Group Camp after 1.0 mile, then a rocky outcropping on the left in another 0.8 mile featuring spectacular views of San Gorgonio Mtn. and the pass below. Pass a junction with the PCT, 0.7 mile beyond the outcrop, then turn right up a hill at a sign for the Fuller Ridge Trailhead. Drive 0.2 mile and park in the clearing.

The Pacific Crest Trail (PCT) follows Fuller Ridge northwest from San Jacinto Peak. The long dirt road by which you arrived reaches the trail at 7720 feet, the highest point to which you can drive on the mountain. This high trailhead might seem to offer an easy route to the summit, but the trail climbs up and down to bypass gendarmes on the rugged ridge, then makes a long detour south around Folly Peak to the Deer Springs area before climbing to the summit by way of Little Round Valley. On the way down, you make the same detour and the same downs and ups, resulting in a surprisingly demanding hike. Your hard work is rewarded with stunning views of Snow Creek carving the dramatic northwest face of San Jacinto. You are likely to enjoy solitude along this little-used section of the PCT.

Hike on the PCT along the north side of Fuller Ridge through a rich forest of sugar pines and white firs. In a mile, pass a saddle on the right. A vast field of wild blue and red currants grows in a clearing here, offering a tasty snack in late summer. Cross the state park boundary in 0.3 mile. In another 0.3 mile, the trail begins climbing steeply and then ascends a series of switchbacks.

VARIATION

Immediately before the first switchback, you may find a cairn on the right side marking a climber's trail up to the spires of Castle Rocks on the ridge. Despite the sheer cliffs atop much of Fuller Ridge, the highest point can be reached without any scrambling or bushwhacking if you care to make the optional detour. This excursion adds 300 feet of climbing in a steep 0.2 mile.

After passing Castle Rocks, the trail reaches a saddle on the ridge. From here, there are terrific views of Snow Creek to the east and the forested slopes to the west. After passing the rocks, the trail contours south and crosses the headwaters of the San Jacinto River before reaching a junction with the Deer Springs Trail 5 miles from the start.

Turn left (northeast) and follow the Deer Springs Trail 1 mile to Little Round Valley Trail Camp situated in a splendid bowl beside the creek. Then climb 1.3 miles to the saddle immediately south of San Jacinto

San Jacinto Mountains National Monument

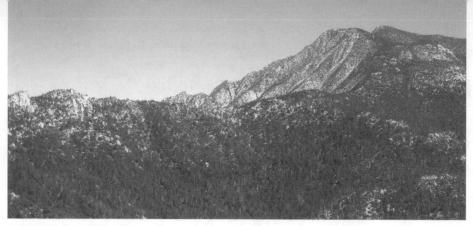

Fuller Ridge from Black Mtn.

Peak, turn left, and climb the last 0.3 mile to the summit.

Return the way you came, or make a longer loop on any of the other fine trails circling the mountain. Although a cross-country descent of upper Fuller Ridge by way of Folly Peak would appear to save substantial distance, the route involves unpleasant wading through a sea of manzanita and buckthorn.

trip 9.4 North Fork of the San Jacinto River

Distance	2 miles (out-and-back)
Hiking Time	2 hours
Elevation Gain	600′
Difficulty	Moderate
Best Times	March–November
Agency	San Bernardino National Forest (Idyllwild Ranger Station)
Recommended Map	Tom Harrison *San Jacinto Wilderness* or *San Jacinto Peak* 7.5′

see map on p. 172

DIRECTIONS From Banning, drive southeast on State Highway 243 to the signed North Fork of the San Jacinto River at mile marker 243 RIV 11.25, 0.7 mile past Fuller Mill Creek Picnic Area. The other end of the trail can also be reached from a bridge just south of the Dark Canyon Public Campground (see Trip 9.5).

The San Jacinto River is fed by small springs dotting the upper reaches of the mountain, which coalesce and flow down the west side. By the time it reaches Highway 243, it has grown into a modest but dependable stream tumbling down between boulders. In the springtime, the banks are lined with wildflowers. Water-loving trees hug the edge, while oaks, incense cedars, and pines grow tall on the slopes above. This part of the river is a great place to take a saunter while visiting the Idyllwild area. Although this is a short hike, it becomes strenuous near the end because the trail can be steep and poorly defined. Wear boots with good traction.

The San Jacinto River is of special biological interest since it is one of the last populated habitats in the San Bernardino National Forest for the endangered mountain yellow-legged frog (*Rana muscosa*). Historically this was one of the most common frogs in Southern California and used to be found in virtually every year-round stream in the mountains, but it has been driven to near extinction recently. Due to the presence of this and other sensitive species, the Forest Service asks visitors to avoid water play, wading, rock hopping, and fishing, and to stay 10 feet from the creek's edge. However, hiking the trail above the creek is still allowed. Watch for signs posted in the area with the latest information or check with the Idyllwild Ranger Station.

The unmarked trail begins on the south side of the highway bridge and leads east upstream. Frequent forks lead down to the water, but stay on the main trail as it

wanders past boulders and trees. In 1 mile, reach a bridge just south of the Dark Canyon Public Campground. If you are lucky, you may find delicious ripe wild raspberries growing below the bridge.

trip 9.5 Seven Pines Trail

Distance	7 miles (out-and-back)
Hiking Time	4 hours
Elevation Gain	2400'
Difficulty	Strenuous
Trail Use	Dogs, suitable for backpacking
Best Times	May–October
Agency	San Bernardino National Forest (Idyllwild Ranger Station) and Mt. San Jacinto State Park
Recommended Map	Tom Harrison *San Jacinto Wilderness, Santa Rosa and San Jacinto Mountains National Monument* or *San Jacinto Peak 7.5'*
Permit	San Jacinto Wilderness Permit Required

see map on p. 172

DIRECTIONS From Highway 243 near mile marker 243 RIV 9.75, 200 yards east of Alandale Ranger Station, turn northeast on the paved Azalea Trails Rd. (4S02). Stay left at a junction in 100 yards and continue 0.8 mile to a junction with the Marion Mtn. Campground Rd. (4S71). Stay left again and continue to the Dark Canyon Campground. Follow the one-way loop road through the campground to rejoin 4S02 just past the top of the loop, where it becomes a fair dirt road. Pass the Azalea Trails Girl Scout Camp and arrive at the signed Seven Pines trailhead (2E13), 4.1 miles from the highway.

The lightly traveled Seven Pines Trail climbs through the spectacular forests, creeks, and rock formations on the western slopes of San Jacinto. It is longer but less steep than the nearby Marion Mtn. Trail. This is a good place to escape when you would like to contemplate the mountain in quiet and solitude.

From the trailhead, the Seven Pines Trail switchbacks up to the northeast, passing north of a small knob before turning south and descending to the San Jacinto River. This stretch of the river headwaters is home to the endangered mountain yellow-legged frog (*Rana muscosa*). To protect the frog and its habitat, the river and its banks are presently closed to all entry. However, crossing the river along the trail is still permitted. Beyond the river, the trail continues upward and twice crosses the intermittent

Snow Plant

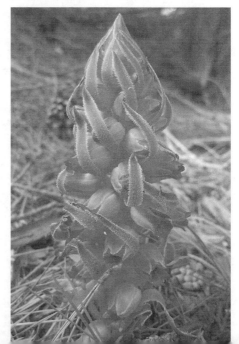

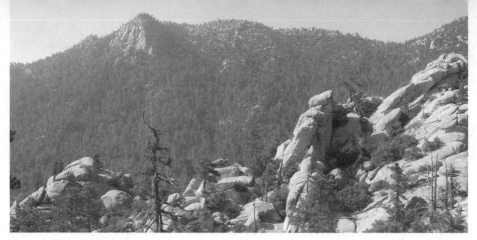

Western slopes of San Jacinto

creek flowing down from Deer Springs before arriving at the PCT. Return the way you came.

VARIATIONS

Many other options are available for a longer trip. You can continue up to San Jacinto Peak. Or, with a 4-mile car or bicycle shuttle, you can descend the nearby Marion Mtn. Trail. Note that the road between the two trails drops 600 feet to cross the San Jacinto River near Dark Canyon before climbing back up, so it is a vigorous bicycle ride in either direction.

trip 9.6 San Jacinto Peak via the Marion Mtn. Trail

Distance	12 miles (out-and-back)
Hiking Time	7 hours
Elevation Gain	4500'
Difficulty	Strenuous
Trail Use	Dogs, suitable for backpacking
Best Times	June–October
Agency	San Bernardino National Forest (Idyllwild Ranger Station) and Mt. San Jacinto State Park
Recommended Map	Tom Harrison *San Jacinto Wilderness, Santa Rosa and San Jacinto Mountains National Monument* or *San Jacinto Peak 7.5'*
Permit	San Jacinto Wilderness Permit Required

see map on p. 172

DIRECTIONS From Highway 243 near mile marker 243 RIV 9.75, 200 yards east of Alandale Ranger Station, turn northeast on the paved Azalea Trails Rd. (4S02). Stay left at a junction in 100 yards and continue 0.8 mile to a junction with the Marion Mtn. Campground Rd. (4S71). Turn right and follow this road for 0.6 mile to the Marion Mtn. trailhead, located between the Fern Basin and Marion Mtn. Campgrounds.

The Marion Mtn. Trail on the western flank of San Jacinto is the shortest route to the summit without taking the tram. This side of the mountain attracts relatively few hikers, so it good for those seeking seclusion. Moreover, its short and direct route is ideal for springtime snow ascents of San Jacinto.

The signed Marion Mtn. Trail (2E14) starts across the road from the parking area and immediately begins switchbacking up the ridge through incense cedars, oaks, firs, pines, and manzanitas. In 0.4 mile, it passes a dirt road, then a signed cutoff trail back down to Marion Mtn. Campground, then another to Stone Creek Campground. (Note that the main trail does not go straight to the campground as shown on the 7.5´ topo map.) The Marion Mtn. Trail continues up the north shoulder of the ridge, offering views into the headwaters of the San Jacinto River. At 1.25 miles, a rocky clearing 50 feet north of the trail offers unobstructed vistas. Shortly before reaching the Pacific Crest Trail (PCT), pass a peculiar gigantic boulder with a "window" near the top.

At 2.8 miles, reach the PCT and turn left. In 100 feet, pass a signed junction for the Seven Pines Trail that leads back down to Dark Canyon Campground (see Trip 9.5). Continue east and then north for 0.5 mile,

crossing the creek coming down from Deer Springs, to another junction where the Deer Springs Trail departs the PCT. Turn right and follow the Deer Springs Trail northeast to the pleasant camp at Little Round Valley (1 mile). This section involves difficult navigation when covered in snow because it can be difficult to pick out landmarks. Switchback another 1.3 miles up to the saddle between San Jacinto and Jean Peaks. Turn left and hike 0.3 mile up to the summit rocks of San Jacinto.

Return the way you came. Or, with a car or bike shuttle, explore any of the multitude of other fine trails girding the mountain.

Window Rock along the Marion Mtn. Trail

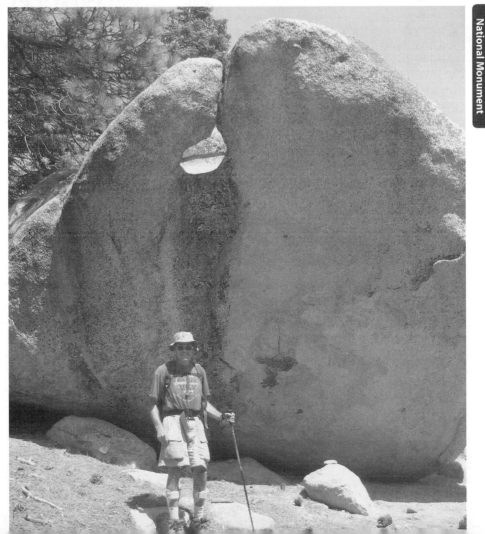

trip 9.7 Webster Trail

Distance	5 miles (out-and-back)
Hiking Time	3 hours
Elevation Gain	2000'
Difficulty	Moderate
Trail Use	Dogs
Best Times	October–June
Agency	San Bernardino National Forest (Idyllwild Ranger Station)
Recommended Map	Tom Harrison *San Jacinto Wilderness* or *Lake Fulmor* and *San Jacinto Peak* 7.5'

see map on p. 172

DIRECTIONS From Pine Cove at the Shell station on State Highway 243, 3 miles from Idyllwild and just north of mile marker 247 RIV 7.25, turn west on Pine Cove Rd. and follow it for 0.8 mile as it curves north to a junction with Forest Roads 5S09 and 5S10. Turn sharp left (southwest) on 5S10 and continue 0.5 mile to a junction at the Lia Hona Lodge. Turn right and descend 0.9 mile on a fair dirt road to the beginning of the Webster Trail, indicated by a wooden sign on the right. Park in the adjacent clearing.

The Webster Trail plunges steeply down a ridge into the secluded canyon carved by the North Fork of the San Jacinto River. The river is a great place to take a dip on a moderately warm day and you will likely have it to yourself. An ideal time to visit is shortly after a good rain in the spring but don't underestimate the steep, shadeless climb on your return. Carry plenty of water and wear boots with good tread or use a hiking pole to help with the loose footing.

The Webster Trail is named for David G. Webster, who established an early ranch in the San Jacinto Valley and drove his cattle up to summer pastures along this trail in the 1870s and 1880s.

The trail descends westward along the ridge, briefly through a forest of Jeffrey pines and oaks, then down through chaparral. It makes a solitary switchback near the bottom to negotiate the final drop into the river canyon.

Hikers cooling their feet at the North Fork of the San Jacinto River

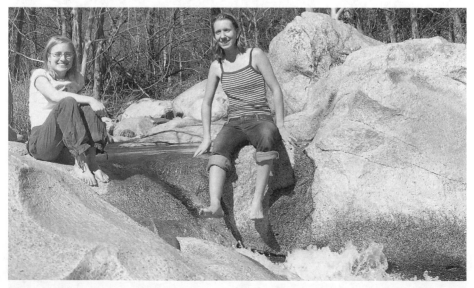

trip 9.8 Suicide Rock

Distance	7 miles (out-and-back)
Hiking Time	3.5 hours
Elevation Gain	1900'
Difficulty	Moderate
Trail Use	Dogs
Best Times	May–October
Agency	San Bernardino National Forest (Idyllwild Ranger Station) and Mt. San Jacinto State Park
Recommended Map	Tom Harrison *San Jacinto Wilderness, Santa Rosa and San Jacinto Mountains National Monument* or *San Jacinto Peak 7.5'*
Permit	San Jacinto Wilderness Permit Required

see map on p. 172

DIRECTIONS From Idyllwild Ranger Station drive west 1 mile on Highway 243. Park on the north side of the road just above the County Park Nature Center and past a sign pointing to Deer Springs Trailhead Parking.

Suicide Rock sits atop the ridge overlooking Strawberry Valley, drawing rock climbers to test their mettle on its steep, clean, granite faces. According to legend, the rock gets its name from two young Native American lovers, who leapt from the top rather than obeying the chief's order to separate. The most straightforward route to the top of the rock is via the Deer Springs Trail from the western edge of Idyllwild.

The Deer Springs Trail itself (3E17) starts on the north side of the road 50 yards east of the parking area. Alternatively, walk up a steep unmarked path above the parking area for 150 yards to a junction with the Deer Springs Trail near some power lines.

Suicide Rock from the Devils Slide Trail

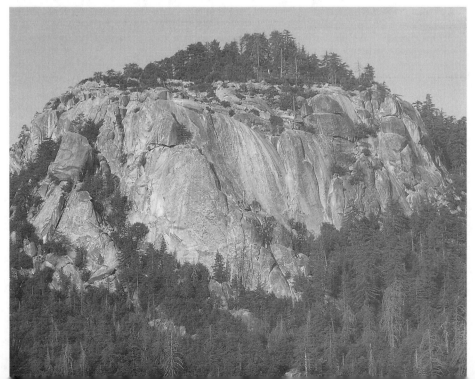

Turn left and proceed uphill, joining the main trail.

The trail climbs north onto the ridge, through stands of huge tree-like manzanita. As you gain altitude, the chaparral gives way to black oak and Jeffrey pine. In 2.3 miles, reach a signed junction and turn right onto the Suicide Rock Trail. The trail contours along the slope, then dips down to cross Marion Creek before climbing back up to Suicide Rock.

Enjoy the views, but take care that children do not stray too far from the trail. The cliffs roll off deceptively before dropping straight down. There is no safe way down to the east without a rope.

ALTERNATIVE FINISH

It is possible to return to the northwest end of Suicide Rock and find a climber's trail that descends the dirt slopes and drops down the steep hill to Fern Valley Rd. at the switchback below Humber Park. The trail can be difficult to follow in places, but with a car or bicycle shuttle, makes for an interesting alternative route.

---

trip 9.9 Tahquitz Rock

Distance	2.2 miles (out-and-back)
Hiking Time	2 hours
Elevation Gain	1600 feet
Difficulty	Moderate
Best Times	May–October
Agency	San Bernardino National Forest (Idyllwild Ranger Station)
Recommended Map	Tom Harrison *San Jacinto Wilderness, Santa Rosa and San Jacinto Mountains National Monument* or *San Jacinto Peak* 7.5′

see map on p. 172

DIRECTIONS From Highway 243 in Idyllwild just south of the ranger station, turn northeast on North Circle Dr. Proceed 0.7 mile, passing Nomad Ventures (a good outdoors and climbing shop). At the four-way intersection, turn right on South Circle Dr. Go 0.1 mile, then turn left on Fern Valley Rd. After 1.7 miles, reach a small parking area for the Ernie Maxwell Scenic Trail. If you reach the large lot and restrooms at Humber Park, you have gone 0.1 mile too far.

Tahquitz Rock, also known as the less imposing sounding Lily Rock, was the birthplace of technical rock climbing in the United States. In the 1930s, Robert Underhill brought modern rope techniques developed in the Alps back to Sierra Club members in California. The massive granite dome of Tahquitz Rock attracted immediate attention. In 1937, Dick Jones and Glen Dawson climbed the Mechanic's Route, which, with a rating of 5.8, was the most difficult route in America at the time. Since then, thousands of climbers have flocked to the rock's sheer walls to hone their skills. Fortunately for hikers, there is an easier route to the summit involving some rock scrambling but no ropes.

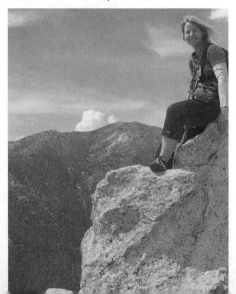
Marion Mtn. from Tahquitz Rock

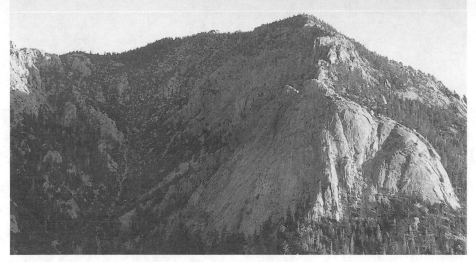
Tahquitz Rock

Hike south on the Ernie Maxwell Scenic Trail through a forest of oaks, white firs, incense cedars, and Jeffrey pines. Immediately descend to cross the east fork of Strawberry Creek, then round a bend and look for a steep and rough climber's trail leading up the hill to your left, 0.2 mile. Climb the trail, staying right of a huge rockslide. In 0.4 mile, reach a large boulder known to climbers as Lunch Rock. Pass around the right side to the base of Tahquitz Rock. Follow the climber's trail to the right around the south and east side of the rock; it can be difficult to follow in places but is worth finding because it avoids the worst of the bushes. When it tops out on a saddle directly east of the summit, climb third-class ramps and boulders to the summit of Tahquitz Rock, 0.5 mile. Return the way you came. This is the only safe way off the summit without a rope.

ALTERNATIVE FINISH

Once back to the saddle, it is also possible to shimmy down the third-class north gully, loop part way around the rock, and follow another climber's trail north back down to Strawberry Creek.

trip 9.10 Ernie Maxwell Scenic Trail

Distance	5 miles (out-and-back)
Hiking Time	2.5 hours
Elevation Gain	700'
Difficulty	Easy
Trail Use	Dogs
Best Times	May–October
Agency	San Bernardino National Forest (Idyllwild Ranger Station)
Optional Map	Tom Harrison *San Jacinto Wilderness, Santa Rosa and San Jacinto Mountains National Monument* or *San Jacinto Peak 7.5'*

see map on p. 172

DIRECTIONS This trail can be accessed from either the south or north end. This description starts at the south end so that the hike is downhill on the way back. From Highway 243 near the south end of Idyllwild next to the Idyllwild School, turn east on Saunders Meadow Rd. Note that Saunders Meadow forms a loop and intersects Highway 243 a second time farther south by the dump. Drive 0.8 mile, turn left (north) on Pine Ave., go 0.2 mile, and turn right on Tahquitz View Dr. Proceed 0.5 mile, passing the South Ridge Trail Rd. junction, to the signed Ernie Maxwell Scenic Trail. Parking is limited to a few wide spots along the road. The north end of the trail is just below Humber Park (see Trip 9.9).

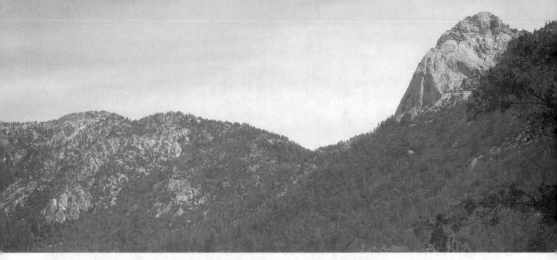

Tahquitz Rock and Strawberry Valley from the Ernie Maxwell Scenic Trail

The Ernie Maxwell Scenic Trail commemorates the founder of the *Idyllwild Town Crier* newspaper and long-time conservationist who greatly influenced the town of Idyllwild. This pleasant trail through the forest above town is a good place to take a stroll while visiting town.

Tahquitz Rock is prominently visible from the southern terminus of the trail. The path leads northeast through a forest of oaks, cedars, pines and firs with occasional glimpses of Strawberry Valley and Suicide Rock through the woods. In the spring, you may see brilliant red snow plants poking up through the ground. In 2.5 miles, pass beneath Tahquitz Rock and reach the northern end at Humber Park. Return the way you came.

trip 9.11 Skunk Cabbage Meadow

Distance	6.5 miles (out-and-back)
Hiking Time	3 hours
Elevation Gain	1700'
Difficulty	Moderate
Trail Use	Dogs, suitable for backpacking
Best Times	May–October
Agency	San Bernardino National Forest (Idyllwild Ranger Station)
Recommended Map	Tom Harrison *San Jacinto Wilderness, Santa Rosa and San Jacinto Mountains National Monument* or *San Jacinto Peak 7.5'*
Permit	San Jacinto Wilderness Permit Required

see map on p. 172

DIRECTIONS From Highway 243 in Idyllwild just south of the ranger station, turn northeast on North Circle Dr. Drive 0.7 mile, passing Nomad Ventures (a good outdoors and climbing shop). At the four-way intersection, turn right on South Circle Dr. Proceed 0.1 mile, then turn left on Fern Valley Rd. After 1.7 miles, pass a small parking area for the Ernie Maxwell Scenic Trail. Continue 0.1 mile up the hill to the outhouse and larger parking area of Humber Park.

The Devils Slide Trail is the main trail out of Idyllwild. Cattle ranchers used to drive their herds up through the loose and dangerous slopes over thorn bushes, boulders, and logs to summer pastures in Tahquitz Valley. The trail is now so well-graded that some have rechristened it *Angel's Glide*, but it nevertheless has a strenuous start if you are hiking with a heavy pack. On the far side of Saddle Junction is a fine conifer forest dotted with a few meadows. This trip leads to one of those meadows, with a pleasant camp centrally located for exploring the plethora of nearby trails.

Take the Devils Slide Trail 2.5 miles to Saddle Junction. It climbs 1600 feet from Humber Park to Saddle Junction. Saddle Junction is a five-way junction. Take the signed fork leading northeast toward Skunk Cabbage Meadow and Willow Creek. Divinely perfumed azaleas grow by some of the springs adjacent to the trail. In 0.6 mile, turn right at another signed junction and hike 0.2 mile to the campsites near the meadow. Wilderness regulations require campsites to be at least 200 feet away from meadows. Water can normally be found between the junction and Willow Creek.

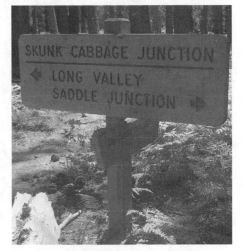

Skunk Cabbage Junction

trip 9.12 Tahquitz Peak via Saddle Junction

Distance	8.5 miles (out-and-back)
Hiking Time	5 hours
Elevation Gain	2400'
Difficulty	Strenuous
Trail Use	Dogs, suitable for backpacking
Best Times	May–October
Agency	San Bernardino National Forest (Idyllwild Ranger Station)
Recommended Map	Tom Harrison *San Jacinto Wilderness, Santa Rosa and San Jacinto Mountains National Monument* or *San Jacinto Peak 7.5'*
Permit	San Jacinto Wilderness Permit Required

see
map on
p. 172

DIRECTIONS From Highway 243 in Idyllwild just south of the ranger station, turn northeast on North Circle Dr. Drive 0.7 mile, passing Nomad Ventures (a good outdoors and climbing shop). At the four-way intersection, turn right on South Circle Dr. Proceed 0.1 mile, then turn left on Fern Valley Rd. After 1.7 miles, pass a small parking area for the Ernie Maxwell Scenic Trail. Continue 0.1 mile up the hill to the outhouse and larger parking area of Humber Park.

Tahquitz Peak (8828') is the second major summit in the San Jacinto Mountains after San Jacinto itself. The summit overlooks Idyllwild and is guarded by dramatic granite buttresses, most notably Tahquitz Rock. Tahquitz Peak is named for a legendary evil Cahuilla shaman who eats the souls of the unwary. Hikers use several pronunciations, but the correct Cahuilla pronunciation is "taw-kwish."

The peak can be reached from either the north or south. This trip follows the more heavily traveled northern route, which starts from the popular Humber Park Trailhead. See Trip 9.17 for the route up the south ridge.

From Humber Park, hike 2.5 miles up the Devils Slide Trail to the five-way Saddle Junction, where you meet the PCT. Take the rightmost fork and hike south on the PCT toward Tahquitz Peak, gradually climbing through the open forest. The trees become smaller and more weather-beaten as you climb. In 1.4 miles, reach the South Ridge

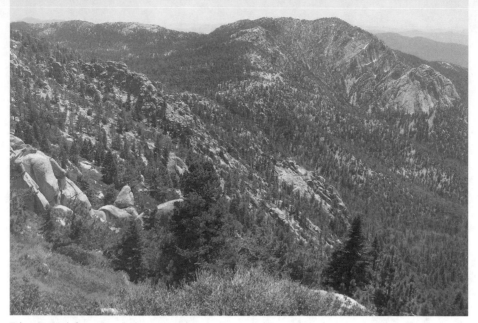

Tahquitz Peak from the north

Trail junction. Take it right (southwest) toward Tahquitz Peak for 0.4 mile, then take a short spur up to the summit.

Tahquitz Peak Fire Lookout is located on the summit, taking advantage of the commanding views in all directions. The remote lookout is staffed during fire season by San Bernardino National Forest Association Fire Lookout Hosts who hike up to their airy post. The friendly and knowledgeable volunteers are happy to point out the sights and talk about the San Jacinto Mountains.

trip 9.13 Caramba

Distance	14 miles (out-and-back)
Hiking Time	7 hours
Elevation Gain	3300′
Difficulty	Strenuous
Trail Use	Dogs, suitable for backpacking
Best Times	May–October
Agency	San Bernardino National Forest (Idyllwild Ranger Station)
Recommended Map	Tom Harrison *San Jacinto Wilderness, Santa Rosa and San Jacinto Mountains National Monument* or *San Jacinto Peak, Palm Springs* 7.5′
Permit	San Jacinto Wilderness Permit Required

see map on p. 172

DIRECTIONS From Highway 243 in Idyllwild just south of the ranger station, turn northeast on North Circle Dr. Drive 0.7 mile, passing Nomad Ventures (a good outdoors and climbing shop). At the four-way intersection, turn right on South Circle Dr. Proceed 0.1 mile, then turn left on Fern Valley Rd. After 1.7 miles, pass a small parking area for the Ernie Maxwell Scenic Trail. Continue 0.1 mile up the hill to the outhouse and larger parking area of Humber Park.

Tahquitz Valley hangs on the southeastern slope of the San Jacinto Mountains, walled in by granite ridges. Tahquitz Creek flows down the gentle valley beneath the white firs and Jeffrey pines until it abruptly drops over a waterfall and plunges down Tahquitz Canyon to the desert near Palm Springs. Caramba Trail Camp sits alongside the creek by the lip of the precipice. *¡Ay, caramba!* is a Spanish expression of surprise, more recently popularized by Bart Simpson. Author John Robinson relates two stories of how the camp got its name. In one, cowboys camping on the rim were spooked by strange noises in the night. In another more prosaic story, the abrupt drop from Tahquitz Valley down to the desert shocked the travelers.

In 1916–1917, Moses Gordon cut a remarkable trail from Palm Springs up Tahquitz Canyon to Caramba and onto Idyllwild to connect his winter home and summer cabin. He stayed at Caramba camp while building the trail. Unfortunately, the Gordon Trail has fallen into disrepair and now the upper reaches of Tahquitz Canyon are nearly impassable because of steep cliffs and heavy brush.

This trip offers a fine tour of Tahquitz Valley and impressive views down Tahquitz Canyon. It is a good backpacking trip and you are likely to have Caramba Camp to yourself even on a fine summer weekend where crowds flock to the less remote camps on San Jacinto. However, water sources are not dependable in the summer.

Grind your way 1600 feet up the Devils Slide Trail for 2.5 miles to the five-way Saddle Junction. Follow a signed trail southeast through the open forest toward Tahquitz Valley and Laws-Caramba. In 0.6 mile, pass a trail junction in Tahquitz Valley. Continue east another 1.6 miles to Law's Camp, where travel writer George Law built a stone summer cabin along Willow Creek in 1915. Beyond, the trail descends to another tributary creek, climbs, and then drops 2 miles to Caramba.

From the camp, you can wander a few yards downstream to the first Tahquitz Creek waterfall, which drops into Tahquitz Canyon. Better yet, scramble up the hillside east of camp for an unobstructed view down into the canyon. There is another beautiful campsite here, although you must haul water up from the creek.

VARIATION

South of Caramba are a pair of bumps on the ridge between Tahquitz and Andreas Canyons. The higher one (7339′) is unofficially known as Sam Fink Peak in honor of the Sierra Club leader who pioneered the trail along the Desert Divide; it is a fun excursion for campers with extra energy. Bring the *Palm Springs* topo map for cross-country navigation. Sam Fink Peak is easily reached from the ridge east of Caramba camp by taking a compass bearing on the saddle between the bumps and traveling a half mile cross-country to the saddle, then turning left (southeast) and hiking up to the summit for a spectacular view.

Caramba Camp

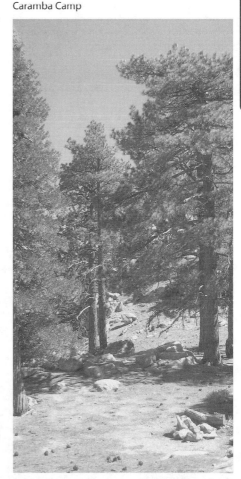

trip 9.14 Strawberry Valley Loop

Distance	10 miles (one way or loop)
Hiking Time	5 hours
Elevation Gain	2600'
Difficulty	Strenuous
Trail Use	Dogs, suitable for backpacking
Best Times	May–October
Agency	San Bernardino National Forest (Idyllwild Ranger Station) and Mt. San Jacinto State Park
Recommended Map	Tom Harrison *San Jacinto Wilderness*, *Santa Rosa and San Jacinto Mountains National Monument* or *San Jacinto Peak 7.5'*
Permit	San Jacinto Wilderness Permit Required

see map on p. 172

DIRECTIONS This loop hike near Idyllwild starts at Humber Park and ends at the Deer Springs trailhead, requiring a 3.6-mile car shuttle. If no shuttle is available, it is possible to descend a climber's trail near Suicide Rock to return to Humber Park, but this demands some cross-country route-finding skill. From Highway 243 northwest of Idyllwild, leave a getaway vehicle at the Deer Springs Trailhead 1 mile west of the ranger station. The poorly marked trailhead is on the north side of the highway just above the County Park Nature Center. To reach Humber Park, continue down Highway 243 toward Idyllwild past the ranger station and turn northeast on North Circle Dr. Proceed 0.7 mile, passing Nomad Ventures (a good outdoors and climbing shop). At the four-way intersection, turn right on South Circle Dr. Go 0.1 mile, then turn left on Fern Valley and follow it 1.8 miles to the large Humber Park lot.

Strawberry Creek carves a scenic valley out of the south slopes of Marion Mtn. and the San Jacinto ridge. The ridges are lushly forested and are decorated with huge granite outcrops, including the famous Tahquitz and Suicide Rocks. This loop climbs the Devils Slide Trail to the east ridge, cuts across the north slopes of the valley, and descends the west ridge past Sui-cide Rock. There are several fine campsites along the way.

The Devils Slide Trail climbs 1600 feet from Humber Park over 2.5 miles to Saddle Junction. The first cattle ranchers used to drive their herds up through the loose and dangerous slopes to summer pastures in Tahquitz Valley. The trail is now so well-graded that some have rechristened

Upper reaches of Strawberry Valley

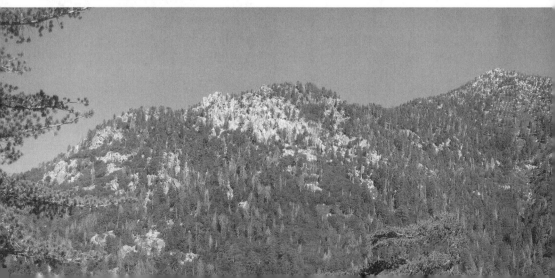

it *Angel's Glide* but it nevertheless has a strenuous start if you are carrying a heavy pack.

The five-way Saddle Junction delimits the west end of the splendid Tahquitz Valley. Creeks flow through the meadows and open forest, and there is good camping at Tahquitz Valley and Skunk Cabbage Meadow. If you have an extra day, consider spending the night in the valley and exploring the trails to Tahquitz Peak or the Caramba Overlook.

Turn left (north) at Saddle Junction and follow the PCT as it climbs the ridge. At a junction in 1.8 miles, turn left (west) and hike across the chaparral-clad slopes forming the north wall of Strawberry Valley. There are magnificent views of Tahquitz and Suicide Rocks from this portion of the trail. Strawberry Creek flows down from its source high on Marion Mtn., and you may be able to refill water here, though the creek dries up in late summer. In 2.2 miles, come to the dry but spectacularly situated Strawberry Junction trail camp beneath the Jeffrey pines and to another trail junction just beyond.

Turn left (south) and leave the PCT, joining the Deer Springs Trail instead. The open forest of pines and firs are some of the most beautiful in Southern California. Follow the trail down the ridge for 1.6 miles to the Suicide Rock turnoff. If a vehicle awaits at the Deer Springs Trailhead, continue straight down the ridge for another 2.1 miles through a "forest" of giant manzanitas to the trailhead. The trail splits beneath some wires at the very end and the right path shortcuts down to the western trailhead parking.

ALTERNATIVE FINISH

If you do not have a shuttle available, turn left at the Suicide Rock turnoff and hike 1.2 miles northeast up to the rock. This adds 600 feet of climbing to the trip. You may wish to continue all the way to the top to enjoy the view. However, the best descent begins back at the northwest end of the rock and skirts the cliffs. Take care not to head down Suicide Rock's sheer face, for obvious reasons. A climber's trail follows the base of the slabs to the east end of the rock, then drops down to the Fern Valley Rd. It can be difficult to follow at times and is quite steep in places. The route eventually meets Forest Haven Dr., then crosses Strawberry Creek and arrives at Fern Valley Rd. just below the water tanks, 1 mile down from the rock. Hike 0.3 mile up the road to the Humber Park lot.

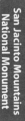

San Jacinto Mountains
National Monument

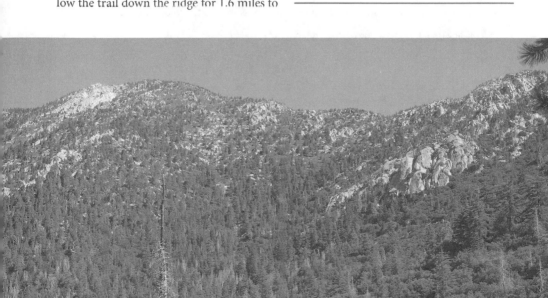

trip 9.15 Idyllwild–Round Valley Loop

Distance	14 miles (loop)
Hiking Time	7 hours
Elevation Gain	3600 feet
Difficulty	Strenuous
Trail Use	Dogs, suitable for backpacking
Best Times	May–October
Agency	San Bernardino National Forest (Idyllwild Ranger Station) and Mt. San Jacinto State Park
Recommended Map	Tom Harrison *San Jacinto Wilderness, Santa Rosa and San Jacinto Mountains National Monument* or *San Jacinto Peak 7.5'*
Permit	San Jacinto Wilderness Permit Required

see map on p. 172

DIRECTIONS From Highway 243 in Idyllwild, just south of the ranger station, turn northeast on North Circle Dr. Drive 0.7 mile, passing Nomad Ventures (a good outdoors and climbing shop). At the four-way intersection, turn right on South Circle Dr. Proceed 0.1 mile, then turn left on Fern Valley Rd. After 1.7 miles, pass a small parking area for the Ernie Maxwell Scenic Trail. Continue 0.1 mile up the hill to the outhouse and parking area of Humber Park.

John Robinson offers a marvelously poetic description of Round Valley in *San Bernardino Mountain Trails*:

> Southeast from San Jacinto's lofty crown, nestled in high hanging valleys ringed by jagged spurs of white granite, is an enchanting wonderland of green. Here, suspended 8000 feet above the desert, pines and firs grow tall and sturdy, lush meadows are waist-high with fern and azalea, lupines spot hillsides in their late-summer bloom of purple and pale mauve, and little singing streams flow clear and cold. In the heart of this high sylvan wilderness is Round Valley, an oval meadow of verdant grass, threaded by an icy-cold brook, surrounded by a dense forest of lodgepole pine. Here is the most popular trail camp in the San Jacinto high country, frequented by dozens of backpackers almost every summer and early fall weekend.

This trip visits Round Valley the hard way, up the Devils Slide from Idyllwild and through Tahquitz valley, offering a fine tour of the southeast side of San Jacinto.

Tahquitz Valley from the south side of the Hidden Divide

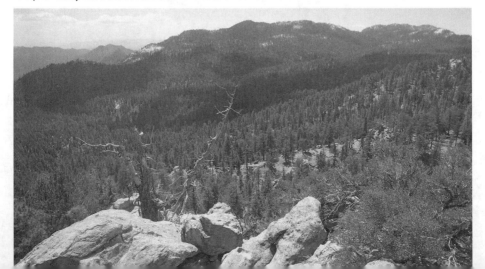

Follow the Devils Slide Trail 2.5 miles as it climbs 1600 feet to the five-way Saddle Junction. Take the signed trail northeast toward Willow Creek and Long Valley. In 0.5 mile, pass a field of ferns and the signed turnoff for Skunk Cabbage Meadow (good camping can be found here). Continue east and drop down to cross Willow Creek, then climb to a trail junction on the north side of a rocky knob in another 1.5 miles. Take the north fork toward Long and Round Valleys. The trail climbs gradually, then passes an intermittent creek to a pleasant shady bench. Beyond, the trail switchbacks up toward the Hidden Divide. Watch for a rocky outcrop where you can scramble up for a fine view of Tahquitz Valley. Reach the saddle on Hidden Divide in 1.7 miles.

The main trail continues north and in 0.3 mile reaches another junction. If you like, you can take the right (north) fork, which leads to the Long Valley Ranger Station and tramway and curves back toward Round Valley, but it is shorter to head directly west for 1 mile. Rejoin the trail from Long Valley continuing west and in 0.2 mile arrive at Round Valley, which is often filled with legions of happy campers who came the short way from the tram.

Your route climbs steadily west for 1 mile to the Wellman Divide, the highest point on the loop. Turn left and hike another mile past the seeping Wellman Cienega to reach a junction with the PCT. Turn left again and hike 1.9 miles south down the ridge back to Saddle Junction, then follow Devils Slide Trail back to the trailhead.

trip 9.16 San Jacinto Peak from Idyllwild

Distance	18–20 miles (loop)
Hiking Time	10 hours
Elevation Gain	4500′
Difficulty	Strenuous
Trail Use	Dogs, suitable for backpacking
Best Times	June–October
Agency	San Bernardino National Forest (Idyllwild Ranger Station) and Mt. San Jacinto State Park
Recommended Map	Tom Harrison *San Jacinto Wilderness, Santa Rosa and San Jacinto Mountains National Monument* or *San Jacinto Peak* 7.5′
Permit	San Jacinto Wilderness Permit Required

see map on p. 172

DIRECTIONS From Highway 243 in Idyllwild just south of the ranger station, turn northeast on North Circle Dr. Drive 0.7 mile, passing Nomad Ventures (a good outdoors and climbing shop). At the four-way intersection, turn right on South Circle Dr. Proceed 0.1 mile, then turn left on Fern Valley Rd. After 1.7 miles, reach a small parking area for the Ernie Maxwell Scenic Trail. Continue 0.1 mile up the hill to the outhouse and larger parking area of Humber Park.

This trip is our favorite tour of the San Jacinto Wilderness high country. This is a land of superlatives: the most dramatic granite faces, most beautiful conifer forests, and second highest mountains in Southern California. Starting at Humber Park in Idyllwild, it makes a counterclockwise loop by way of Saddle Junction and over the Wellman Divide, then to the very pinnacle

of San Jacinto Peak, before descending through Little Round Valley and returning along the PCT. It is a great way to get to know the San Jacinto Peak area. Several beautifully situated trail camps along the route offer tempting backpacking options.

From Humber Park, take the strenuous Devils Slide Trail to Saddle Junction climbing 1600 feet in just over 2.5 miles. Along

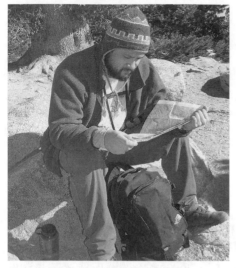

Consulting a map on the Wellman Divide

the way, enjoy spectacular views of Suicide and Tahquitz Rocks, which are swarming with bold climbers on pleasant days. Backpackers can find good camping just east of Saddle Junction in Skunk Cabbage Meadow and Tahquitz Valley, but our trip turns sharply left at Saddle Junction and joins the northbound PCT as it climbs the ridge overlooking Strawberry Valley.

In 1.9 miles, the trail reaches a junction. The PCT turns west toward Strawberry Junction (see Trip 9.14), but we continue north for another mile past the swampy Wellman Cienega and up through chaparral and boulders to the Wellman Divide. Here another trail descends east to the campsites of Round Valley and down to the Palm Springs Aerial Tramway.

Continue north along the chaparral-clad east slope of Jean Peak. The prominent pyramid to the northeast is Cornell Peak (see Trip 9.20). After one big switchback, the trail reaches the saddle south of San Jacinto Peak in 2.4 miles. Turn right and hike north 0.3 mile to the granite summit boulders. Along the way, pass a stone hut, which offers emergency shelter (although it is not recommended in an electrical storm). The final yards to the summit involve hopping up the big talus.

After returning to the saddle, continue west and descend 1.3 miles to Little Round Valley, with splendid camping beneath the Jeffrey pines along a seasonal stream. This is about the halfway point of the trip, although all of the strenuous climbing is now behind you.

Descend another mile to rejoin the PCT. Follow it west for 0.5 mile to junctions with the Seven Pines and Marion Mtn. trails, then south through beautiful open forest of Jeffrey pines and white firs. In 2.3 miles, reach Strawberry Junction. A small dry trail camp with panoramic views is situated just east of the junction.

Here you have three return options: via the PCT, Suicide Rock, or Deer Springs. The 6.7-mile PCT option is the simplest choice, leading east across the head of Strawberry Valley, then turning south and retracing your earlier route to Saddle Junction and the Devils Slide Trail to Humber Park.

ALTERNATIVE FINISHES

The 4.2-mile Suicide Rock option requires plenty of daylight and involves difficult cross-country travel that is only recommended for experienced hikers with light packs. Take the Deer Springs Trail south for 1.8 miles, then turn left and follow the Suicide Rock Trail 1.0 mile to the 7528-foot summit for an outstanding view. Retrace your steps to the northwest end of the rock, where you can find a climber's trail skirting the edge. Do not be tempted to descend the cliffs directly; there is no safe route without a rope. Follow the faint and often confusing climber's trail, which is occasionally marked with cairns. It passes along the base of the rock, then steeply descends for a mile to Forest Haven Dr. and back to Fern Valley Rd. Hike uphill for 0.4 mile back to Humber Park.

The Deer Springs option is the shortest, but requires a car shuttle. Simply hike 4.1 miles down the ridge to the trailhead, located 1 mile west of the Idyllwild Ranger Station on Highway 243 (see Trip 9.8).

trip 9.17 Tahquitz Peak via the South Ridge Trail

Distance	7 miles (out-and-back)
Hiking Time	4 hours
Elevation Gain	2400'
Difficulty	Strenuous
Trail Use	Dogs
Best Times	May–October
Agency	San Bernardino National Forest (Idyllwild Ranger Station)
Recommended Map	Tom Harrison *San Jacinto Wilderness, Santa Rosa and San Jacinto Mountains National Monument* or *Idyllwild, San Jacinto Peak 7.5'*
Permit	San Jacinto Wilderness Permit Required

see map on p. 172

DIRECTIONS From Highway 243 on the south edge of Idyllwild next to the Idyllwild School, drive up Saunders Meadow Rd. for 0.8 mile. Turn left on Pine Ave., drive 0.2 mile, then turn right on Tahquitz View Dr. for 0.3 mile. Just before the road becomes dirt, turn right on South Ridge Rd. (5S11). Proceed 0.9 mile, passing several minor side roads, to the signed South Ridge Trail (3E08) parking area.

Tahquitz Peak (8828´) is the second major summit in the San Jacinto Mountains after San Jacinto itself. The summit overlooks Idyllwild and is guarded by dramatic granite buttresses, most notably Tahquitz Rock. The peak can be reached from either the north or south. This trip follows the shorter and more secluded route up the beautiful south ridge. See Trip 9.12 for the northern route.

Follow the trail as it climbs to the ridge crest, then zigzags up the divide through rich forest. In 1.4 miles, pass a curious "window" in the rock framing a splendid view of the Desert Divide to the east. Continue through a field of massive boulders for 0.3 mile to a flat clearing about halfway to your destination, a good rest stop. Beyond, you climb on the steep west face below the rocky ridge. Pass through chinquapin thickets, scattered lodgepole pines, and towering granite gendarmes. The views continue to open up, with Tahquitz Rock and the San Jacinto massif to the north, Suicide Rock and the San Gabriel Mountains to the northwest, Idyllwild and Santiago Peak to the west, and the Garner Valley, Desert Divide, and Toro Peak to the south. Just below the summit, reach a junction. Turn right and walk a short distance to the summit lookout, 3.6 miles from the start.

Tahquitz Peak Fire Lookout stands on the summit, taking advantage of the commanding views in all directions. The remote lookout is staffed during fire season by San Bernardino National Forest Association Fire Lookout Hosts who hike up to their airy post. The friendly and knowledgeable volunteers are happy to point out the sights and talk about the San Jacinto Mountains. Return the way you came.

ALTERNATIVE FINISH

For a terrific 11-mile loop, continue east to the PCT, follow it north to Saddle Junction, descend the Devils Slide Trail, and hike back along the Ernie Maxwell Trail and South Ridge Rd.

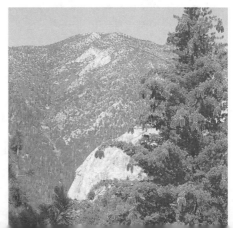

Sugar Pine, Tahquitz Rock, and Marion Mtn. from the South Ridge Trail

San Jacinto Mountains National Monument

trip 9.18 Desert View Loop

Distance	1.6 miles (loop)
Hiking Time	1 hour
Elevation Gain	350'
Difficulty	Easy
Trail Use	Good for children
Best Times	May–October
Agency	Mt. San Jacinto State Park
Optional Map	Tom Harrison *San Jacinto Wilderness, Santa Rosa and San Jacinto Mountains National Monument* or *San Jacinto Peak 7.5'*

see map on p. 172

DIRECTIONS From State Highway 111, 8.5 miles south of Interstate 10 at the northern edge of Palm Springs, turn west up Tramway Rd. and drive 4 miles to Valley Station, the lower terminus of the Palm Springs Aerial Tramway. The tram operates daily, starting at 10 A.M. Monday–Friday, 8 A.M. Saturday, Sunday, and holidays. The last tram return is 9:45 P.M. The tram closes for annual maintenance, typically in September. Round-trip tickets are $21.95. Check www.pstramway.com or call (888) 515-TRAM for the most current information.

This family-friendly hike is an easy introduction to the pleasures of Mt. San Jacinto State Park. It tours forest, meadow, and creek, as well as taking you to impressive vista points looking into the desert from the sheer east slopes of San Jacinto. There is a short Desert View Loop Trail and an even shorter Nature Loop Trail. Interpretive signs along the path explain some of the flora and fauna, while park volunteers periodically lead guided tours; ask at the Long Valley Ranger Station for more information. Kids may enjoy scrambling on the rocks and fallen logs; teach them not to trample the inviting but fragile meadow.

From Mountain Station, proceed 0.2 mile down the cement walkway to the Long Valley Picnic Area. Look for the sign marking the start of the Desert View Trail to the left (south). If you reach the ranger station, you have gone 0.1 mile too far.

You can take the loop in either direction, but this description follows a counterclockwise direction. At a fork beyond the sign, veer right and cross a small bridge at the end of a meadow. Long Valley Creek runs through this area until August during a normal year, though it may dry up by July in a drought year. Look and listen for the many species of birds that inhabit the meadow and the adjoining forest of Jeffrey pines and white firs.

In 0.25 mile, the Nature Trail veers left to loop back to the start, but the main Desert View Loop continues. In another 0.1 mile, come to a vista point above a granite dome. The loop curves around and climbs an open slope dotted with Jeffrey pines to a second vista point, where you can admire the Santa Rosa Mountains and Toro Peak on the skyline at the head of Palm Canyon. It then passes a third and fourth outlook with views into the desert. Occasionally the trail may become poorly defined, but choose the path that looks most heavily traveled. Pass a second junction with the Nature Trail loop, and soon return to the start near the bridge.

Desert View Nature Trail

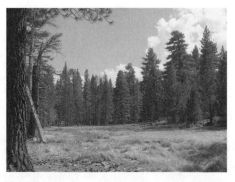

trip 9.19 Round Valley

Distance	4.5 miles (out-and-back)
Hiking Time	2.5 hours
Elevation Gain	700'
Difficulty	Easy
Trail Use	Good for children, suitable for backpacking
Best Times	May–October
Agency	Mt. San Jacinto State Park
Recommended Map	Tom Harrison *San Jacinto Wilderness, Santa Rosa and San Jacinto Mountains National Monument* or *San Jacinto Peak 7.5'*
Permit	Mt. San Jacinto State Wilderness Permit Required

see map on p. 172

DIRECTIONS From State Highway 111, 8.5 miles south of Interstate 10 at the northern edge of Palm Springs, turn west up Tramway Rd. and drive 4 miles to Valley Station, the lower terminus of the Palm Springs Aerial Tramway. The tram operates daily, starting at 10 A.M. Monday–Friday, 8 A.M. Saturday, Sunday, and holidays. The last tram return is 9:45 P.M. The tram closes for annual maintenance, typically in September. Round-trip tickets are $21.95. Check www.pstramway.com or call (888) 515-TRAM for the most current information.

The Palm Springs Aerial Tramway provides rapid access to the high country in the San Jacinto State Park Wilderness. From the tram station, it is an easy walk down to the Long Valley Ranger Station, then up along Long Valley Creek through the woods to the campground at Round Valley. This is a popular destination in the summer for picnics, family campouts, and Boy Scout hikes. In the winter there is easy access to snow, and it is a great place for cross-country skiers and snowshoers.

From the rear of the tram station, walk 0.3 mile west down to the Long Valley Ranger Station, passing the signed turnoff to the left for the Desert View Trail. Get a wilderness permit at the ranger station and continue west. In 0.1 mile, arrive at another signed junction. The left trail leads to the Hidden Divide, but your trail continues straight ahead through the forest of pines and firs dotted with granite boulders. The Long Valley Creek nearby usually runs until August, though in a dry year it may stop in July. Look for a meadow with corn lilies before reaching another trail junction in 1.4 miles. A lateral trail turns hard left back toward the Hidden Divide, but the main trail again continues straight. Pass another meadow on the north side of the trail with good views of the pointy Cornell Peak beyond. In 0.4 mile more, arrive at the Round Valley Campground.

This is a good place to explore and have lunch. An outhouse is nearby. A trail leads north for 0.5 mile to Tamarack Valley. Numerous fine campsites are scattered along side trails in Round and Tamarack Valleys. Return the way you came. Or, for a longer trip, continue up to San Jacinto Peak (see Trip 9.21) or Cornell Peak (Trip 9.20).

San Jacinto Mountains National Monument

trip 9.20 Cornell Peak

Distance	6.5 miles (out-and-back)
Hiking Time	4 hours
Elevation Gain	1400'
Difficulty	Moderate
Trail Use	Suitable for backpacking
Best Times	June–October
Agency	Mt. San Jacinto State Park
Required Map	Tom Harrison *San Jacinto Wilderness, Santa Rosa and San Jacinto Mountains National Monument* or *San Jacinto Peak* 7.5'
Permit	Mt. San Jacinto State Wilderness Permit Required

see map on p. 172

DIRECTIONS From State Highway 111, 8.5 miles south of Interstate 10 at the northern edge of Palm Springs, turn west up Tramway Rd. and drive 4 miles to Valley Station, the lower terminus of the Palm Springs Aerial Tramway. The tram operates daily, starting at 10 A.M. Monday–Friday, 8 A.M. Saturday, Sunday, and holidays. The last tram return is 9:45 P.M. The tram closes for annual maintenance, typically in September. Round-trip tickets are $21.95. Check www.pstramway.com or call (888) 515-TRAM for the most current information.

Cornell Peak is an impressive pyramid-shaped peak with a rocky summit block overlooking Round Valley. This hike is relatively short but requires some cross-country navigation and some airy rock climbing at the very top. It is, by far, the most enjoyable summit in the San Jacinto area.

From the tramway station, descend to the Long Valley Ranger Station to get a wilderness permit, then hike west 2.2 miles to Round Valley, and follow the side trail north 0.5 mile to the northernmost campsite in Tamarack Valley (see Trip 9.19). Along the way, keep an eye out for the distinctive peak and assess the best route to the top.

From Tamarack Valley, hike cross-country up steep slopes to the north, threading your way around bands of manzanita. You may find some use trails and animal paths, but it is hard to distinguish the best one from the others. Your goal is to reach the summit ridge between Cornell Peak and the rounded rock pile immediately to the east. Once on the ridge, turn west and follow it to the summit rocks.

The final 20 feet of climbing is tricky third class. Many hikers stop at the base rather than risk climbing the steep rock. The easiest ascent scales a wide crack with a chockstone, then shimmies along the summit block to the highest point. Getting down is harder than getting up.

VARIATIONS

If you wish to climb some more, there are two more small peaks nearby. The 9520+' rock pile on the ridge just east of Cornell is locally known as Harvard Peak. The more interesting 9360+' pinnacle southeast of Harvard Peak is called Yale Peak.

Cornell Peak's airy summit block

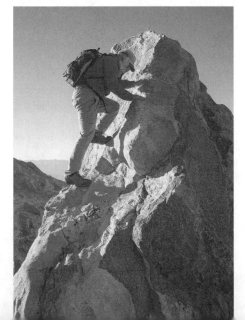

Descend the way you came, heading southeast until it is easy to walk down through the trees. Do not be tempted to head directly south or west from the summit; steep cliffs block all of these paths. Once off the summit, it is possible to take a shortcut cross-country to the southeast to rejoin the main trail halfway back to Long Valley. The route follows a good use trail along the north bank of the north fork of Long Valley Creek. You rejoin the main trail in 0.6 mile at a switchback where the trail crosses the creek. Then follow the main trail 0.5 mile back to the Long Valley Ranger Station.

trip 9.21 San Jacinto Peak from the Palm Springs Aerial Tramway

Distance	10 miles (out-and-back)
Hiking Time	6 hours
Elevation Gain	2600'
Difficulty	Strenuous
Trail Use	Suitable for backpacking
Best Times	June–October
Agency	Mt. San Jacinto State Park
Recommended Map	Tom Harrison *San Jacinto Wilderness*, *Santa Rosa and San Jacinto Mountains National Monument* or *San Jacinto Peak 7.5'*
Permit	Mt. San Jacinto State Wilderness Permit Required

see map on p. 172

DIRECTIONS From State Highway 111, 8.5 miles south of Interstate 10 at the northern edge of Palm Springs, turn west up Tramway Rd. and drive 4 miles to Valley Station, the lower terminus of the Palm Springs Aerial Tramway. The tram operates daily, starting at 10 A.M. Monday–Friday, 8 A.M. Saturday, Sunday, and holidays. The last tram return is 9:45 P.M. The tram closes for annual maintenance, typically in September. Round-trip tickets are $21.95. Check www.pstramway.com or call (888) 515-TRAM for the most current information.

This is the easiest route to the summit of San Jacinto, but it is still a strenuous and rewarding hike.

From the tramway station, descend to the Long Valley Ranger Station to obtain a wilderness permit, then hike west 2.2 miles to Round Valley (see Trip 9.19). Continue 1 mile west to meet a trail junction on the Wellman Divide. Turn right (north) and gradually climb across the east face of Jean Peak through interminable fields of chinquapin, then switchback up to a saddle south of San Jacinto Peak in 1.7 miles. Turn right (north) and follow a trail 0.3 mile to the summit, passing an emergency shelter along the way. The cabin was constructed by the California Conservation Corps around 1933 and is cared for by volunteers; if you visit or must use it in a storm, leave it better than you found it. The final stretch involves scrambling up boulders to the summit rocks. For those who have hiked Half Dome in Yosemite this final stretch is reminiscent of the last part of the Half Dome Trail immediately below the cables.

Emergency shelter near San Jacinto Peak

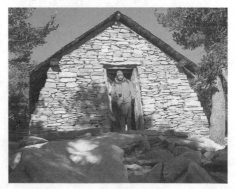

Peer over the north edge of the summit to admire Snow Creek, which drops more than 8000 feet to the desert below in scarcely 3 miles. The precipice is especially impressive when covered with snow in the spring and early summer. Venturing along Snow Creek is only suitable for an advanced mountaineer with ice and rock gear; more than one casual hiker has perished here. The Desert Water Agency owns a critical section of land at the base of Snow Creek and unfortunately does not grant permits to hikers, making access to the route difficult. Return the way you came.

trip 9.22 Seven Peaks of the San Jacinto Wilderness

Distance	15 miles (loop)
Hiking Time	11 hours
Elevation Gain	5400'
Difficulty	Very strenuous
Trail Use	Suitable for backpacking
Best Times	June–October
Agency	Mt. San Jacinto State Park
Required Map	Tom Harrison *San Jacinto Wilderness, Santa Rosa and San Jacinto Mountains National Monument* or *San Jacinto Peak 7.5'*
Permit	Mt. San Jacinto State Wilderness Permit Required

see map on p. 172

DIRECTIONS From State Highway 111, 8.5 miles south of Interstate 10 at the northern edge of Palm Springs, turn west up Tramway Rd. and drive 4 miles to Valley Station, the lower terminus of the Palm Springs Aerial Tramway. The tram operates daily, starting at 10 A.M. Monday-Friday, 8 A.M. Saturday, Sunday, and holidays. The last tram return is 9:45 P.M. The tram closes for annual maintenance, typically in September. Round-trip tickets are $21.95. Check www.pstramway.com or call (888) 515-TRAM for the most current information.

This challenging trip explores all of the officially named summits of the San Jacinto high country; visiting the summits of Marion Mtn., Jean Peak, Newton Drury Peak, Folly Peak, San Jacinto, Miller Peak, and Cornell Peak. This excursion is primarily composed of cross-country hiking as opposed to traveling a well-used trail. The high country here is as reminiscent of the Sierra Nevada as any location in Southern

San Jacinto high country from Luella Todd Peak

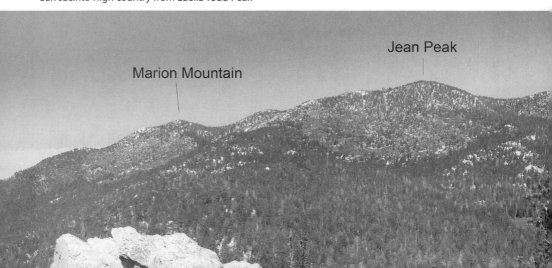

Marion Mountain

Jean Peak

California. The Jeffrey pine and white fir forests give way to lodgepole and limber pines as you climb. San Jacinto's south-facing slopes are heavily overgrown with chinquapins, manzanitas, and buckthorns. The central objective in this trip is to pick a path that minimizes the bushwhacking. Some of the summits involve stimulating third-class climbing on excellent granite. You should be intimately familiar with the area before attempting this adventure. If you are doing it as a dayhike, plan to take the 8 A.M. tram up. Bring a headlamp and be sure to return before the tram closes at 9:45 P.M. Water sources along the route are unreliable, so it is best to carry at least 4 quarts.

From the tram station, hike down to the Long Valley Ranger Station and obtain a wilderness permit. Follow the trail to Round Valley, then up to Wellman Divide. The direct route from the Divide to Marion Mtn. is unbearably brushy. Instead, turn south and follow the trail 0.5 mile, descending several switchbacks to reach Wellman Cienega, in a huge field of ferns and corn lilies. Turn right (northwest) and pick a path up the unlikely-looking slope toward the saddle. This unfortunately involves tramping through the tall plants for a short distance; beware of rattlesnakes. Stay toward the right side of the corn lilies and you will soon find a ducked climber's path where

the chinquapin has been beaten down. This is crucial to the route; the alternatives are quite unpleasant. The route eventually shifts right onto a shallow ridge with Jeffrey and lodgepole pines mixed with chaparral, then bears left into a better-defined gully, and left again onto an open-forested slope that leads up to the saddle.

Marion Mtn. is the westernmost high point along the ridge to your southwest. The top of the ridge is dotted with large boulders, so the best route is to contour west before climbing south. Again, you may find a ducked climber's trail. The summit boulders are immense; they can be climbed from the northeast by starting at a dead tree, scaling a short crack, jogging right, and then turning left again and ascending a third-class chimney. Marion has arguably the best view of any peak in the San Jacinto Mountains. The summit towers above the trees, offering a 360-degree panorama and a particularly good view of the next four peaks that you are about to climb. It is worth studying the map and planning your routes to Jean, Newton Drury, Folly, and San Jacinto.

The easiest path to Jean Peak is nearly a straight line, staying just west of Peak 10388′. Navigation is tricky in the forest, but simply head for the high point after passing Peak 10388′; there are no false sum-

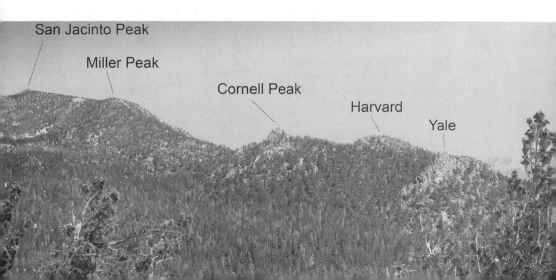

San Jacinto Peak

Miller Peak

Cornell Peak

Harvard

Yale

mits near Jean. Although Jean is the second highest peak in the area, views from it are obstructed by the forest.

Newton Drury Peak is the next destination. The peak was named for one of the most successful 20th Century American conservationists. He led the Save the Redwoods League of California, served for more than a decade as director of the National Park Service, and arranged the 1930 land swap with the Southern Pacific Railroad that created San Jacinto State Park. The bump is puny for a man of such great stature, but it is covered in a beautiful limber pine forest and great granite slabs. There is a shallow ridge connecting Drury to Jean. The south side of the ridge is brushy. The best route from Jean is to hike north toward a saddle before turning west toward Drury. Descend to another saddle immediately east of Drury, then scamper the short way up to the summit.

Folly Peak is another insignificant bump on the scenic and rocky Fuller Ridge, which drops northwest from San Jacinto. To reach Folly, return to the saddle east of Drury, then follow easy slopes northwest down to Little Round Valley Campground. You may find water here, though the source dries up early in the season in some years. Follow the San Jacinto Trail up seven switchbacks to the 10,000-foot contour, where you leave the trail and trudge north toward the ridge, weaving back and forth to avoid the worst of the chinquapin and boulders. Some bushwhacking is inevitable. There are several bumps on the ridge of nearly equal height to Folly Peak. Folly is the westernmost bump; below it is a boulder field dropping down into the upper reaches of Snow Creek.

Follow the ridge from Folly up to San Jacinto. You may find a climber's trail in places just south of the ridgeline. The tectonic forces that thrust upward and shattered these massive granite blocks to build San Jacinto are nearly inconceivable. On a pleasant summer afternoon, you are very likely to surprise dayhikers relaxing on the summit.

Follow the trail down from San Jacinto, past the emergency shelter, heading south to the saddle, then northeast to a major switchback. Miller Peak is scarcely a stone's throw away. Take an easy walk up and across a sandy clearing before scrambling up the dark summit boulders. The bump on the ridge is named for Frank A. Miller, the founder of Riverside's famous Mission Inn. He was a prominent advocate of Boy Scouting and world peace. The peak was dedicated in 1936 by 22 scout troops who simultaneously ignited bonfires atop summits all over Southern California. A plaque on the summit commemorates Miller and the Scout Oath.

Follow the San Jacinto Trail south to Wellman Divide and back down to Round Valley. A historic trail once shortcut directly down to Tamarack Valley, but it was closed to protect a sensitive deer fawning area. If daylight permits, continue on to Cornell Peak. This dramatic granite pyramid is the lowest but most exhilarating of the seven summits. From Round Valley follow the trail north to Tamarack Valley, then pick a path among the numerous use trails up to the top (see Trip 9.20). The summit register is located immediately below the summit rocks. Climbers will enjoy the third-class scramble up a crack and an airy shimmy to the highest block. Descend the way you came; staying too far east leads to some tricky climbing.

For your return it is possible to hike east cross-country from Tamarack Valley to shortcut back to the main trail. The route follows a good use trail along the north bank of the north fork of Long Valley Creek. It rejoins the main trail in 0.6 mile at a switchback where the trail crosses the creek. Then you follow the main trail 0.5 mile back to the Long Valley Ranger Station, and finally stumble up the paved walkway to the tram.

VARIATIONS

There are obviously many possible variations for this loop, and you may add or subtract peaks according to your tastes. Jean Peak can also be reached without too much bushwhacking by climbing its northeast slope from the San Jacinto Trail or by running the ridge from San Jacinto. The west ridge of Folly Peak looks like a convenient shortcut down to the PCT on Fuller Ridge, but it is not recommended because of heavy brush. The 9520+′ rockpile immediately east of Cornell is locally known as Harvard, and the more attractive 9360+′ summit southeast of that is called Yale. Peak 9356′ on the Hidden Divide is sometimes called Luella Todd or Landells Peak, and features a grand view of San Jacinto's east side.

Desert Divide

The Desert Divide is a remote and lonely mountainous backbone running south from San Jacinto and Tahquitz Peak to Highway 74. It overlooks the tranquil Garner Valley to the west and the deep Palm Canyon to the east. The northern section is rugged, studded with massive granite outcrops, while the southern section is rounded and gentler.

Much of the Divide is covered in dense chaparral. The legendary Sam Fink, a Santa Ana fire captain and Sierra Club leader, spent nearly a decade in the 1960s and 1970s chopping a route along the crest of the Divide. The Pacific Crest Trail (PCT) now follows much of the Sam Fink Trail's original route. Constructing the PCT along the Divide required three years of drilling, blasting, and cutting, making it the most difficult stretch to build in Southern California. The well-engineered trail now offers hospitable access to this formerly inaccessible country.

The Desert Divide is a great place to visit if you are seeking solitude. It can be suitable for hiking year round, but tends to be hot in the summer, and sometimes the northern exposures are icy well into the spring. If you plan to visit the higher elevations before the middle of April, an ice axe and crampons may be necessary.

The entire Desert Divide is within the Santa Rosa and San Jacinto Mountains National Monument, which was established by Congress in 2000. The portions of the Desert Divide north of Fobes Saddle are in San Jacinto Wilderness. A wilderness permit is required to enter wilderness areas. The permits can be obtained in person or by mail, at no charge, from the Idyllwild Ranger Station. At the time of this writing, the Devils Slide Trail is the only trailhead with a quota.

On April 29, 2008, a thoughtless hiker discarded a lit cigarette on the trail. The resulting Apache fire burned 784 acres on Apache Peak and the upper reaches of Murray and West Palm canyons. Over 700 firefighters hiked in and chopped their way through dense chaparral to contain the blaze.

Desert Divide from the east

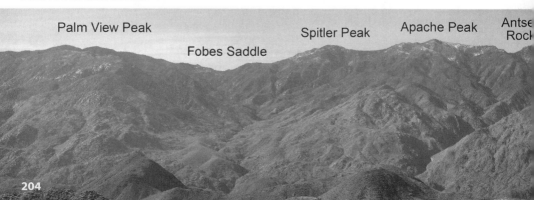

Palm View Peak Fobes Saddle Spitler Peak Apache Peak Antse Rock

trip 10.1 Antsell Rock

Distance	4 miles (out-and-back)
Hiking Time	4 hours
Elevation Gain	2300'
Difficulty	Strenuous
Best Times	April–June, October–November
Agency	San Bernardino National Forest (Idyllwild Ranger Station)
Recommended Map	Tom Harrison *San Jacinto Wilderness, Santa Rosa and San Jacinto Mountains National Monument* or *Idyllwild, Palm View Peak* 7.5'
Permit	San Jacinto Wilderness Permit Required

see map on p. 206

DIRECTIONS From State Highway 74, 3.4 miles southeast of Mountain Center and just before mile marker 074 RIV 62.75, turn left (east) onto Apple Canyon Rd. Proceed 3.3 miles to its end at Pine Springs Ranch. Immediately before entering the ranch, veer right onto a good private dirt road leading to the Zen Mountain Center. In 1.1 miles, park in a small dirt lot on the left just before entering the Zen Center.

Antsell Rock is the jewel of the Desert Divide. Edmund Perkins, of the USGS, named it for an artist at the Keen Camp Resort who was painting the peak. Antsell Rock stands high above the Divide and its stony buttresses make an impressive sight from most directions. It is also one of the few mountaineers' peaks in Southern California requiring more than the usual plodding to reach the third-class summit. While this trip is short, it is certainly not easy.

Access to the Desert Divide is plagued by private property inholdings within the San Bernardino National Forest. However, the Zen Mountain Center graciously allows hikers to cross their property and follow a spectacular trail that leads directly to the Divide. Please help retain this privilege by being a courteous trail user. Avoid bringing large groups or large numbers of vehicles. Keep your voice down while crossing the center so as not to disturb meditation. Dogs are not permitted. This trail is not shown on topographic maps and is not regularly maintained.

Antsell Rock from the north

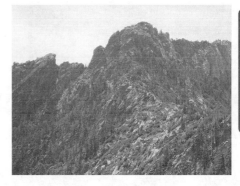

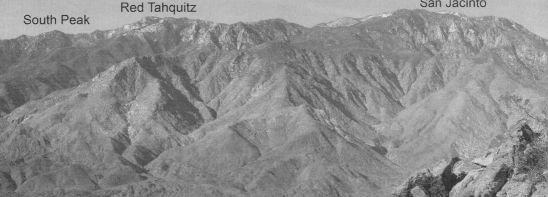

South Peak   Red Tahquitz   San Jacinto

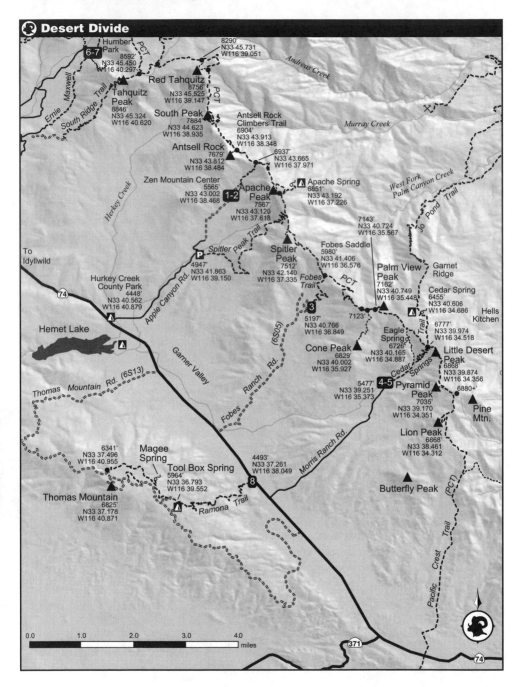

Desert Divide

Humber Park
6-7
8592'
N33 45.450
W116 40.297

8290'
N33 45.731
W116 39.051

Andreas Creek

Red Tahquitz
8756'
N33 45.525
W116 39.147

Tahquitz
Peak
8846'
N33 45.324
W116 40.620

South Peak
7884'
N33 44.623
W116 38.935

Antsell Rock
Climbers Trail
6904'
N33 43.913
W116 38.348

Murray Creek

Antsell Rock
7679'
N33 43.812
W116 38.484

6937'
N33 43.665
W116 37.971

Zen Mountain Center
5565'
N33 43.002
W116 38.468

Apache Spring
6851'
N33 43.192
W116 37.226

West Fork
Palm Canyon Creek

Apache
Peak
1-2
7567'
N33 43.120
W116 37.618

Jo Pond Trail

7143'
N33 40.724
W116 35.567

Spitler Peak Trail

Spitler
Peak
7512'
N33 42.140
W116 37.335

Fobes Saddle
5980'
N33 41.406
W116 36.576

Palm View
Peak
7162'
N33 40.749
W116 35.448

Garnet
Ridge

To
Idyllwild

4947'
N33 41.863
W116 39.150

Fobes
Trail

PCT

Cedar Spring
6455'
N33 40.606
W116 34.686

Hells
Kitchen

Hurkey Creek
County Park
4448'
N33 40.562
W116 40.879

74

Apple Canyon Rd.

5197'
N33 40.766
W116 36.849

7123'

3

6777'
N33 39.974
W116 34.518

Cedar Springs Trail

Hemet Lake

Garner Valley

(6S05)

Ranch

Rd.

Cone Peak
6829'
N33 40.002
W116 35.927

Eagle
Spring
6726'
N33 40.165
W116 34.887

Little Desert
Peak
6868'
N33 39.874
W116 34.356

6880'+

Thomas Mountain Rd. (6S13)

Fobes

5477'
N33 39.251
W116 35.373

4-5
Pyramid
Peak
7035'
N33 39.170
W116 34.351

Pine
Mtn.

6341'
N33 37.496
W116 40.955

Magee
Spring

Morris Ranch Rd.

Lion Peak
6868'
N33 38.461
W116 34.312

Tool Box Spring
5964'
N33 36.793
W116 39.552

4493'
N33 37.261
W116 38.049

8

Ramona Trail

Butterfly Peak

Thomas Mountain
6825'
N33 37.178
W116 40.871

Pacific   Crest   Trail

(PCT)

0.0   1.0   2.0   3.0   4.0
miles

371

74

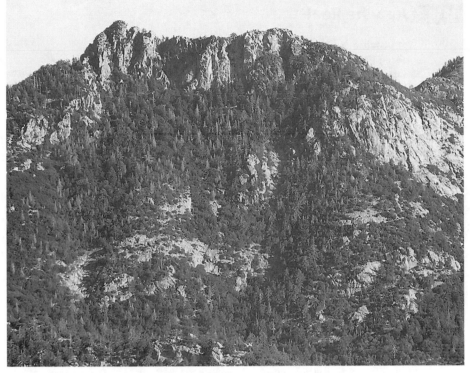

Antsell Rock from the south ridge of Tahquitz Peak

From the parking area, continue up the dirt road through the gate. Stay left at a fork by the office, then left again at a fork near the cabins. Continue up the dirt road toward the low point on the Desert Divide. In 0.3 mile, pass two water tanks. The unsigned trail begins here where the road switchbacks. It follows the spectacular canyon along a seasonal creek beneath enchanting incense cedars and black oaks. In 0.1 mile, a spur on the right leads to the creek while the main trail begins climbing steeply to the left. Watch for Coulter pines with their enormous cones. The trail ascends the chaparral-clad slopes and reaches the crest in another 0.8 mile.

Turn left (west) and follow the PCT along the northeast side of Antsell Rock. In 0.5 mile, look for a gully marked with cairns in a grove of black oaks. A use trail up this gully leads to the summit of Antsell Rock. The jaunt is only 0.3 mile as the crow flies, but involves 800 feet of strenuous climbing. The steep and loose gully leads up to a prominent notch to the right of the rocky peak. The summit register can be found in this notch, so those uncomfortable with rock scrambling may stop here. For one of the more delightful mountaineering experiences in Southern California, continue up to the true summit. Scramble up a weakness in the rock above the notch, and then go left around the corner to another tree-filled gully leading to the rocky summit ridge. Some third-class climbing is required.

Return the way you came. Or, for a longer trip, continue southeast on the PCT to Apache Peak (see Trip 10.2).

trip 10.2 Apache Peak

Distance	6 miles (out-and-back), or 8.5 miles (loop)
Hiking Time	5 hours
Elevation Gain	2100'
Difficulty	Strenuous
Trail Use	Suitable for backpacking
Best Times	April–June, October–November
Agency	San Bernardino National Forest (Idyllwild Ranger Station)
Recommended Map	Tom Harrison *San Jacinto Wilderness, Santa Rosa and San Jacinto Mountains National Monument* or *Idyllwild, Palm View Peak* 7.5'
Permit	San Jacinto Wilderness Permit Required

see map on p. 206

DIRECTIONS From State Highway 74, 3.4 miles southeast of Mountain Center and just before mile marker 074 RIV 62.75, turn left (east) onto the Apple Canyon Rd. In 2.6 miles, pass a turnout at the signed Spitler Peak Trailhead on the right. If you plan to make a loop trip, you may wish to leave a shuttle vehicle here. Continue 0.7 mile to the end of Apple Canyon Rd. at Pine Springs Ranch. Immediately before entering the ranch, veer right onto a good private dirt road leading to the Zen Mountain Center. In 1.1 miles, park in a small dirt lot on the left just before entering the Zen Center.

Apache Peak stands high on the Desert Divide, guarded on the north and west by sheer rock walls. Surprisingly, the summit itself is merely a rounded bump covered in chaparral. Whatever the peak may lack in rugged beauty, however, is compensated for by its 360-degree views of the entire Desert Divide, Santa Rosa Mountains, and Coachella and Garner Valleys. Backpackers will enjoy the nearby Apache Spring, with a reliable water source and good camping. The trip can be done as an out-and-back hike from the Zen Center, or with a short shuttle, as a loop down the scenic Spitler Peak Trail. Apache Peak is a seemingly strange name for the peak, which is located in the middle of Cahuilla Indian territory.

Access to the Desert Divide is plagued by private property inholdings within the San Bernardino National Forest. However, the Zen Mountain Center graciously allows hikers to cross their property and follow a spectacular trail that leads directly to the Divide. Please help retain this privilege by being a courteous trail user. Avoid bringing large groups or large numbers of vehicles. Keep your voice down while crossing the center so as not to disturb meditation. Dogs are not permitted. This trail is not shown on topographic maps.

The 2008 Apache Fire scorched the east side of the Desert Divide between Apache Peak and Antsell Rock and closed the PCT for more than a month. Fortunately, Apache Spring is still running well. The Forest Service recommends treating the water before drinking.

From the parking area, continue up the dirt road through the gate. Stay left at a fork by the office, then left again at a fork near the cabins. Continue up the dirt road toward the low point on the Desert Divide. In 0.3 mile, pass two water tanks. The unsigned trail begins here where the road switchbacks. It follows the spectacular canyon along a seasonal creek beneath incense cedars and black oaks. In 0.1 mile, a spur on the right leads to the creek while the main trail begins climbing steeply to the left. Watch for Coulter pines with their enormous cones. The trail ascends the chaparral-clad slopes and joins the PCT at the crest in another 0.8 mile.

Turn right (east) on the PCT and follow the trail as it climbs through the red cliffs. In 0.4 mile, round a corner at a rocky promontory to get your first views of Apache Peak. It is worth following a faint use trail onto the promontory for terrific views of the northern Desert Divide, San Jacinto massif, and the mountains and desert to the east.

Continue south for 0.8 mile to reach the north slope of Apache Peak. The stately fir forest on this slope burned and now has been replaced by a buckthorn thicket. The trail loops around the east side of the peak. In 0.4 mile, where the trail reaches the summit plateau and abruptly turns left, look for a faint use trail leading through the chaparral toward the peak. Two hills are visible to the northwest; Apache Peak's highest point is the one on the left, 0.2 mile from the PCT. Enjoy the wide-ranging views from the top.

On the PCT 100 yards south of the turn-off for the summit trail is a sign marking a turnoff for Apache Spring. The year-round spring is located 0.5 mile northeast of the main trail and 500 feet down the slope. The Forest Service recommends boiling the water before drinking it. There are several good camping sites on a knob just east of the spring, so this is a popular stop for PCT hikers. Return the way you came.

ALTERNATIVE FINISH

If you would like to make a worthwhile loop, continue 0.6 mile south from Apache Peak along the PCT to the saddle between Apache and Spitler Peaks. There are fine views to the east from the saddle into West Fork Canyon, over the Palisades on Garnet Ridge, and into the Santa Rosa Mountains. Follow the Spitler Peak Trail down as it makes gratuitously long and flat switchbacks through the oak and chaparral between the cliffs of the adjacent peaks. In 1 mile, reach a seasonal creek shaded by a diverse and gorgeous forest of incense cedars, Coulter pines, sugar pines, firs, and oaks. The trail then makes a long and gradual descent into the chaparral and crosses a splendid field of ribbonwood trees before reaching the paved road in another 3.7 miles. If you have left a car or bicycle here, your trip is complete. Alternatively, you can walk 1.8 miles up the road to the Zen Center trailhead.

Hikers on the PCT nearing Apache Peak

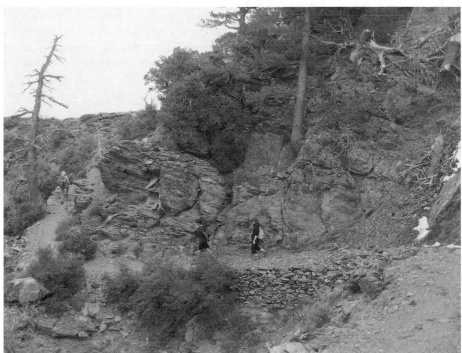

trip 10.3 Palm View Peak

Distance	8 miles (out-and-back)
Hiking Time	5 hours
Elevation Gain	2100'
Difficulty	Strenuous
Trail Use	Dogs
Best Times	October–June
Agency	San Bernardino National Forest (Idyllwild Ranger Station)
Recommended Map	*Santa Rosa and San Jacinto Mountains National Monument* or *Palm View Peak* 7.5'

see map on p. 206

DIRECTIONS From State Highway 74, 6.8 miles southeast of Mountain Center and just past mile marker 074 RIV 66.00, turn left (northeast) onto the fair dirt Fobes Ranch Rd. (6S05). Stay left at a fork in 0.4 mile, then follow it across the Garner Valley for 3.2 miles to another junction. The main road goes north to Fobes Ranch (private); you turn right and proceed 0.4 mile to the signed Fobes Trailhead. Parking is limited to three or four vehicles; you may have to park a short distance below the trailhead.

The Fobes Saddle and Palm View Peak offer a gentler hike to sample the pleasures of the Desert Divide. This southern region is lower in elevation, and is a good place to visit in the winter when the high country is buried under snow. Enjoy this hike for the journey more than for the destination. Palm View Peak itself is the least attractive part of the entire hike; the summit is lost in dense woods and offers neither palms nor views.

From the trailhead, follow the seemingly never-ending switchbacks through the chaparral toward Fobes Saddle. This section of the trail passes through large stands of aptly named ribbonwoods (the bark hangs in shreds), also called red shanks (*Adenostama sparsifolium*). In 0.5 mile, the trail forks; take the right fork. In another mile, reach the PCT junction at the Fobes saddle on the crest of the Divide.

Turn right and follow the PCT southeast, first on the east side of the ridge, then on the west, and finally switchbacking up the crest. The trail levels out and passes a small outcrop, then enters a clearing 2.4 miles from the saddle. Turn left and leave the trail, making a short cross-country excursion through white firs and black oaks to the summit of Palm View Peak. The proper departure point from the PCT can be difficult to identify because the summit is heavily wooded. If the trail starts to go downhill, you have gone too far. A small pile of rocks and a summit register marks the high point. Unfortunately, the peak is hemmed in by trees, so there are no views. Return to the clearing because the other sides of the summit are blocked by dense brush.

After enjoying the summit, retrace your steps to the car. There are many other peaks and trailheads along the Desert Divide, so numerous variations can be considered if a car shuttle is available.

Happy hikers on Fobes Saddle Trail

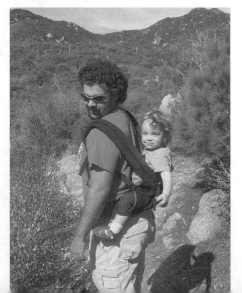

trip 10.4 Cone Peak

Distance	11 miles (out-and-back)
Hiking Time	7 hours
Elevation Gain	3600'
Difficulty	Strenuous
Best Times	April–June, October–November
Agency	San Bernardino National Forest (Idyllwild Ranger Station)
Required Map	*Santa Rosa and San Jacinto Mountains National Monument,* or *Palm View Peak* 7.5'

see map on p. 206

DIRECTIONS From State Highway 74, 8.6 miles south of Mountain Center in the Garner Valley and just beyond mile marker 074 RIV 67.75, turn left (northeast) onto the paved Morris Ranch Rd. (6S53). Follow it up 3.7 miles, passing the Joe Sherman Girl Scout Camp, to the signed Cedar Spring Trailhead (4E17) on the right. There is a large parking area on the side of the road 0.1 mile south of the trailhead.

Cone Peak is one of the more dramatic and challenging summits of the southern Desert Divide. Its rocky turrets look foreboding from the Cedar Spring Trailhead, but the dense chaparral proves to be tougher than the clean granite. Although the peak is quite close to the trailhead, a ranch lies in between the two, so the direct route is closed to hikers even if they wished to brave the nearly impenetrable brush. Instead, this hike takes a circuitous approach east up the Cedar Spring Trail to the saddle, then northwest along the PCT, then southwest cross-country along a ridge to Cone Peak. The summit rocks involve some third-class scrambling. Those who are uncomfortable rock climbing may choose to sign the register at the base. Be particularly aware of rattlesnakes when hiking cross-country.

Follow the Cedar Spring Trail for 2.3 miles to a four-way junction on a saddle (see Trip 10.5). Turn left (northwest) and follow the PCT for 1.7 miles, passing several humps along the way. There are some good views of Cone Peak along the way. The trail levels out near its high point beside the densely forested Palm View Peak. Just beyond, it reaches a saddle next to Point 7123'; to the left, you will see a grassy slope and ridge leading south-southwest.

Cone Peak from the South

Desert Divide

The following GPS waypoints may be helpful in the cross-country navigation. Depart the PCT here (N33 40.712 W116 35.722). Your goal is to follow the ridge to Cone Peak; this is easier said than done. The crest of the ridge is covered in brush and rock, so stay left (southeast) of the crest at first. Look for faint traces of an old trail (N33 40.657 W116 35.705); the walking should be easy and you are off-route if it is not. Soon the trail becomes somewhat better defined and gains the crest just above a large rock formation. (N33 40.521 W116 35.677) It weaves along the crest, then drops down the left side again (at N33 40.408 W116 35.744). When in doubt, look for cairns or saw marks to pick the proper path. The trail vanishes as it reaches a gully below a saddle on the crest (N33 40.247 W116 35.764). Turn right and ascend the gully, then veer left as you reach brush near the top. Emerge near some rocks marked with cairns at the south side of the saddle (N33 40.274 W116 35.826). Follow cairns south along the ridge around rocks and through some dense buckthorns, manzanitas, and scrub oaks; this may be easy if somebody has recently pruned the chaparral, or quite a bushwhack if not. The summit has several granite teeth. The southernmost is the highest, so stay below the summit boulders until you reach it. Return the way you came.

ALTERNATIVE FINISHES

Devoted peak baggers may take an excursion to the underwhelming Palm View Peak on the return (see Trip 10.3). The turnoff to Palm View from the PCT is located 0.2 mile east of the Cone Peak turnoff. Another alternative involves taking a shortcut back to the Cedar Spring Trailhead by way of an unmaintained trail to Eagle Spring. This unmarked trail, cut through the manzanitas, departs from the PCT near the saddle that is found 0.7 mile northwest of the main saddle at the top of the Cedar Spring Trail. Yet another possibility, with a car shuttle, is to follow the PCT 2.7 miles north to Fobes Saddle, then another 1.5 miles down to the Fobes trailhead.

trip 10.5 Cedar Spring

Distance	6.5 miles (out-and-back)
Hiking Time	3.5 hours
Elevation Gain	1700'
Difficulty	Moderate
Trail Use	Dogs, suitable for backpacking
Best Times	March–June, September–November
Agency	San Bernardino National Forest (Idyllwild Ranger Station)
Recommended Map	*Santa Rosa and San Jacinto Mountains National Monument,* or *Palm View Peak 7.5'*

see map on p. 206

DIRECTIONS From State Highway 74, 8.6 miles south of Mountain Center in the Garner Valley and just beyond mile marker 074 RIV 67.75, turn left (northeast) onto the paved Morris Ranch Rd. (6S53). Follow it up 3.7 miles, passing the Joe Sherman Girl Scout Camp, to the signed Cedar Spring Trailhead (4E17) on the right. There is a large parking area on the side of the road 0.1 mile south of the trailhead.

PCT hikers on the lengthy Desert Divide depend on small springs as their only source of water. One of the most attractive of these is Cedar Spring, situated on the desert slopes east of the Divide beneath a fine grove of incense cedars and black oaks. The best time to visit is in the spring, when the water is reliable, the temperatures

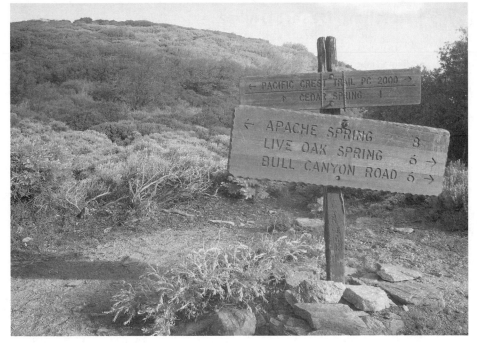

Saddle atop Cedar Spring Trail

are moderate, and the wildflowers are in bloom. This is a popular destination for Boy Scout troops.

Hike up the road from the parking area 0.1 mile to the signed Cedar Spring Trail (4E17) on your right. The first part of this trail follows a narrow fenced corridor through private property; please respect the property owners by staying on the trail so that the path will remain open to hikers in the future. Pass through a gate at the start and close it behind you. The valley is filled with a diverse ribbonwood, manzanita, scrub oak, and yucca chaparral. Hike past a water tank, and through a second gate in 0.4 mile, and a third gate in another 0.4 mile. Just beyond, the trail turns left to join an old dirt road. In 0.2 mile, pass some picnic tables near the head of the valley as the road narrows back to a trail again. Here, the relentless switchbacks begin, climbing 1.3 miles to a saddle and four-way junction with the PCT.

The PCT crosses this saddle en route from Mexico to Canada, but our trail con-

tinues straight down the other side of the saddle through more chaparral. Parts of this area burned some time back, but the scrub oak is vigorously regenerating. There are breathtaking views down into Palm Canyon and out over the Santa Rosa Mountains. In 0.9 mile, the trail abruptly rounds a bend and enters a shady grove where you can find Cedar Spring and plenty of fine campsites.

Return the way you came. There is 400 feet of climbing on the way back to the saddle.

VARIATION

Cedar Spring can also be reached from Palm Canyon by way of the arduous Jo Pond Trail (see Trip 11.12). The two trips can be combined into a lengthy one-way hike from the Garner Valley to Palm Canyon. Remember that the gate to Palm Canyon closes at 5 P.M.; plan to meet your get-away vehicle outside the gate unless you arrive before the gate closes.

trip 10.6 **Northern Desert Divide**

Distance	11 miles (one-way)
Hiking Time	6 hours
Elevation Gain	2000' (without peaks)
Difficulty	Strenuous
Trail Use	Suitable for backpacking
Best Times	April–June, October–November
Agency	San Bernardino National Forest (Idyllwild Ranger Station)
Recommended Map	Tom Harrison *San Jacinto Wilderness, Santa Rosa and San Jacinto Mountains National Monument* or *San Jacinto Peak, Idyllwild,* and *Palm View Peak* 7.5'
Permit	San Jacinto Wilderness Permit Required

see map on p. 206

DIRECTIONS Park a getaway vehicle at the Zen Center trailhead, then drive back to the Devils Slide Trailhead at Humber Park Trailhead. To reach the Zen Center trailhead, take State Highway 74. 3.4 miles southeast of Mountain Center, and just before mile marker 074 RIV 62.75, turn left (east) onto the Apple Canyon Rd. In 3.3 miles, reach the end of the paved road at Pine Springs Ranch. Immediately before entering the ranch, veer right onto a good private dirt road leading to the Zen Mountain Center. In 1.1 miles, park in a small dirt lot on the left just before entering the Zen Center. To reach Humber Park drive back to Mountain Center, then north on Highway 243 to Idyllwild (see the map on p. 172). Just south of the ranger station, turn right (northeast) on North Circle Dr. Drive 0.7 mile, to a four-way intersection, where you turn right on South Circle Dr. Proceed 0.1 mile, then turn left on Fern Valley Rd. Proceed 1.8 miles to the large Humber Park Trailhead parking at the end of the road.

The northern stretch of the Desert Divide is one of the most rugged and spectacular ridges in Southern California. The well-built PCT runs along the Divide, and offers fine hiking along this otherwise inaccessible terrain. This one-way trip starts in Idyllwild and ends in the scenic Garner Valley. Many variations are possible, including climbing some of the peaks along the way and extending the hike in either direction (see Trip 10.7).

Access to the Desert Divide is plagued by private property inholdings within the San Bernardino National Forest. However, the Zen Mountain Center graciously allows hikers to cross their property and follow a spectacular trail that leads directly to the Divide. Please help retain this privilege by being a courteous trail user. Avoid bringing large groups or large numbers of vehicles. Keep your voice down while crossing the center so as not to disturb meditation. Dogs are not permitted. This trail is not shown on topographic maps.

From Humber Park, hike 2.5 miles up the Devils Slide Trail to the five-way Saddle

Junction, where you meet the PCT. Take the southeast fork 0.6 mile to Tahquitz Valley, where you can find the best camping available along this route. Turn south and hike 0.8 mile to meet the PCT in Little Tahquitz Valley.

Follow the PCT east along the forested north slope of Red Tahquitz Peak. In 1.4 miles, the trail rounds the east end of the mountain overlooking Andreas Canyon and turns south, marking the beginning of your adventures along the Desert Divide. Stands of Jeffrey pines, white firs, and incense cedars cling to the steep ridge. Hike south for 1.8 miles across the head of Murray Canyon to South Peak. The trail skirts the peak on the east side, then switchbacks down the rocky slope and continues south toward the formidable obstacle of Antsell Rock. The PCT bypasses this difficult stretch on the northeast side by switchbacking down below the cliffs. In 2.1 miles, the trail enters a grove of black oaks at the base of a gully. Cairns mark a steep climber's trail up the gully to the summit (see Trip 10.1). But the PCT continues southeast for another

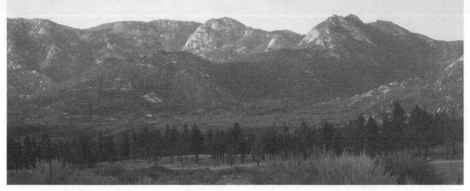
Northern Desert Divide overlooking Garner Valley. Antsell Rock on the right.

0.5 mile to a saddle. The 2008 Apache Fire burned through the steep chaparral on the east side of the Divide here.

From here, the easiest way off the Divide is to descend the steep trail to the southwest, reaching the Zen Center in 1.2 miles.

ALTERNATIVE FINISH

Alternatively, continue along the PCT past Apache Peak, then follow the long but scenic Spitler Peak Trail down to Apple Canyon Rd. See Trip 10.2 for direction to parking at Spitler Peak Trailhead. This adds 5.7 miles to the trip.

trip 10.7 Nine Peaks of the Desert Divide

Distance	21 miles (without peaks), or 26.5 miles (with nine peaks, one-way)
Hiking Time	11–15 hours
Elevation Gain	5700′ (without peaks), or 9000′ (with nine peaks)
Difficulty	Very strenuous
Trail Use	Suitable for backpacking
Best Times	April–June, October–November
Agency	San Bernardino National Forest (Idyllwild Ranger Station)
Required Map	*Santa Rosa and San Jacinto Mountains National Monument*, Tom Harrison *San Jacinto Wilderness* (only covers northern part of route) or *San Jacinto Peak, Idyllwild,* and *Palm View Peak* 7.5′
Permit	San Jacinto Wilderness Permit Required

see map on p. 206

Desert Divide

DIRECTIONS Park a getaway vehicle at the Cedar Spring Trailhead, then drive back to the Devils Slide Trailhead at Humber Park. To reach the Cedar Spring Trailhead from State Highway 74, 8.6 miles south of Mountain Center in the Garner Valley and just beyond mile marker 074 RIV 67.75, turn left (northeast) onto the paved Morris Ranch Rd. (6S53). Follow it up 3.7 miles, passing the Joe Sherman Girl Scout Camp, to the signed Cedar Spring Trailhead (4E17) on the right (GPS SB81). (If you reach Morris Ranch, you've driven 0.25 mile too far.) The best parking is at a large lot on the east side of the road 0.1 mile before reaching the trailhead. To reach Humber Park, drive back to Mountain Center, then north on Highway 243 to Idyllwild. Just below the ranger station, turn northeast on North Circle Dr. Drive 0.7 mile to a four-way intersection, where you turn right on South Circle Dr. Proceed 0.1 mile, then turn left on Fern Valley Rd. Proceed 1.8 miles to the large Humber Park trailhead parking at the end of the road.

This challenging hike is one of the most rewarding in Southern California, offering a grand tour of the rugged and unique Desert Divide. It follows the PCT along the crest from Tahquitz Peak south to Cedar Spring, with optional excursions to nine nearby summits along the way: Tahquitz, Red Tahquitz, South Peak, Antsell Rock,

Apache Peak, Spitler Peak, Palm View Peak, Little Desert, and Pyramid Peak. The northern stretch is extraordinarily rugged, while the southern part becomes more gentle and rolling. It is especially enjoyable in April, when flowers are in bloom and when you may meet a parade of PCT through-hikers starting their long northbound journeys. By the end of this trip, you are guaranteed to be tired, hungry, and fully satisfied.

Good route-finding skills are essential to locate the easiest ways to many of the summits. There is no convenient water along this route, so bring at least 4 quarts on a cool day and more if it will be warm. A headlamp and enough clothing to survive an unplanned night out are also strongly advisable. Those looking for a somewhat easier trip through the best part of the Desert Divide with *only* four or five peaks may

Aerial view of the Desert Divide from the south. Fobes Saddle in the foreground, with San Jacinto at the far end, and the tall ridge of San Gorgonio looming on the horizon.

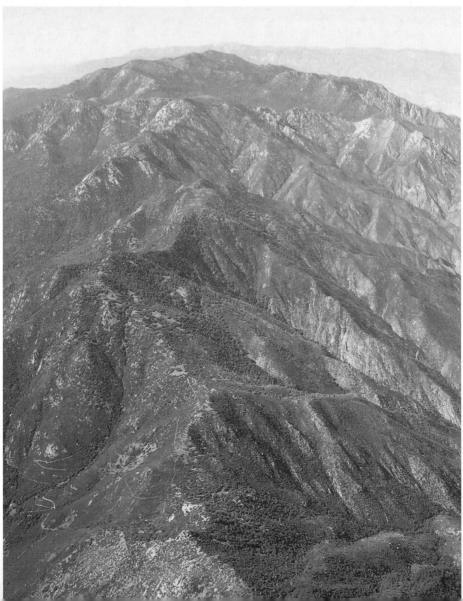

plan to exit the Spitler Peak or Fobes Trail instead (see Trips 10.2 or 10.3).

From Humber Park, hike 2.5 miles up the Devils Slide Trail to the five-way Saddle Junction, where you meet the PCT. Take the rightmost fork and hike south toward Tahquitz Peak, gradually climbing through the open forest. The granite slopes of Red Tahquitz come into view and the trees become smaller and more weather-beaten as you climb. In 1.4 miles, reach a junction with the South Ridge Trail. Follow this right toward Tahquitz Peak 0.4 mile, then take a short spur to the summit. From the top, study the granite-toothed Desert Divide leading south and the summits of Toro and Rabbit Peaks beyond, then return to the PCT.

Hike back east along South Ridge Trail, pass the junction of PCT that you came in on, continuing east and then north on the PCT, descending in 0.8 mile to another junction with a side trail leading north to Tahquitz Valley. Continue 0.8 mile on the PCT as it leads east beneath the white north walls of Red Tahquitz, and pass just below and south of a small rocky knob, then in 0.2 mile more, come to a draw. This is one of the weaknesses in Red Tahquitz's defenses and the shortest way to the summit. Turn south and hike 0.3 mile uphill through the forest until you reach the mountain top. Red Tahquitz sits on the border between the high-quality white granite of the San Jacinto/Tahquitz region and the band of distinctive red granite farther south. Although it is tempting to take a shortcut down to the east, you are better off returning the way you came because the brush and cliff bands make an eastern descent difficult.

Follow the PCT east around a knob overlooking Andreas Canyon, then south across the head of Murray Canyon. The Desert Divide takes on its most rugged and interesting character between here and Apache Peak. Along the high part of the divide, Jeffrey pines, white firs, and incense cedars are common, though some chaparral also clings to the parched cliffs. In 2.4 miles, from Red Tahquitz pass along the east side of South Peak. At the corner where the trail turns west across the south side of the peak look for a use trail, sometimes marked with cairns, that leads 0.1 mile up to the nearby summit.

The PCT switchbacks down the ridge and the dark imposing hulk of Antsell Rock looms large ahead. The PCT drops to cross the east face below the cliffs. In 2.1 miles, look for a gully marked with cairns in a grove of black oaks. In this gully is a use trail to the summit of Antsell Rock. It is only 0.3 mile as the crow flies, but involves 800 feet of strenuous climbing. The steep and loose gully leads up to a prominent notch to the right of the rocky peak. The summit register can be found in this notch, so those uncomfortable with rock scrambling may stop here. But for one of the most fun mountaineering experiences in Southern California, continue up to the true summit. Scramble up a weakness in the rock, then go around the corner to another tree-filled gully that leads to the rocky summit ridge. Some third-class climbing is required. Return the way you came.

From the PCT continuing southeast in 0.5 mile, reach a saddle on the Desert Divide. Here, an unmarked trail leads up from the Zen Center in Apple Canyon (see Trip 10.1). Continue south on the PCT beneath the red battlements on the north wall of Apache Peak. The 2008 Apache Fire burned the east side of the Desert Divide in this area. From the junction with the Zen Center trail in 0.4 mile consider following a use trail to a vista point atop the wall just before the trail rounds a corner. In another 0.8 mile, cross a burn zone on north slope of Apache Peak. It is possible to take a shortcut to the summit of Apache by bushwhacking up a gully to the skyline, then turning right and walking a few yards to the summit. Otherwise, follow the PCT as it loops 0.4 mile around the east side to reach the summit plateau of Apache Peak, where a faint use trail branches off. Two hills are visible to the northwest from the junction; Apache Peak's highest point is the one on the left, 0.2 mile from the PCT. The unimposing summit has terrific views.

In less than 0.1 mile farther south on the PCT, come to a signed junction with a trail leading east 0.5 mile and 500 feet down to the reliable Apache Spring. The Forest Service recommends treating water from this spring. A few tent sites with excellent views are available here.

Continue south on the PCT 0.6 mile to a junction with the Spitler Peak Trail coming up from Apple Canyon; this is an escape route if you have a vehicle parked below. Otherwise, Spitler Peak is the next challenge on the Divide. It has two use trails marked with cairns. One climbs the serpentine north ridge from a point just south of the Spitler Peak Trail/PCT junction; the other rises almost straight up from a point 0.5 mile farther along the PCT, almost due east of the summit. It would be appealing to ascend the north ridge and descend to the east, but the summit is choked with vegetation and finding the eastern route from above can be difficult.

Spitler Peak marks the end of the rocky section of the Desert Divide. Farther south, the ridges and peaks are lower and more rounded. Pines and firs give way to oaks, manzanitas, buckthorns, and the striking ribbonwood. In 1.5 miles, reach Fobes Saddle, where a trail comes up from Fobes Canyon (another escape route). The PCT makes a long switchback, crosses over to the west side of the Divide, and climbs 2.3 tedious miles to a flattish area. Palm View Peak is 0.2 mile to the east, hidden in a dense grove of oaks and firs. The summit is difficult to find because it is rather flat and concealed in the vegetation. If you begin to descend on the PCT, you have gone too far and now have a thicket blocking your path to the peak. The name is misleading; there are views of nothing but the trees you have just thrashed through. This is decidedly the least enjoyable peak on your route.

Return to the PCT and continue 1.4 miles southeast over some rolling hills and along a boulevard cut through the manzanita to reach the Cedar Spring Trail junction. If daylight and energy remain, follow the PCT 0.2 mile farther over the top of the unimpressive Little Desert Peak and 1 mile beyond to Pyramid Peak to round out your nine summits for the day. There is a climber's path up to the summit of Pyramid from the saddle south of Pyramid Peak. Then return to the Cedar Spring junction. Switchback down the Cedar Spring Trail to the southwest, then pass through a gate and reach some picnic benches in 1.3 miles. The trail becomes a dirt road for a while, then veers off to the right again and passes through several gates in a corridor between fenced properties. After a seemingly unending mile, complete your adventure at the signed trailhead.

ALTERNATIVE FINISH

Truly ambitious peak baggers can finish out the Desert Divide by following the PCT south past Pine Mtn. and Lion Peak all the way to where the trail crosses Highway 74 at a signed trailhead. This stretch is 10.5 miles from the Cedar Spring junction, so it increases the total trip to 32 miles and 11 peaks. Pine Mtn. has a ducked trail from the PCT that starts 100 yards north of the saddle at the south end of Peak 6880+ and leads over the small peak, then east to the saddle and up the southwest slope of Pine Mtn. The path can be horribly overgrown with chaparral unless somebody has trimmed the path recently. Many hikers skip the summit monolith, which involves moderate fifth-class climbing and a rappel descent on a 50-meter rope. Lion Peak has a climber's trail starting from the PCT at the saddle on the northeast side of the peak.

trip 10.8 Thomas Mtn.

Distance	13 miles (out-and-back)
Hiking Time	7 hours
Elevation Gain	2400'
Difficulty	Strenuous
Trail Use	Dogs, equestrians, cyclists, suitable for backpacking
Best Times	April–June, October–November
Agency	San Bernardino National Forest (Idyllwild Ranger Station)
Recommended Map	*Anza* 7.5' (roads and trails have changed somewhat since the 1996 printing)

see map on p. 206

DIRECTIONS From State Highway 74, in Garner Valley 8.1 miles south of Mountain Center and just south of mile marker 074 RIV 67.25, turn west into the Ramona Trail parking area.

Optionally, cut the trip in half by arranging to leave a shuttle vehicle at the top. From Highway 74 at mile marker 074 RIV 64.25, turn west onto the fair dirt Thomas Mtn. Rd. (6S13). Drive 7.4 miles up to the junction with 6S13C near yellow post campsite #6 just north of the summit. Park where you do not obstruct traffic.

Thomas Mtn.'s long ridge forms the western side of the beautiful Garner Valley. It is perfectly situated to offer fantastic views of the Desert Divide and San Jacinto Wilderness. The lower slopes are covered in delightful stands of ribbonwoods. On the top of the ridge, cool breezes blow through the rich forest of Jeffrey pines, white firs, and incense cedars. Wildflowers are abundant in the spring and early summer. The mountain is named for Charles Thomas, a pioneer who founded a ranch in the valley in 1861. The valley was also known as Thomas Valley until the ranch was sold to Robert Garner, who gave the valley its present name.

The Ramona Trail, named for Helen Hunt Jackson's tragic heroine, climbs to the ridge from Garner Valley. The dirt Thomas Mtn. Rd. runs along the top of the ridge, providing access to numerous fine yellow-post camping spots and also offering an alternative descent if you choose to make a one-way hike.

The good trail (3E26) starts at the west end of the Ramona Trail parking area and switchbacks up the slope through stands of ribbonwoods, manzanitas, and mountain mahoganys. In 2.5 miles, the chaparral yields to forest on the upper flanks of the

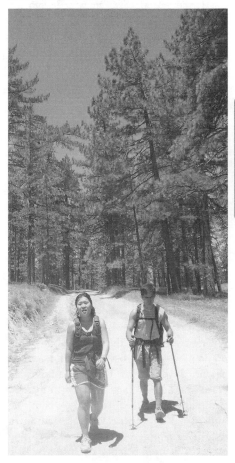

Hikers on Thomas Mtn. Rd.

Desert Divide

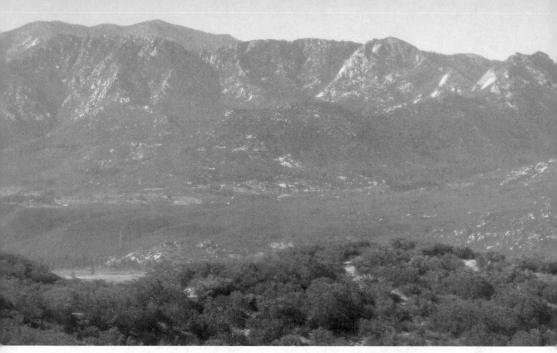

The Northern Desert Divide from San Jacinto to Apache Peak, viewed from Thomas Mtn.

mountain. In another 1.0 mile, reach an unmarked fork. The main trail continues right, but a side trail leads left 100 yards up a draw to Toolbox Springs shaded under the cedars and Jeffrey pines. The concrete trough here is suitable for watering stock, but is unappealing to hikers. Just above the spring is the quiet Tool Box Spring Campground located at the bottom end of a dirt road.

In 0.1 mile on the Ramona Trail, reach a second unmarked junction. Both trails lead to dirt roads and up to Thomas Mtn. Rd., but the right fork is the shorter way to go. In 0.2 mile, the right fork reaches a dirt road near yellow-post campsite #9. This trip follows the dirt road from here to the summit.

VARIATION

The trail crosses the dirt road at a trail marker by yellow-post site #9 and continues northwest. It can be hard to follow in places because it passes many unmarked cow paths. The first major cow path, 0.6 mile from the campsite, leads 0.1 mile down to Magee Spring, marked by a watering trough. The trail reaches Thomas Mtn. Rd.

in 2.1 miles at an unlabeled trail marker where the road makes a hairpin turn north of Thomas Mtn. Turn left and hike 0.2 mile back to 6S13C to rejoin the main route 0.4 mile below the summit.

Turn left up the road and follow it 0.3 mile to Thomas Mtn. Rd. Turn right and follow Thomas Mtn. Rd. northwest along the ridge. Although hiking on a fire road might sound unappealing, the forest and wildflowers are delightful and the walking is pleasant. Pass yellow-post site #8, then a logging road on the left, then yellow-post sites #7 and #6. In 1.8 miles, just beyond site #6, reach a road junction on the north side of Thomas Mtn. Turn left and take the switchbacking road, 6S13C, 0.4 mile up to the summit of the mountain, where concrete foundations mark the site of the former fire lookout. From here, there are fabulous views south and west over Anza Valley and Cahuilla Mtn., and north to San Gorgonio, as well as the panoramas of the Desert Divide that you have enjoyed all along.

If you left a shuttle vehicle near the summit, your trip is done. Otherwise, return the way you came.

trip 10.9 Cahuilla Mtn.

Distance	6 miles (out-and-back)
Hiking Time	3 hours
Elevation Gain	1400'
Difficulty	Moderate
Trail Use	Dogs, suitable for backpacking
Best Times	October–June
Agency	San Bernardino National Forest (Idyllwild Ranger Station)
Recommended Map	*Cahuilla Mountain 7.5'*

DIRECTIONS From Interstate 15 in Temecula, go east on Highway 79 for 17 miles to Aguanga, then turn left on Highway 371. In 11.25 miles, near mile marker 371 RIV 68.0 and the sign for Cahuilla Mtn. Trail (2E45), turn left (north) onto Cary Rd., which eventually changes name to Tripp Flats Rd. At a signed junction in 3.6 miles, turn left onto the dirt Forest Service Road 6S22. In 0.8 mile, reach Trip Flats Fire Station at a fork. Stay left on 6S22 and continue 1.6 mile to the signed Cahuilla Mtn. Trail (2E45), on your left, close to phone lines overhead. Park in the small clearing on your right.

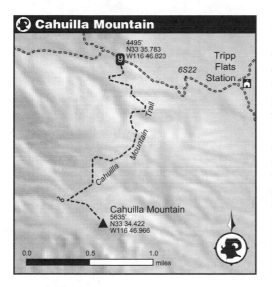

Cahuilla (pronounced "ka-wee-ah") Mtn. stands by itself, well to the west of the Desert Divide and Thomas Mtn. It overlooks the Anza Valley and a Cahuilla tribal reservation. Cahuilla Mtn. is in a proposed Wilderness area. Although seldom visited today, is was the setting of Helen Hunt Jackson's famous 1884 novel, *Ramona*, about the injustices faced by Native Americans. At the height of the novel's popularity, tourists came by the wagonload to visit the scene and meet Ramona Lubo and visit the grave of her husband Juan Diego. The novel is inspired by a true story. After a misunderstanding, a white man murdered Juan Diego, and a white judge acquitted the murderer. This is a good trip for those with

Desert Divide

Cahuilla Mountain

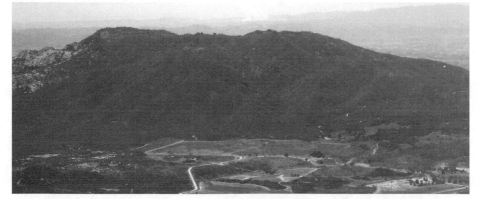

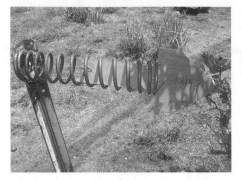

Spring—a young man's fancy

a vivid imagination who can conjure up the events of the past and contemplate the current state of American justice.

The trail leads up the northeast side of the mountain through the chaparral. It then follows the summit ridge through a forest of black oaks and Jeffrey and Coulter pines. In 2.5 miles, pass a signed trail on the right leading 0.1 mile down to a small spring where water is usually available in the wet season. There are several bumps of nearly equal height along the ridge. The trail leads to the southeastern summit, which at 5635 feet is the high point of the mountain.

chapter 11

Palm Springs and the Indian Canyons

Over time, the San Andreas Fault has thrust an enormous block of granite into the sky, forming the San Jacinto Mountains. Along the mountains' east and north faces, the elevation rises from below sea level in the Coachella Valley to 10,834 feet on San Jacinto Peak, forming the tallest vertical wall in the United States outside Death Valley. The Palm Canyon Fault, a spur of the San Andreas Fault system, slices a trench between the San Jacinto and Santa Rosa Mountains. The pulverized rock in the fault

forms an impermeable layer. Desert streams that ordinarily run underground cannot penetrate this rock and are forced to the surface at a series of springs. Native California fan palm (*Washingtonia filifera*) oases are found here and in many of the nearby canyons. Since ancient times, the Agua Caliente Band of Cahuilla (pronounced "ka-wee-ah") Indians has made their home in these canyons and in the nearby mountains, hunting and gathering the native animals and plants. Spanish missionaries

Palm Canyon and Murray Hill from the West Fork Trail

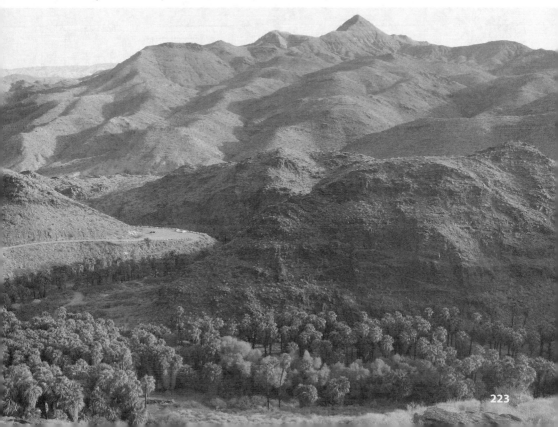

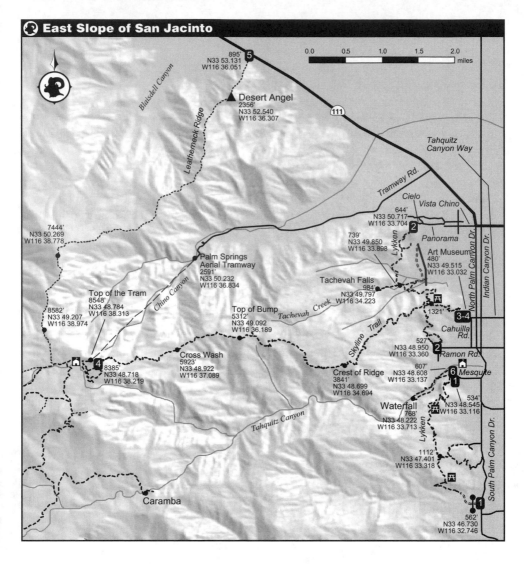

East Slope of San Jacinto

895'
N33 53.131
W116 36.051

Blaisdell Canyon

Leatherneck Ridge

0.0   0.5   1.0   1.5   2.0
⌐▬▬▬▬▬▬▬▬▬▬▬▬▬▬▬▬▬┐ miles

Desert Angel
2356'
N33 52.540
W116 36.307

111

Tahquitz
Canyon Way

Tramway Rd.

Cielo
644'
N33 50.717
W116 33.704

Vista Chino

739'
N33 49.850
W116 33.898

Panorama

7444'
N33 50.269
W116 38.778

Lykken

Art Museum
480'
N33 49.515
W116 33.032

Palm Springs
Aerial Tramway
2591'
N33 50.232
W116 36.834

Tachevah Falls
984'
N33 49.797
W116 34.223

North Palm Canyon Dr.

Indian Canyon Dr.

Top of the Tram
8548'
N33 48.784
W116 38.313

Chino Canyon

Top of Bump
5312'
N33 49.092
W116 36.189

Tachevah Creek

1321'

Cahuilla
Rd.

8582'
N33 49.207
W116 38.974

8385'
N33 48.718
W116 38.219

Cross Wash
5923'
N33 48.922
W116 37.089

Skyline Trail

527'
N33 48.950
W116 33.360

Ramon Rd.

4

Crest of Ridge
3841'
N33 48.699
W116 34.694

607'
N33 48.608
W116 33.137

Mesquite

534'
N33 48.545
W116 33.116

Waterfall
768'
N33 48.222
W116 33.713

Lykken

Tahquitz Canyon

1112'
N33 47.401
W116 33.318

South Palm Canyon Dr.

Caramba

562'
N33 46.730
W116 32.746

brought farming, "civilization," and disease. A smallpox epidemic reduced the tribe to 70 individuals by the late 1800s.

In 1877, the Southern Pacific Railroad was completed, following a line near where Interstate 10 presently runs. As an incentive for rail construction, the Federal government granted Southern Pacific every other square mile section of land forming a checkerboard extending 10 miles on either side of the tracks. Southern Pacific, in turn, began selling land to private owners. In 1884, Judge John McCallum and

his family became permanent settlers in the Palm Springs area. He built an irrigation canal from the Whitewater River to Palm Springs. Shortly after, hotels began to open, first catering to tuberculosis patients who sought the warm dry weather and the hot springs, but soon drawing the rich and famous from all over the West. Golf courses and resorts followed. By the 1980s, development reached a frenetic pace; the number of resorts and houses doubled in the decade and started to push into the pristine mountains. People became aware of the need to protect the wilderness for the enjoyment of future generations and for the survival of the desert bighorn sheep and other species. In 1990, portions of the area were designated the Santa Rosa Mountains National Scenic Area under management of the BLM. In 2000, Congress established the Santa Rosa and San Jacinto Mountains National Monument, protecting 272,000 acres including most of the hills surrounding Palm Springs. The Agua Caliente Band of Cahuilla Indians owns Palm Canyon and the surrounding area, and opens the canyon to hikers and equestrians for day use.

This chapter describes hikes around Palm Springs on the eastern desert flank of San Jacinto and in the Indian Canyons. Chapter 12 covers other hikes in the Santa Rosa Mountains, while Chapter 9 covers hikes near San Jacinto Peak and Chapter 10 covers those along the Desert Divide overlooking Palm Canyon.

Many of the hikes in this section are in the Indian Canyons. The canyons are part of the tribal lands of the Agua Caliente Band of Cahuilla Indians. The tribe welcomes dayhikers into the canyon, but an admission fee is charged and hours are strictly enforced. Admission fees support the maintenance of the excellent network of trails within the canyons. You will receive a trail map when you pay your admission at the entrance station on South Palm Canyon Dr. More information is available at the Trading Post store and information center on Hermits Bench at the southern terminus of Palm Canyon Dr. The Trading Post and the Tahquitz Canyon Visitor Center sell a detailed Indian Canyons topographic map of the trails for a nominal charge. At the time of this writing, the Indian Canyons are open daily from 8 A.M. to 5 P.M. During the heat of the summer months, the canyons are open Friday through Sunday and only the shortest hikes are enjoyable. Admission is $8, and discounts are available for students, seniors, and children. For more information, call (760) 323-6018 or visit www.theindiancanyons.com. Mountain bikes are prohibited, partly due to irresponsible behavior of a minority of riders in the past. Pets and rock climbing are also prohibited. The land is sacred to the tribe, so treat it as you would your own place of worship.

Tribal rangers lead short but informative tours of Palm Canyon and Tahquitz Canyon; call for the schedule. Wranglers from the Smoke Tree Stables in Palm Springs also organize hourly horseback excursions into Palm Canyon; for more information, visit www.smoketreeranch.com/smoketreestables.html or call (760) 327-1372.

Entrance to Palm Canyon

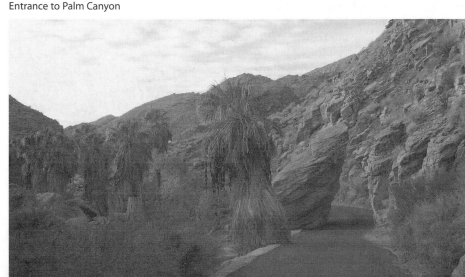

trip 11.1 South Lykken Trail

Distance	4.5 miles (one-way)
Hiking Time	2.5 hours
Elevation Gain	1100'
Difficulty	Moderate
Best Times	October–April, day use only
Agency	Santa Rosa and San Jacinto Mountains National Monument
Optional Map	*Santa Rosa and San Jacinto Mountains National Monument* or *Palm Springs 7.5'*

see map on p. 224

DIRECTIONS From Interstate 10, take Highway 111 south into Palm Springs. The road changes name to North Palm Canyon Dr., then South Palm Canyon Dr. Most lanes turn left to become East Palm Canyon, but stay right (straight) and continue on South Palm Canyon Dr. for 1.7 miles. Park at a turnout on the west side of the road, 0.1 mile beyond Canyon Heights Dr. This is the south end of the South Lykken Trail.

If you plan to do this as a one-way hike, it is possible to arrange a shuttle at the north end of the trail at Mesquite Ave. Mesquite is located 0.5 mile north of the East Palm Canyon/South Palm Canyon split. Mesquite leads west from North Palm Canyon Dr. for 0.4 mile, then abruptly turns north toward the Tahquitz Canyon Visitor Center. The trailhead is at this corner, but the only parking is back down the hill along Mesquite Ave. just west of South Palm Canyon Dr.

The Lykken Trail is named in fitting tribute to Carl Lykken, a pioneering Palm Springs businessman and the city's first postmaster. There are two separate legs of the Lykken Trail, designated South and North. Both trails start on the outskirts of Palm Springs, at city elevation. The trails ascend the slopes of the San Jacinto Mountains that border the city to the west, providing unparalleled views of Palm Springs and the Coachella Valley. From the ridges above the city one can truly appreciate Palm Springs as a beautiful green oasis set against the forbidding Colorado Desert. Camping is not permitted along this trail.

The South Lykken Trail features a spectacular overlook from the curving lip of Tahquitz Canyon and also offers great views of the jets coming and going below you at Palm Springs International Airport. This trip can be done as a one-way hike. If you haven't arranged a car or bicycle shuttle, you can make a loop by taking a somewhat unpleasant 2.5-mile walk back on the shoulder of Palm Canyon Dr. For an out-and-back alternative, hike the first 3 miles to the dramatic Josie Johnson Vista, then retrace your steps, or descend the side trail midway and walk back along Palm Canyon Dr.

VARIATION

For a longer one-way hike, join up with the North Lykken Trail (see Trip 11.2). The direct link between the two trails is conspicuously missing, but a brief detour on city streets will connect you to the other leg of the trail. Follow Mesquite Road east to Palm Canyon Dr., then go north to Ramon Rd. and back west.

South Lykken Trail picnic tables

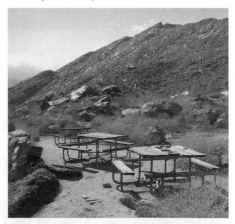

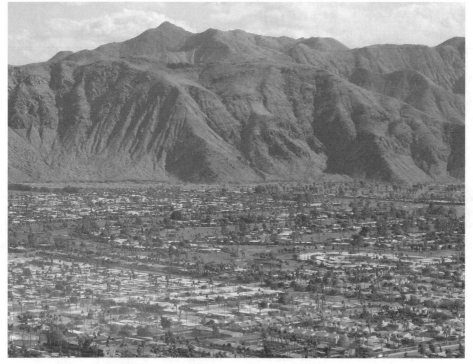

Murray Hill from South Lykken Trail

From the unsigned trailhead on the side of South Palm Canyon Dr., follow a closed gravel road east 0.4 mile along the north side of a wash to the signed start of the Lykken Trail. The footpath begins switchbacking north up the toe of the mountain, reaching the Simone Kennett Vista Point in 0.7 mile. From here, there are memorable views of Palm Springs, Murray Hill, and the northern Santa Rosa Mountains, and Palm Canyon. The trail begins contouring north across the tilted slopes of San Jacinto. In 0.6 mile, it reaches a junction marked by a cairn.

VARIATION

The right fork descends a mile to the city. It splits a third of the way down. The left (north) path leads to a dirt parking area in a residential neighborhood at the corner of Camino Descanso and Camino Barranca. The right (south) path descends to the Desert Riders Park, then joins a dirt road that emerges at a gate near the top of Cahuilla Hills Dr., a steep private road with no hiker parking.

Continue north on the Lykken Trail from the junction for another 1.4 miles past barrel and cholla cacti to picnic tables at the Josie Johnson Vista Park on the lip of Tahquitz Canyon. From here, there are impressive views down the steep walls of the canyon and out over the city. Aviation enthusiasts will also enjoy the steady stream of jets landing and departing from Palm Springs International Airport below.

The trail begins descending along the east rim of the canyon. In 0.1 mile, a spur trail leads left for 100 yards to another impressive viewpoint on the canyon lip. This is a good place to admire Tahquitz Falls during the wetter months. The main trail switchbacks steeply down 1.3 miles farther to finish the south leg of the trail at Mesquite Rd. near the Tahquitz Canyon Visitor Center.

trip 11.2 North Lykken Trail

Distance	4 miles (one-way)
Hiking Time	2.5 hours
Elevation Gain	1500′
Difficulty	Moderate
Best Times	October–April, day use only
Agency	Santa Rosa and San Jacinto Mountains National Monument
Recommended Map	*Santa Rosa and San Jacinto Mountains National Monument* or *Palm Springs* 7.5′ (trail incompletely marked)
Permit	See below

see map on p. 224

DIRECTIONS From Interstate 10, take Highway 111 south into Palm Springs. The road changes name to North Palm Canyon Dr., then South Palm Canyon Dr. In 11.7 miles from the interstate, turn west on Ramon Rd. and drive to the trailhead at the end.

If you plan to do this as a one-way hike, first arrange a shuttle at the north end of the trail. Go back north 2.0 miles to Vista Chino (Palm Canyon is one-way south in this area, so go east one short block and follow the one-way north Indian Canyon Dr. instead). Take Vista Chino west for 0.2 mile, then turn right on Via Norte, proceed 0.1 mile, turn left on Chino Canyon Rd. In 0.2 mile, the road hits a T. Turn left and follow Panorama 0.3 mile, then stay left on Cielo Dr. In 0.1 mile, turn left on an unnamed spur to the trailhead parking between a tennis court and an impressive cactus garden.

The Lykken Trail is named in fitting tribute to Carl Lykken, a pioneering Palm Springs businessman and the city's first postmaster. There are two separate legs of the Lykken Trail, designated South and North. Both trails start on the outskirts of Palm Springs, at city elevation. The trails ascend the slopes of the San Jacinto Mountains that border the city to the west, providing unparalleled views of Palm Springs and the Coachella Valley. From the ridges above the city one can truly appreciate Palm Springs as a beautiful green oasis set against the forbidding Colorado Desert. Camping is not permitted along this trail.

VARIATIONS

The North Lykken Trail features a short side trip to the imposing Tachevah Falls. There are some unmarked and unauthorized side trails, so this hike requires good navigational skills to stay on the correct path. This trip can be done as a one-way hike with a car or bicycle shuttle. Alternatively, hike halfway, then descend the Museum Trail (see Trip 11.3) and follow Cahuilla Rd. 0.5 mile south back to Ramon Rd.

From Ramon Rd. a dirt road leads north from the trailhead for 200 feet. When it turns right, look for the unmarked but well-built trail that begins climbing unrelentingly northwest. Barrel cacti cling tenaciously to the rocky soil. In 0.4 mile, reach a signed junction with another trail to the right that returns to the dirt road where you started. Stay left and continue up the Lykken Trail for 0.9 mile to a second junction marked with a large cairn. The Museum Trail forks right and descends to the Palm Springs Art Museum at Tahquitz Canyon Way (see Trip 11.3), but the Lykken Trail continues north. The National Monument plans to require free self-issued wilderness permits to hike the northern segment of the North Lykken Trail. When this permit requirement goes into effect, the permits will be available at a kiosk alongside the trail. If a wilderness permit kiosk has been established by the time you do this hike, you will be required to obtain a free permit for travel beyond this point. The permits will allow the National Monument to track the number of hikers using this area and assess their impact on the endangered peninsular bighorn sheep.

In another 200 feet at a sign painted on a boulder, the Skyline Trail forks to the left and climbs 8 arduous miles to Long Valley (see Trip 11.4), but the Lykken Trail again continues north, rounds the corner of the ridge, and switchbacks down to the valley floor in 1.1 miles. After completing the final switchbacks, look for an easy-to-miss trail junction. The right fork leads down to the spillway on a large levee and ends at a fence, but you stay on the left fork. In another 0.1 mile, reach a second junction near a huge boulder. Again, stay left rather than descending to the spillway.

VARIATION

In 100 yards, reach yet another unmarked junction. The left fork is a worthy side trip, although it is only open legally for travel from October to December. It leads 0.4 mile up the narrow Tachevah Canyon to a spectacular slab topped by a lone palm tree. A thin waterfall trickles down the slab during the wet season. The rocky trail braids in and out of the wash and there are many ways to go. Beware of the long-thorned mesquite bushes near the end. Rock climbers have established numerous moderate to difficult routes up the cliffs. Return to the junction after you have finished exploring.

The Lykken Trail continues north through the boulders at the wide mouth of the next canyon. It then climbs past creosote bushes and rounds a hill. An unmarked side trail leads right and down into the basin beside the levee, but this trail is not recommended because it crosses private property belonging to the Riverside County Flood Control District. Instead, stay on the main trail, which once again climbs steeply up the next ridge to picnic tables at a flat area with fine vistas, then descends steeply to the north trailhead near Cielo Dr., 1.6 miles from Tachevah Canyon.

Dedication of the Lykken Trail. From left to right: Mayor Bill Foster, Jane Lykken Hoff (Carl Lykken's daughter), Scooter (Art Smith's horse), and Art Smith.

Photograph courtesy of Doug Evans, Desert Riders

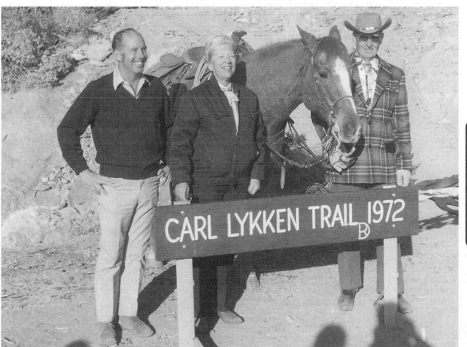

trip 11.3 Museum Trail

Distance	2 miles (out-and-back)
Hiking Time	1.5 hours
Elevation Gain	1000'
Difficulty	Moderate
Best Times	October–April, or by moonlight in the summer
Agency	Santa Rosa and San Jacinto Mountains National Monument
Optional Map	*Santa Rosa and San Jacinto Mountains National Monument* or *Palm Springs* 7.5' (trail not marked)

see map on p. 224

DIRECTIONS From Interstate 10, take Highway 111 south into Palm Springs. The road changes name to North Palm Canyon Dr. In 11.2 miles from the interstate, turn right (west) on Tahquitz Canyon Way and go 0.2 mile, then turn right on Museum Rd. There is no public parking at the Palm Springs Art Museum, but you may find limited parking on Museum Rd.

The Museum Trail is a short but steep trail leading from the Palm Springs Art Museum up the western flank of San Jacinto. It offers great views of Palm Springs and is a popular exercise trail, either by itself or as a loop with the North Lykken Trail. Camping is not permitted along this trail.

The signed trailhead is partially hidden behind trees and landscaping in the northwest corner of the museum parking lot. Immediately cross a private road. The trail switchbacks steeply up the hillside. There are numerous unmarked shortcuts along the way. However, these paths increase erosion; try to stay on the most heavily used trail.

The trail climbs westward on the south side of the ridge for 0.4 mile, then crosses over to the north side, descending 50 feet to bypass some rocks along the way. In another 0.4 mile, pass an outcrop and come to picnic tables at a four-way junction. Sometimes, you may find a trail register to sign. Enjoy the magnificent views of saddle-backed Toro Peak at the head of Palm Canyon, the sheer sickle-shaped gorge of Tahquitz Canyon immediately south, the ridges and canyons of the Santa Rosa Mountains to the east, and the Little San Bernardino Mountains to the north, along with the city of Palm Springs immediately below.

ALTERNATIVE FINISH

Return the way you came. Or, if you prefer to make a loop with a more gradual descent, continue straight ahead for 0.1 mile to a cairn marking the junction with the North Lykken Trail (see Trip 11.2). Turn left and descend the trail to Ramon Rd., then follow Cahuilla Rd. north back to the Museum Trailhead. This option adds a mile of walking.

Sunrise over the Santa Rosa Mountains and Palm Springs from the Museum Trail

trip 11.4 Cactus-to-Clouds

Distance	10 miles (one-way)
Hiking Time	9 hours
Elevation Gain	8000'
Difficulty	Very strenuous
Best Times	October–November
Agency	Santa Rosa and San Jacinto Mountains National Monument
Required Map	*Santa Rosa and San Jacinto Mountains National Monument* or *Palm Springs, San Jacinto* 7.5' (trail not marked)
Permit	See below

see map on p. 224

DIRECTIONS If you plan to descend via the tram, you may wish to leave a vehicle at the Palm Springs Aerial Tramway station. From State Highway 111, 8.5 miles south of Interstate 10 at the northern edge of Palm Springs, turn west up Tramway Rd. and drive 4 miles to Valley Station, the lower terminus of the Palm Springs Aerial Tramway. The tram operates daily, starting at 10 A.M. Monday–Friday, 8 A.M. Saturday, Sunday, and holidays. The last tram return is 9:45 P.M. The tram closes for annual maintenance, typically in September. Round-trip tickets are $21.95. Check www.pstramway.com or call 888-515-TRAM for the most current information.

To reach the trailhead, continue 3.2 miles south on Highway 111. The road changes name to North Palm Canyon Dr. Turn right (west) on Tahquitz Canyon Way and go 0.2 mile, then turn right on Museum Rd. There is no public parking at the Palm Springs Art Museum, but you may find limited parking on Museum Rd.

Cactus-to-Clouds, also known as the Skyline Trail, is a classic Southern California hike. It is the only trail in the United States to directly climb 8000 feet, scaling the sheer east ridge of San Jacinto from Palm Springs to the upper Aerial Tramway station. Most hikers stop at the station, but diehards continue on to bag the summit of San Jacinto. The Civilian Conservation Corps built the trail the during the Great Depression. It had fallen into obscurity for decades, but is now heavily traveled. The trail also features some of the most varied and interesting scenery and plant life found anywhere in Southern California. Camping is not permitted along this trail.

The National Monument plans to require free self-issued wilderness permits for the Skyline Trail. When this permit requirement goes into effect, the permits will be available at a kiosk alongside the trail.

Some trail runners can make the enormous ascent in less than 5 hours, but a normal fit hiker should plan for double that. The trail is scorched by the sun at the bottom for most of the year and is covered

in ice at the top after the first winter snows, so late fall is an ideal season for the climb. Several hikers have died on this route, and others have required rescue. Bring 4–6 quarts of water. After the first storm of the

Dire warnings at the start of the Skyline Trail

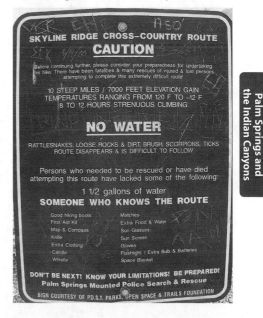

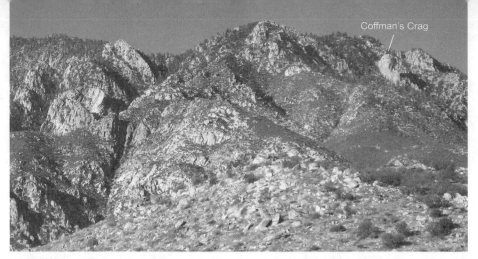
Coffman's Crag

Upper Skyline Ridge

season, the upper part of the route is usually covered in snow and becomes unsuitable for hikers who do not already know the route and who lack ice axe, crampons, and adequate snow mountaineering experience.

The first mile of this hike climbs up the Museum Trail (see Trip 11.3). The signed trailhead is partially concealed behind trees and landscaping in the northwest corner of the museum parking lot. Immediately cross a private road. The trail switchbacks steeply up the hillside. There are numerous unmarked shortcuts along the way. However, these paths increase erosion; stay on the most heavily-used trail. The trail climbs westward on the south side of the ridge for 0.4 mile, then crosses over to the north side, descending 50 feet to bypass some rocks along the way. In another 0.4 mile, pass a rock outcrop and come to picnic tables at a four-way junction with good views. Continue straight for 0.1 mile to a cairn marking the junction with the North Lykken Trail (see Trip 11.2). Turn right and go 200 feet, then turn left where a sign painted on a rock indicates the trail to Long Valley. A sign near the start warns of the perils of the trail.

Follow the Skyline Trail for 8.3 miles and another incredible 7000 feet of elevation gain to reach Long Valley near the Tram Station. As you climb, observe how the vegetation transitions through many different zones. At the bottom, brittle bushes, creosote bushes, and barrel cacti are common.

After climbing the ridge and east slopes, the trail momentarily levels out, then crosses to the right side of the ridge, offering great views into Tachevah Canyon to the north. The desert vegetation begins changing. Junipers, ribbonwoods, scrub oaks, valley cholla cacti, and Mojave yuccas start dotting the hillside. The trail briefly flattens again, then gains the crest of the ridge. After surmounting the next hill, a great view of the granite ramparts of the upper mountain comes into view. You can pick out most of the route from here. Look for the prominent Coffman's Crag on the right side of the ridge; this is the largest monolithic rock on the east face. Eagle-eyed climbers may notice the Palm Springs Aerial Tramway passing immediately north of the crag. The trail follows the top of the narrowing ridge between Chino Canyon to the north and Tahquitz Canyon to the south, then switchbacks through the dense band of chaparral, then climbs into the forest and ascends the gully on the south side of Coffman's Crag.

The next stretch of desert vegetation is especially lush, with several species of yuccas dotting the landscape. Views of the dramatic upper ridge continue to improve. As the ridge narrows, you are briefly treated to breathtaking glimpses of the zebra-striped cliffs in Chino Canyon. At 6000 feet, the trail crosses a dry wash above a small granite-slab waterfall. The vegetation abruptly changes to dense chaparral, including scrub oaks, manzanitas, and ribbonwoods. Travel would be horrendous were it not for the well-built trail snaking through the brush. In another 1000 feet, Jeffrey pines begin to appear, followed by cedars and live oaks. Enjoy the impressive cliffs of Coffman's Crag as you pass directly along side it, then suddenly pop over the lip of the ridge into the flat valley beyond.

You have emerged on the Desert View Nature Trail in Long Valley. From here, you have several options. You can return the way you came, take the tram down (a one-way ticket purchase is required), or get a wilderness permit and hike to the summit

of San Jacinto. To reach the summit of San Jacinto, follow the directions in Trip 9.21. This adds 10 miles and 2600 feet of elevation gain to your monumental adventure and typically demands a very early start. For the later two options, follow the Desert View Trail west and north to a signed junction with the paved trail coming down from the aerial tramway. To reach the tram, turn right and hike up the switchbacks. If you do not have a vehicle waiting at the tram station, the information desk can call a taxi to take you back to the Museum Trailhead (about $25).

trip 11.5 Leatherneck Ridge

Distance	8 miles (one-way)	
Hiking Time	11 hours	
Elevation Gain	9000'	
Difficulty	Very strenuous	see map on p. 224
Best Times	October–November, closed January–September	
Agency	Santa Rosa and San Jacinto Mountains National Monument	
Required Map	*Santa Rosa and San Jacinto Mountains National Monument*, Tom Harrison *San Jacinto Wilderness* or *Desert Hot Springs, Palm Springs, San Jacinto* 7.5'	

DIRECTIONS From Interstate 10, turn south on Highway 111 and proceed 5.5 miles, passing Windy Point and the mouth of Blaisdell Canyon. Park off the highway at the toe of the ridge. On your return the easiest way down is by way of the Palm Springs Aerial Tramway; arrange for a car or bicycle shuttle from the tram station, or plan to take a short taxi ride back.

San Jacinto's great north face is carved with deep canyons and great ridges rising almost 2 vertical miles from the desert floor to the summit. After driving past these magnificent formations enough times, a mountaineer inevitably begins to wonder if they can be climbed. This hike takes you up one of the long ridges, known to locals as Leatherneck Ridge, which starts on Highway 111 between Blaisdell and Chino Canyons. It climbs over the rocky point named Desert Angel (an enjoyable destination itself), then continues all the way up, terminating near the tram station. This route is cross-country all the way, following ridges and the occasional deer track. Cross-country travel is only legal

from October–December to protect the endangered peninsular bighorn sheep. Fire burned the ridge in August 2005 and most of the worst brush is temporarily gone, but the vegetation is not as lush or varied as on Cactus-to-Clouds. (Three campers in Blaisdell Canyon accidentally started the 5000-acre inferno when their campfire burned out of control. The campers were held responsible for more than $1.7 million in firefighting costs.)

Although it is the easiest of the huge cross-country routes on the north and east sides of the mountain, Leatherneck Ridge is substantially more demanding than Cactus-to-Clouds (see Trip 11.4) and should only be undertaken by strong and experienced mountaineers. The best season for this trip is the late fall. Earlier in the year it is unbearably hot at the bottom. Later in the year, ice covers the upper ridge and makes travel excessively difficult.

From the toe of the ridge where you parked your car, climb onto the crest of the ridge and hike up the talus, slabs, and dirt. After 0.8 mile of steep climbing and 1500 feet of elevation gain, reach the boulders atop Desert Angel, where you can admire your progress so far. Continue up the undulating ridge, watching as the vegetation changes. Beware of rattlesnakes in the deep grass. Beyond Desert Angel, there are few signs of human passage, but the deer and sheep have blazed a passable set of trails through the low brush.

At about 4200 feet, Leatherneck Ridge briefly levels out. Great views open up to the south into zebra-striped Chino Canyon. At 5500 feet, the ridge rises steeply westward again toward the forested skyline. This next stretch is one of the most difficult as you pick a path between the brush and big boulders. After gaining another hard-earned 2000 feet of elevation, reach the crest and peer over at the massive granite ramparts of Falls and Snow Creeks. You have covered 4.5 strenuous miles from Desert Angel. If conditions do not look good ahead, this is a good place to turn around or to turn north and descend Windy Point Ridge, which reaches Highway 111, 1.6 miles northwest of where you started.

Otherwise, turn south and follow the ridge 1.5 miles toward the upper part of the mountain, passing several bumps and many breathtaking views along the way. This stretch is again difficult, with boulders and fallen logs slowing your travel along the narrow ridge. Finally, top out at a pine-covered clearing.

An inspection of a map would suggest that you could hike directly to the tram station. Unfortunately, the ridge is stacked with huge granite blocks, making the travel difficult. A faster alternative is to stay west of these obstacles, following a gentle shallow drainage that tends southward. In 0.7 mile, reach the Long Valley Trail. Turn left (east) and head 0.3 mile toward the ranger station, passing the Hidden Divide Trail forking off to the south. Then follow the paved trail up to the tram station.

Upper Leatherneck Ridge

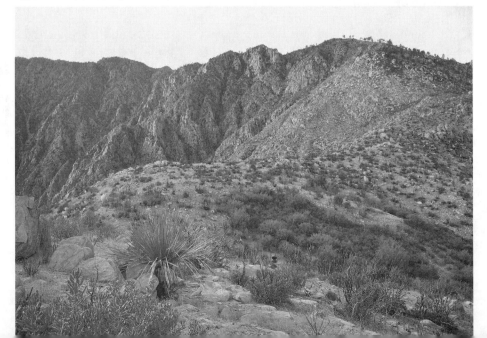

trip 11.6 Tahquitz Canyon

Distance	2 miles (loop)
Hiking Time	2.5 hours
Elevation Gain	350'
Difficulty	Easy
Best Times	September–May, 7:30 A.M.–5 P.M.
Agency	Agua Caliente Band of Cahuilla Indians
Optional Map	none

see map on p. 224

DIRECTIONS From North Palm Canyon Dr. 0.5 mile south of Ramon Rd. in Palm Springs, turn west on Mesquite Ave. Follow Mesquite as it winds up to the Tahquitz Canyon Visitor Center at 500 W. Mesquite.

Native peoples have inhabited Tahquitz Canyon for over 3000 years. According to Cahuilla Indian legend, Tahquitz was the tribe's first shaman. Tahquitz was powerful, but he abused his might. Driven from the village by his people, he transformed himself into a green ball of fire and flew into the sky. According to legend, he now abducts people in order to eat their souls. Some members of the tribe still refuse to venture into Tahquitz Canyon alone. Hikers use several pronunciations, but the correct Cahuilla pronunciation is "taw-kwish."

The canyon was overrun by hippies in the 1970s, but it has been cleaned up and is now open to hikers from 7:30 A.M. to 5 P.M. Excellent 2.5-hour ranger-guided tours depart daily at 8, 10, 12, and 2. The admission fee is presently $12.50 for adults and $6 for children. Schedules may change, so call (760) 416-7044 or visit www.tahquitzcanyon.com for information and reservations. Admission to the Indian Canyons may come with a $2.50 discount to Tahquitz Canyon, so if you are planning to explore both, consider visiting the Indian Canyons first.

The trail starts behind the Tahquitz Canyon Visitor Center and makes a figure-eight pattern up the canyon. On the guided hike rangers point out many native plants along the way that were used for food or medicine, including barrel and cholla cactus, creosote bush and brittlebush, mesquite, and cat's claw acacia. A stream flows for most of the year in the upper portion of the

canyon. The creek plunges over Tahquitz Falls at the top of the trail into a deep pool, 1 mile uphill from the visitor center. The Cahuilla people believe that this is a place of power that rejuvenates and energizes. After enjoying the waterfall, continue back along the loop trail.

Waterfall at the top of the Tahquitz Canyon trail

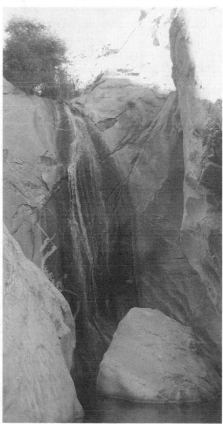

trip 11.7 Andreas Canyon

Distance	1 mile (loop)
Hiking Time	30–45 minutes
Elevation Gain	200′
Difficulty	Easy
Trail Use	Good for children
Best Times	September–May, 8 A.M.–5 P.M.
Agency	Agua Caliente Band of Cahuilla Indians
Optional Map	*Indian Canyons* or *Santa Rosa and San Jacinto Mountains National Monument*

see map on p. 237

DIRECTIONS From Interstate 10, take Highway 111 south into Palm Springs. The road changes name to North Palm Canyon Dr., then South Palm Canyon Dr. Most lanes turn left to become East Palm Canyon, but stay right (straight) and continue on South Palm Canyon Dr. Follow South Palm Canyon Dr. 2.8 miles to the Indian Canyons tollgate. Beyond the gate, immediately turn right and follow Andreas Canyon Rd. for 0.8 mile to its end at the Andreas Canyon parking area.

Andreas Canyon contains the world's second largest California fan palm oasis and is the ancestral home of the Paniktum clan of the Agua Caliente Band of Cahuilla Indians. This short trail follows Andreas Creek through the palm-filled canyon for a half mile, then returns along the south rim with views into the canyon. Friday through Sunday at 1 P.M., rangers lead interpretive hikes through the canyon for a nominal fee. Inquire at the entrance station for more information and to confirm times.

Before starting the hike, make sure to examine the rock mortars in which the Cahuilla Indians once ground their food; they are located adjacent to the parking lot. The trail leads west from the parking lot along the creek beneath the dramatic

California Fan Palms (*Washingtonia filifera*) in Andreas Canyon

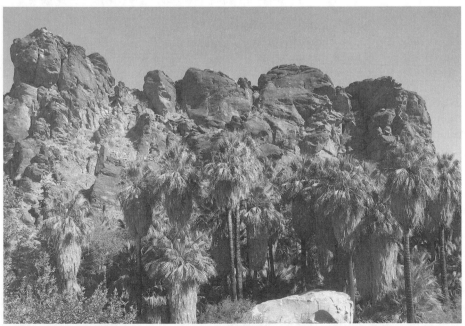

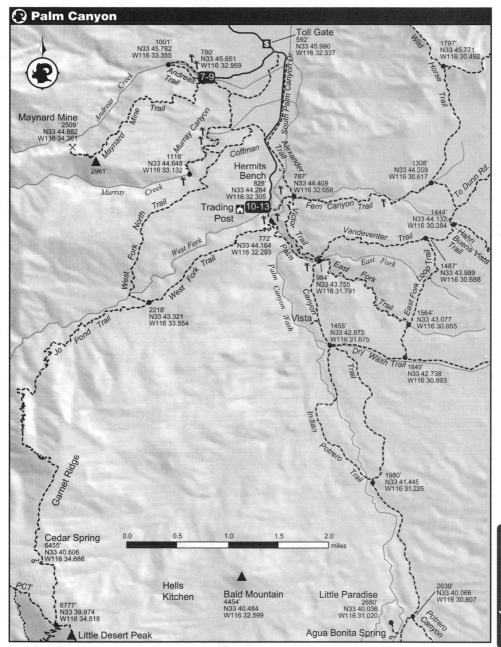

Palm Canyon

Toll Gate
592'
N33 45.990
W116 32.337

1001'
N33 45.782
W116 33.355

780'
N33 45.651
W116 32.959

7-9

Andreas
Trail

1797'
N33 45.771
W116 30.492

Wild Horse Trail

Andreas Creek

Trail

Maynard Mine
2509'
N33 44.882
W116 34.361

Maynard Mine Trail

Murray Canyon

Coffman

1118'
N33 44.648
W116 33.132

2961'

Hermits
Bench
828'
N33 44.284
W116 32.305

Alexander Trail

787'
N33 44.409
W116 32.058

1308'
N33 44.559
W116 30.617

To Dunn Rd.

Murray Creek Trail

Trading
Post

10-13

Fern Canyon Trail

1444'
N33 44.132
W116 30.384

Hahn Buena Vista Trail

West Fork North Trail

West Fork

772'
N33 44.164
W116 32.293

Victor Trail

Palm

Vandeventer Trail

East Fork Loop Trail

1487'
N33 43.989
W116 30.688

West Fork Trail

Palm Canyon Wash

East Fork

East Fork

984'
N33 43.755
W116 31.791

Trail

1564'
N33 43.077
W116 30.855

2218'
N33 43.321
W116 33.554

Jo Pond Trail

Vista

Canyon

1455'
N33 42.873
W116 31.675

Dry Wash Trail

1649'
N33 42.738
W116 30.893

Trail

Indian Potrero Trail

1980'
N33 41.445
W116 31.225

Garnet Ridge

Cedar Spring
6455'
N33 40.606
W116 34.686

0.0   0.5   1.0   1.5   2.0
miles

PCT

Hells
Kitchen

Bald Mountain
4454'
N33 40.484
W116 32.599

Little Paradise
2680'
N33 40.036
W116 31.020

2639'
N33 40.066
W116 30.807

6777'
N33 39.974
W116 34.518

Little Desert Peak

Agua Bonita Spring

Potrero Canyon

metamorphic schist cliffs making up the north wall of the canyon. In 0.1 mile, steps lead down to the left to a seductively charming pool. Continue 0.4 mile to a fence marking the abrupt end of the trail. The trail then crosses the creek and climbs onto the south flank of the canyon where there are lovely views, and then returns to the parking area.

trip 11.8 Murray Canyon

Distance	4 miles (out-and-back)
Hiking Time	2 hours
Elevation Gain	500 feet
Difficulty	Moderate
Trail Use	Equestrians
Best Times	October–May, 8 A.M.–5 P.M.
Agency	Agua Caliente Band of Cahuilla Indians
Optional Map	*Indian Canyons* or *Santa Rosa and San Jacinto Mountains National Monument*

see map on p. 237

DIRECTIONS From Interstate 10, take Highway 111 south into Palm Springs. The road changes name to North Palm Canyon Dr., then South Palm Canyon Dr. Most lanes turn left to become East Palm Canyon, but stay right (straight) and continue on South Palm Canyon Dr. Follow South Palm Canyon Dr. 2.8 miles to the Indian Canyons tollgate. Beyond the gate, immediately turn right and follow Andreas Canyon Rd. for 0.8 mile to the Andreas Canyon parking area. Turn left., cross a bridge, pass the Bent Palm Picnic Area, and park at the Murray Canyon trailhead in 0.2 mile.

Murray Canyon is named for the Scottish rancher, Welwood Murray, who founded the Palm Springs Hotel in 1887 and brought attention to the area as a spa and resort. The canyon cuts a groove down the rugged eastern slope of the Desert Divide. The trail ends at the Seven Sisters, a series of stone pools with a 12-foot waterfall. Murray Creek runs through the winter and spring. The trail crosses the creek a dozen times and the rocks can be slippery so a trekking pole is helpful; this trip is not recommended for those unsure of their balance. Murray Canyon is one of our favorite hikes of its length in the area. The falls are a great destination for a picnic, but don't expect to find solitude on this popular trail.

Follow the trail south across the desert at the base of a ridge past brittlebushes and creosote. In 0.2 mile, pass the Andreas Canyon South trail on your left. In another 0.5 mile, make a switchback down to cross Murray Creek at a palm oasis. On the far side, pass another junction on the left with the West Fork North Trail. In 0.3 mile, reach the mouth of Murray Canyon.

The trail follows the winding canyon, repeatedly crossing the creek. The California fan palms and honey mesquite bushes growing along the creek were important sources of food for the Cahuilla Indians. In 0.4 mile, reach a junction on the left with the Coffman Trail, which leads over the ridge out of the canyon. Just beyond, find a hitching line. Equestrians should leave their horses here because the last half mile of the canyon is unsuitable for riding. After negotiating some steep climbs and slick rocks, arrive at the waterfall at trail's end.

Waterfalls in Murray Canyon

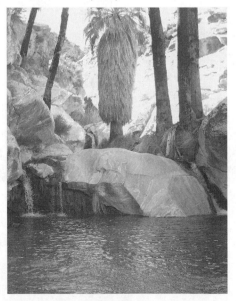

trip 11.9 Maynard Mine

Distance	6 miles (out-and-back)
Hiking Time	4 hours
Elevation Gain	2400 feet
Difficulty	Strenuous
Best Times	October–April, 8 A.M.–5 P.M.
Agency	Agua Caliente Band of Cahuilla Indians
Optional Map	*Indian Canyons* or *Santa Rosa and San Jacinto Mountains National Monument*

see map on p. 237

DIRECTIONS From Interstate 10, take Highway 111 south into Palm Springs. The road changes name to North Palm Canyon Dr., then South Palm Canyon Dr. Most lanes turn left to become East Palm Canyon, but stay right (straight) and continue on South Palm Canyon Dr. Follow South Palm Canyon Dr. 2.8 miles to the Indian Canyons tollgate. Beyond the gate, immediately turn right and follow Andreas Canyon Rd. for 0.8 mile to its end at the Andreas Canyon parking area.

Jim Maynard established a small tungsten mine on the narrow ridge between Andreas and Murray Canyons during World War II. This trip makes a steep climb to the mine site, offering a vigorous workout and sweeping views. Go on a cool day.

From the parking area, hike south across a bridge over Andreas Creek. Immediately beyond, the road turns left, but a sign marks the Maynard Mine Trail leading straight. The trail passes through a grove of honey mesquite, then switchbacks unrelentingly up the brittlebush-covered slopes. In 2.5 miles, it passes along the north side of Peak 2961′. The trail then plunges almost 500 feet down the narrow ridge to the west to its signed terminus.

Turn right and walk about 100 feet down the north slope toward Andreas Canyon to the site of Maynard's excavation. You will find the small adit in the hillside above a clearing. The gasoline engine nearby was brought to the site in pieces on muleback.

Maynard Mine

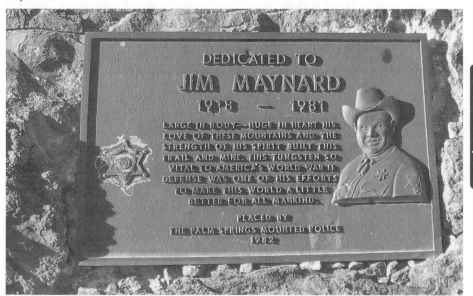

trip **11.10** Lower Palm Canyon

Distance	2.6 miles (loop)
Hiking Time	1.5 hours
Elevation Gain	500′
Difficulty	Easy
Trail Use	Good for children
Best Times	September–May, 8 A.M.–5 P.M.
Agency	Agua Caliente Band of Cahuilla Indians
Recommended Map	*Indian Canyons* or *Santa Rosa and San Jacinto Mountains National Monument*

see map on p. 237

DIRECTIONS From Interstate 10, take Highway 111 south into Palm Springs. The road changes name to North Palm Canyon Dr., then South Palm Canyon Dr. Most lanes turn left to become East Palm Canyon, but stay right (straight) and continue on South Palm Canyon Dr. Follow South Palm Canyon Dr. 2.8 miles to the Indian Canyons tollgate. Beyond the gate, continue 2.5 miles and park at Hermits Bench adjacent to the Trading Post.

Palm Canyon contains the world's largest California palm oasis and is the ancestral home of the Atcitcem Clan of the Agua Caliente Band of Cahuilla Indians, who have lived here for countless centuries. The oasis is one of the most spectacular sights in the Palm Springs vicinity. If you can only see only one of the many oases described in this book, choose Palm Canyon. The tribe charges a modest admission fee, which supports rangers and trail maintenance. Palm Canyon extends 15 miles all the way up to Highway 74 high in the Santa Rosa Moun-

tains, but the first mile has many of the best sights. This loop starts at the road's end on Hermits Bench, follows the floor of the canyon south for 1 mile through the palms, and then returns via the Victor Trail along a ridge overlooking the canyon.

There is a fine view of Palm Canyon from the trailhead on Hermits Bench near the Trading Post. Follow the Palm Canyon Trail that switchbacks down into the canyon to the south. You can enjoy a snack at the picnic tables beneath the magnificent trees. As you explore, keep an eye out for the

Lower Palm Canyon

stone mortars where Cahuilla women once ground their food near the stream's edge.

In 0.2 mile, reach a signed junction with the West Fork Trail at the south end of the main oasis. Continue south on the Palm Canyon Trail along the stream, passing a warm spring. In 1 mile, come to a second large oasis and a complex trail junction. Palm Canyon continues south. If you want a longer ramble, you can follow it as far as you choose before returning. But this loop turns hard left and joins the Victor Trail, which climbs up on to the ridge immediately east of Palm Canyon. Watch for trail signs and take care not to mistakenly follow the Vandeventer or East Fork trails instead.

The stunning Victor Trail was dedicated in 1974 in memory of John Victor, father of the dedicated Desert Rider, Laine Victor.

The vegetation abruptly changes as you climb out of the canyon. Teddy bear cholla and barrel cacti are scattered among the creosote bushes and brittlebushes on the dry hillsides. The rocky trail leads north for a mile overlooking Palm Canyon, then descends to another junction with the Fern Canyon and Alexander Trails. Turn left (west) and follow a trail across the creek. At the next junction with the Palm Canyon Trail, turn right and climb to the Trading Post parking area.

trip 11.11 Fern Canyon

Distance	6.5 miles (loop)
Hiking Time	3 hours
Elevation Gain	1000'
Difficulty	Moderate
Trail Use	Equestrians
Best Times	October–May, 8 A.M.–5 P.M.
Agency	Agua Caliente Band of Cahuilla Indians
Recommended Map	Indian Canyons or Santa Rosa and San Jacinto Mountains National Monument

see map on p. 237

DIRECTIONS From Interstate 10, take Highway 111 south into Palm Springs. The road changes name to North Palm Canyon Dr., then South Palm Canyon Dr. Most lanes turn left to become East Palm Canyon, but stay right (straight) and continue on South Palm Canyon Dr. Follow South Palm Canyon Dr. 2.8 miles to the Indian Canyons tollgate. Beyond the gate, continue 2.5 miles and park at Hermits Bench adjacent to the Trading Post.

Fern Canyon is named for a wall where seeping water once supported a vertical garden of maidenhair ferns. In this drier time, there are fewer ferns, but the canyon is still home to a pleasant oasis. This loop hike is a good way to see many of Palm Canyon's most notable attractions with only a moderate amount of hiking. In addition to the sandy wash and oasis of Fern Canyon, this trip features views down into the huge Palm Canyon oasis and a ridge hike through fields of barrel and teddy bear cholla cacti.

From Hermits Bench, walk east on a gated dirt road to a kiosk marking the start of the Fern Canyon, Victor, and Alexander Trails. Follow the trail north and east to a T-junction. The right fork leads to the main Palm Canyon Oasis, but this trip turns left, crosses Palm Canyon, and climbs over a low ridge to a four-way junction at a bend in Wentworth Canyon, 0.4 mile from Hermits Bench. The Victor Trail leads to the right. The Alexander Trail, used mostly by equestrians, leads left. But this trip goes straight ahead up Wentworth Canyon, which is now better known as Fern Canyon.

The Fern Canyon Trail follows the sandy wash east up the canyon. It then briefly

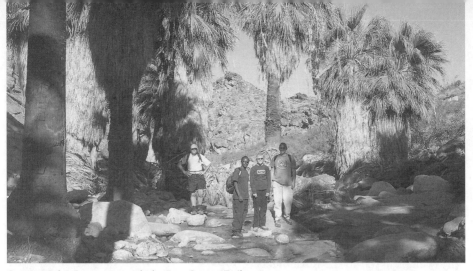

Crossing Palm Canyon to reach the Fern Canyon Trail

leaves the wash and climbs steeply up a ridge before dropping down to the fern wall near another small oasis. There are also good views of Murray Hill to the north.

Reach a series of signed junctions with connector trails. At each junction, stay right and wind around to the south, then west. Pass the Wild Horse Trail, Dunn Road Trail, Hahn Buena Vista Trail, and East Fork Loop Trail as you climb out of the wash and onto a broad ridge studded with spectacular cactus. Your trail changes its name to Vandeventer, and finally descends to a trail junction above a large palm oasis.

You can choose either of two paths back to the Trading Post. The 1-mile Palm Canyon Trail follows the canyon bottom through the enormous oasis, while the 1.6-mile Victor Trail follows the east rim of the canyon and offers sweeping vistas.

To take the Palm Canyon Trail (see Trip 11.10), turn left, walk 220 feet to a second junction, then turn right and descend Palm Canyon for a mile. At a picnic area in the main oasis, follow a path up the hill to the Trading Post.

To take the Victor Trail, turn right and follow the trail along the ridgeline for 1.2 miles, then down into a dry wash where you reach a junction with the Fern Canyon and Alexander Trails where you started this trip. Turn left (west) and follow signs 0.4 mile back to the Trading Post.

Vandeventer Trail

photo by Joe Sheehy

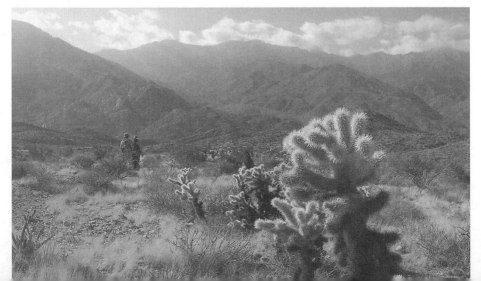

trip 11.12 **Pines-to-Palms**

Distance	15 miles (one-way)
Hiking Time	7 hours
Elevation Loss	3500'
Difficulty	Strenuous
Trail Use	Equestrians, suitable for backpacking
Best Times	October–March
Agency	Agua Caliente Band of Cahuilla Indians
Required Map	*Santa Rosa and San Jacinto Mountains National Monument* or *Palm View Peak, Butterfly Peak, Toro Peak 7.5'*

see maps on pp. 237, 248 & 270

DIRECTIONS This trip requires a car shuttle between Pinyon Pines and Hermits Bench. Unfortunately, Hermits Bench and the Indian Canyons are only open 8 A.M.–5 P.M., so unless you can arrange for somebody else to pick you up or leave your car outside the tollgate, you must hike quickly.

Position one car where you will emerge at Hermits Bench. From Interstate 10, take Highway 111 south into Palm Springs. The road changes name to North Palm Canyon Dr., then South Palm Canyon Dr. Most lanes turn left to become East Palm Canyon, but stay right (straight) and continue on South Palm Canyon Dr. Follow South Palm Canyon Dr. 2.8 miles to the tollgate at the entrance to the Indian Canyons. Notify the ranger at the gate if you expect that you might be out after 5 P.M. Beyond the gate, continue 2.5 miles to Hermits Bench.

To reach the upper trailhead, return to the tollgate and continue north up South Palm Canyon Dr. until you can turn right on East Palm Canyon Dr., which becomes Highway 111. Go east and southeast 11 miles to Highway 74, then turn right and follow Highway 74 for 18 miles. Just past mile marker 074 RIV 77.85, turn right on Pine View Dr. and proceed 0.2 mile to the end of the paved road. This shuttle takes about 45 minutes.

Palm Canyon should be on the to-do list of every serious Southern California hiker. The canyon separates the San Jacinto Mountains and Desert Divide on the west from the Santa Rosa Mountains on the east and offers magnificent scenery in all directions. As the canyon descends from the pinyon pines of the mountains to the cacti of the desert, it takes you past most of the Seussian plant life of the Upper and Lower Sonoran zones. The enormous palm oasis at the bottom of the trail is a fitting conclusion to the long but rewarding day. Some hikers prefer doing this trip in the uphill direction for more exercise. This can also be done as a backpacking trip, but there is no camping in the northern half of the canyon on Reservation land. The boundary between National Forest and Reservation land is about a mile north of Agua Bonita Spring.

See the *Toro Peak* map on page 270 for details about the southern end of the trail. From the parking area on Pine View Dr.,

walk north up a dirt road. In 0.1 mile, veer right at a blank steel trail marker. Hike north through ribbonwoods and chaparral, enjoying the sweeping views of the upper reaches of Palm Canyon. In 1.3 miles reach a signed four-way junction. A dirt road leads right. A trail leads left down into the bottom of Palm Canyon, while jeep tracks leads straight north along the ridge. The ridge route north is preferable because the canyon trail is overgrown and more difficult to follow.

The trail hugs the rolling ridgeline, then switchbacks northeast down into Omstott Canyon. Turn left and follow the trail down the canyon. (If you are doing this hike in the opposite direction, beware: this junction can be hard to spot. It is easy to miss the point where the trail leaves Omstott Canyon. If you find yourself wandering up the canyon bottom, you've missed the turnoff.) Go around a bend and rejoin the canyon bottom trail at a post on the floor

Palm Springs and the Indian Canyons

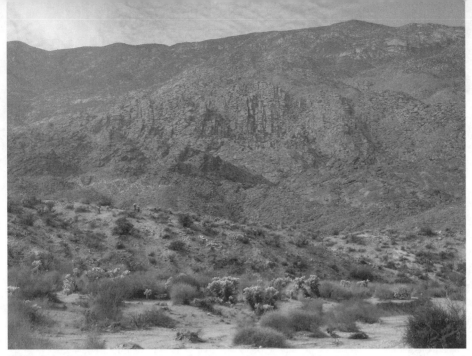

Middle Palm Canyon

of Palm Canyon, 2.5 miles from where the trails originally forked.

The next stretch of trail along Palm Canyon is narrow and faint in places. This land is used for cattle ranching and several gates control the cattle; close them behind you. Stay on Palm Canyon Trail. Within 0.2 mile, pass a fork with the unmaintained Live Oak Canyon Trail leading west. The Dutch Charlie Trail then cuts east to Dunn Rd., and soon after, the faint Oak Canyon Trail veers off southwest through the mesquite, rounds a bend to Hidden Falls, and eventually joins the Live Oak Canyon Trail. However, this trip continues north on the main Palm Canyon Trail.

The next section of the trail is notable for the abundance of yuccas that grow here. In 1.7 miles, reach a signed junction. Agua Bonita Spring is on the canyon bottom below to the west. Water is available here much of the year. Look for bedrock mortars where the Cahuilla once ground their food.

VARIATION

Adventurous hikers may scramble down to the creek at Agua Bonita and walk upstream for a few dozen paces until it is possible to trudge up the west slope, then turn right and follow a rocky draw north to Little Paradise. Unfortunately, Little Paradise is now a misnomer; all that remains after the Palm Canyon Fire are a dead palm tree and some prickly bushes.

Past Agua Bonita Spring 0.3 mile, the Potrero Canyon Trail veers off to the right. Stay in Palm Canyon as it becomes deeper and takes on a rugged appearance. The rocks on the west side have a scale-like look as if they once belonged to a gigantic stone reptile; this area is known as Hell's Kitchen. In another 2 miles, come to a junction with the Indian Potrero Trail. Both Indian Potrero and Palm Canyon trails lead north, one on each side of Palm Canyon, and both are enjoyable. The Indian Potrero and Palm Canyon trails rejoin in 2 miles at a junction with the aptly named Dry Wash Trail, which leads east; the Palm Canyon Trail continues north.

In 1.0 mile past the Dry Wash Trail, come to an enormous palm oasis at the junction with the Victor, Vandeventer, and East Fork Trails. Stay left on the Palm Canyon Trail for another mile, passing many more palms before climbing up to Hermits Bench.

trip 11.13 Jo Pond Trail

Distance	16 miles (out-and-back), or 11.5 miles (one-way to Cedar Spring Trailhead)
Hiking Time	9 hours (out-and-back)
Elevation Gain	6200'
Difficulty	Strenuous
Trail Use	Equestrians
Best Times	October–November, March–April, 8 A.M.–5 P.M.
Agency	Agua Caliente Band of Cahuilla Indians
Recommended Map	*Santa Rosa and San Jacinto Mountains National Monument* or *Palm View Peak* 7.5'

see map on p. 237

DIRECTIONS From Interstate 10, take Highway 111 south into Palm Springs. The road changes name to North Palm Canyon Dr., then South Palm Canyon Dr. Most lanes turn left to become East Palm Canyon, but stay right (straight) and continue on South Palm Canyon Dr. After paying your admission fee at the Indian Canyons tollgate, drive south for 2.5 miles and park at the end of the road at Hermits Bench. If you are doing a one-way hike, start by arranging to leave a second vehicle at the Cedar Spring Trailhead. To reach the trailhead, drive east on Highway 111, then south, west, and back north on Highway 74 to the Garner Valley. Near mile marker 74 RIV 67.75, turn right (northeast) onto the paved Morris Ranch Rd. (6S53) and proceed 3.7 miles to the signed Cedar Spring Trailhead (4E17) on the right. If you reach Morris Ranch, you went 0.25 mile too far. The drive between the trailheads takes about one hour. (See Trip 10.5 and the map on page 206.)

The Jo Pond Trail, completed in 1994, connects Palm Canyon to the Desert Divide, relentlessly climbing Garnet Ridge to Cedar Spring. It does not pass a lake; rather, it was named for Mr. Pond, a member of the Desert Riders and a trail advocate in the Coachella Valley. Some consider it to be one of the most spectacular trails in the region. Beyond its length and steepness, the trail presents substantial logistical challenges. The tollgate at the Indian Canyons is only open from 8 A.M. to 5 P.M., so hiking up and back demands speed as well as stamina. By arranging a car shuttle from

Salton Sea and Santa Rosa Mountains from the Jo Pond Trail

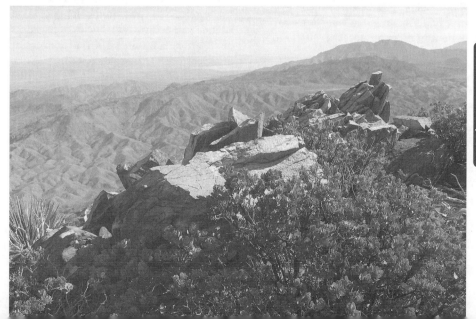

Palm Springs and the Indian Canyons

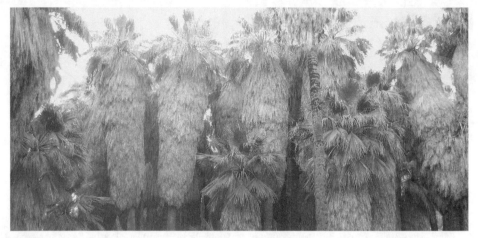

Palm Canyon Oasis

the Cedar Spring Trail, you can slightly shorten the trip and avoid the knee-pounding descent, but you must still leave time for the drive back to retrieve your vehicle before the gate is locked. Let a tribal ranger know about your plans because a search is initiated if vehicles are still present when the gate closes. If you are unsure of your ability to get back in time, notify the tribal rangers at (760) 699-6800. Also, pay special attention to the weather conditions. While Palm Canyon is roasting under an unrelenting sun, the Desert Divide may be covered in snow and ice. The north-facing Garnet Ridge holds snow at surprisingly low altitudes after a winter storm. An ice axe and crampons may be necessary if the upper part of the trail is icy.

From the trailhead, look southwest and identify the massive Garnet Ridge extending toward you from the Desert Divide. The prominent cliffs on the ridge are called the Palisades. Hike south from behind the Trading Post on the Palm Canyon Trail, descending into the enormous palm oasis in Palm Canyon. In 0.2 mile, reach a signed junction at the south end of the oasis. Turn right and switchback up the West Fork Trail. Good views of Palm Canyon and of the pointy Murray Hill open up as you climb. The boulders prominently show desert varnish, a mixture of clay with iron

and manganese oxide formed by chemical reactions on the surface of hot dry rocks. The hills are studded with barrel and cholla cacti. The trail climbs to the rim of the canyon and in 2 miles arrives at a signed junction.

Take the left fork, which is the start of the Jo Pond Trail. The trail is less-used and takes more care to follow. It follows a creek for another mile, then gradually veers away from the canyon and onto the toe of Garnet Ridge. Watch how the vegetation zones change from cactus to chaparral as you switchback up the ridge. Eventually, the grade relents as you gain the upper portion of the ridge and you cross fields of red rocks amidst the manzanitas. The trail then enters an open forest of black oaks and white firs, then arrives at Cedar Spring. The spring usually has water in the wetter months and there is room to camp beneath the shady trees. At this point, you have hiked 8.2 miles and gained 5900 feet of elevation.

If you left your car at Hermits Bench, retrace your steps. Alternatively, if you have a car shuttle, hike south another mile and 300 feet up to the crest of the Desert Divide, to a four-way junction. Take the Cedar Spring Trail straight ahead going southwest 2.3 miles down to your vehicle (see Trip 10.5).

chapter 12

Santa Rosa Mountains
National Monument

The Santa Rosa Mountains tumble south and east from Palm Springs toward the Salton Sea. The deep Palm Canyon separates the Santa Rosas from the San Jacinto Mountains. Toro Peak (8716´) crowns the range and is clad in a white snowy mantle for most of the winter. At first glance, the range might appear hot, dry, and desolate, but closer inspection reveals the Santa Rosas to be undiscovered gems of Southern California: the mountainsides are dotted with marvelous cacti and are home to the endangered peninsular bighorn sheep (*Ovis canadensis cremnobates*). Whether you have an hour at sunrise to jog the hills or a day in the fall or winter to trace ancient Indian footpaths across this remote wilderness, you will come to love this range more each visit.

Congress established the Santa Rosa and San Jacinto Mountains National Monument in 2000 to protect the outstanding natural and cultural resources of these mountains and to provide enduring opportunities for recreation. Spanning 272,000 acres, the land is administered by a wide variety of governmental agencies, the Agua Caliente Band of Cahuilla Indians, and private landowners. In general, the Forest Service is responsible for the higher mountains, the Bureau of Land Management is responsible for the desert regions, and the Agua Caliente band is responsible for Palm Canyon. Major portions of the Santa Rosa and San Jacinto Mountains are designated wilderness areas.

This chapter focuses on hikes in the Santa Rosa Mountains. The range is split

by Highway 74. North of the highway, an extensive trail network provides access from the Coachella Valley. The Desert Riders, an active equestrian organization, constructed many of the trails. Some trails trace the routes once followed by the Indians who crossed the mountains in search of food and commerce. Unfortunately, the region has lacked strong management to post signs, make maps, and concentrate traffic on well-defined routes; hence, a maze of unmarked social trails has developed over the years, making navigation challenging for those not familiar with the area. This is beginning to improve and the publication of the *Santa Rosa & San Jacinto Mountains National Monument* trail map in 2008 was a watershed event for hikers.

South of Highway 74 are the biggest peaks, notably Toro and Rabbit. The top of Toro Peak is on private tribal land and is closed to the public. It is of little interest anyway, because it has been bulldozed flat to mount a large antenna farm accessible by road. Rabbit Peak, on the other hand, is as wild and difficult as any peak in Southern California, and draws a steady flow of hardy hikers wishing to test their desert mettle. A few ancient Indian footpaths cross the wild country in the Southern Santa Rosas and are described in this chapter. There are other worthy peaks in the area, including Martinez Mtn., Sheep Mtn., and Rosa Point, accessed by long cross-country hikes; finding the best route is left to your ingenuity.

The Santa Rosa Mountains are one of the remaining homes for the endangered

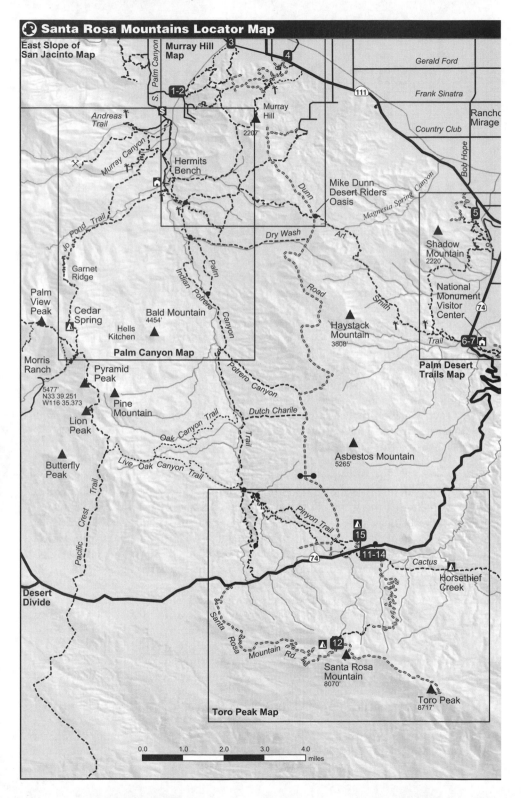

Santa Rosa Mountains Locator Map

East Slope of
San Jacinto Map

Murray Hill
Map

S. Palm Canyon

3

4

111

Gerald Ford

Frank Sinatra

1-2

Andreas
Trail

S

Murray
Hill
2207'

Country Club

Rancho
Mirage

Murray Canyon

Hermits
Bench

Mike Dunn
Desert Riders
Oasis

Dunn

Magnesia Spring Canyon

Bob Hope

5

Jo Pond Trail

Garnet
Ridge

Dry Wash

Art

Shadow
Mountain
2220'

National
Monument
Visitor
Center

74

Palm
View
Peak

Cedar
Spring

Bald Mountain
4454'

Hells
Kitchen

Palm Canyon Map

Indian Potrero

Palm

Canyon

Road

Smith

Haystack
Mountain
3808'

Trail

6-7

Palm Desert
Trails Map

Morris
Ranch

5477'
N33 39.251
W116 35.373

Pyramid
Peak

Pine
Mountain

Lion
Peak

Potrero Canyon

Oak Canyon Trail

Dutch Charile

Trail

Butterfly
Peak

Live Oak Canyon Trail

Pacific Crest Trail

Asbestos Mountain
5265'

Pinyon Trail

15

11-14

Cactus

Horsethief
Creek

Desert
Divide

74

Santa Rosa Mountain Rd.

12

Santa Rosa
Mountain
8070'

Toro Peak
8717'

Toro Peak Map

0.0   1.0   2.0   3.0   4.0
miles

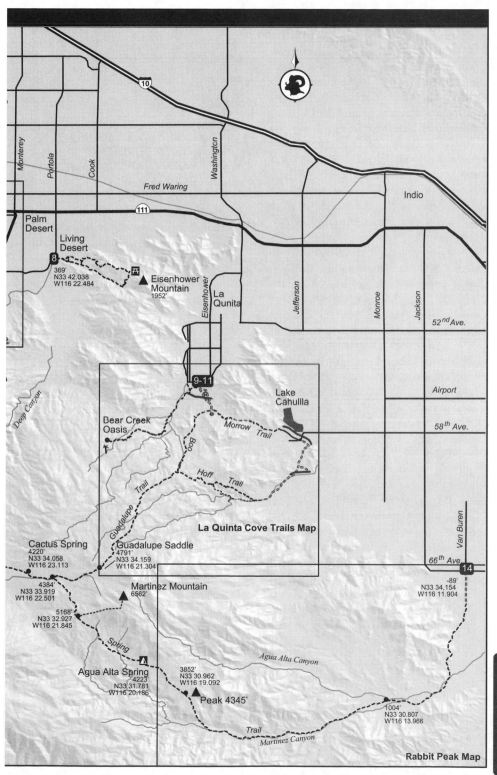

Palm Desert

Living Desert

8

369'
N33 42.038
W116 22.484

▲ Eisenhower Mountain
1952'

Fred Waring

111

Indio

La Quinta

Monterey

Portola

Cook

Washington

Eisenhower

Jefferson

Monroe

Jackson

52nd Ave.

9-11

Lake Cahullla

Airport

58th Ave.

Deep Canyon

Bear Creek Oasis

Morrow Trail

Boo

Hoff Trail

Guadalupe Trail

Van Buren

La Quinta Cove Trails Map

Cactus Spring
4220'
N33 34.058
W116 23.113

Guadalupe Saddle
4791'
N33 34.159
W116 21.304

66th Ave.

14

4384'
N33 33.919
W116 22.501

-89'
N33 34.154
W116 11.904

5168'
N33 32.927
W116 21.845

▲ Martinez Mountain
6562'

Spring

Agua Alta Canyon

Agua Alta Spring
4223'
N33 31.781
W116 20.186

3852'
N33 30.962
W116 19.092

▲ Peak 4345'

1004'
N33 30.807
W116 13.966

Trail

Martinez Canyon

Rabbit Peak Map

peninsular bighorn sheep. An estimated 350 of the majestic but shy animals roam the rocky desert slopes. Count yourself fortunate if you catch a fleeting glimpse of one during a season of hiking in these mountains. Their numbers had been steadily declining as human development encroached on their habitat; sustained efforts in recent years are starting to reverse this decline. Government agencies, including the Fish and Wildlife Service, BLM, and the California Department of Fish and Game, are researching ways to better protect the sheep. For more information about the peninsular bighorn sheep, visit www.bighorninstitute.org.

Hiking regulations in the National Monument have been changing in the past several years and are now based on the Coachella Valley Multiple Species Habitat Conservation Plan, adopted in 2008 to protect 240,000 acres of open space and 27 species, especially the bighorn sheep. Specific rules are detailed in each trip description. Most trails are now open year-round. A few trails that pass sensitive watering spots for bighorn sheep are closed during the hot season, June 15–September 30. Cross-country travel and camping are only allowed October 1–December 31 to avoid disturbing sheep during lambing season and the hot months. Dogs are prohibited on most trails because the sheep fear them as predators. Motorized vehicles are not allowed in the wilderness areas or on Dunn Rd. Travelers on trails entering sensitive areas will require free self-issued wilderness permits, available at the trailheads. These permits allow scientists to track trail use and its impact on sheep. At the time of this writing, the permit kiosks have not yet been

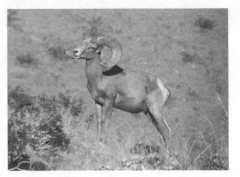

Peninsular bighorn sheep
Photograph reprinted with permission of the Bighorn Institute

constructed. Once they are built, there will be no quotas but failure to carry a permit can result in a citation. All of this information is subject to change based on on-going bighorn sheep research. Check at the trailheads for updated regulations.

The Sonoran Desert around the Coachella Valley is one of the hottest and driest zones in the United States. The Santa Rosa Mountains are similarly hot and dry; they are best visited from late fall through early spring. When much of the Inland Empire shivers under gloomy clouds or rain, the Santa Rosas are usually sunny and mild, perfect for hiking. Nevertheless, be ready for any weather. The desert is known for rapid changes of weather, and for rare but intense showers that will chill the unprepared and unleash flash floods down the narrow canyons. During hotter parts of the year, many of the shorter Santa Rosa hikes are still ideal at dawn, at sunset, and by full moon.

For more information, contact the Santa Rosa and San Jacinto Mountains National Monument Visitor Center. The visitor center also organizes hikes and wildflower walks; call for the current schedule of activities.

trip 12.1 Garstin Trail

Distance	2.5–3.6 miles (out-and-back, or loop)
Hiking Time	2 hours
Elevation Gain	1000'
Difficulty	Moderate
Trail Use	Equestrians
Best Times	October–April
Agency	Santa Rosa and San Jacinto Mountains National Monument
Optional Map	*Santa Rosa and San Jacinto Mountains National Monument* or *Palm Springs* 7.5' (trail not marked)

see map on p. 252

DIRECTIONS From Interstate 10, take Highway 111 south into Palm Springs. The road changes name to North Palm Canyon Dr., then South Palm Canyon Dr. Most lanes turn left to become East Palm Canyon, but stay right (straight) and continue on South Palm Canyon Dr. for 1.9 miles. Turn left on E. Bogart Trail and follow it 0.9 mile over the bridge across Palm Canyon Wash, then immediately turn left on Barona Rd. and park at the end.

The Garstin Trail is a short but steep trail that climbs from Palm Canyon Wash up to a stunning plateau beneath Murray Hill. It offers a vigorous workout and great views of the San Jacinto Mountains. It can be done as an out-and-back hike, or a slightly longer loop. Or you can link to any of the numerous trails on the plateau for an endless variety of longer rambles.

The trails in this area are conveniently located near the Smoke Tree Stables. Many of the trails were built by and named for members of the Desert Riders. The Garstin Trail is named for trail boss D.V. Garstin. The Henderson Trail is named for past president Earl Henderson. The Shannon Trail is named for Shannon Corliss, daughter of past president Ray Corliss. All of the trails are steep; beginning riders are better off staying in Palm Canyon Wash.

The trail starts at an unmarked post at the end of Barona and leads east. In 150 yards, it reaches a signed fork. The Henderson Trail veers left and heads northeast along the toe of the ridge, but turn right and follow the Garstin Trail up steep switchbacks hewn from the hillside. Your efforts are rewarded by steadily widening views to the west.

Shortly before reaching the top of the hill, the trail forks. Both paths run parallel and rejoin in 0.1 mile; the right fork follows the ridgeline and is recommended for its views. (This fork and merge is not shown on the map; the two parallel paths run too close together to distinguish.) Soon after, 1.2 miles from the start, come to a major junction with the Berns Trail on top of the ridge. Many hikers turn around here.

Top of the Garstin Trail

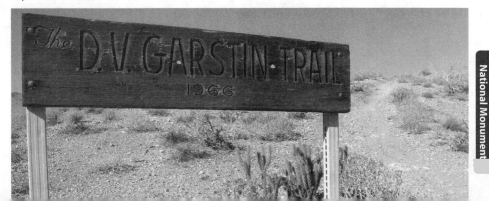

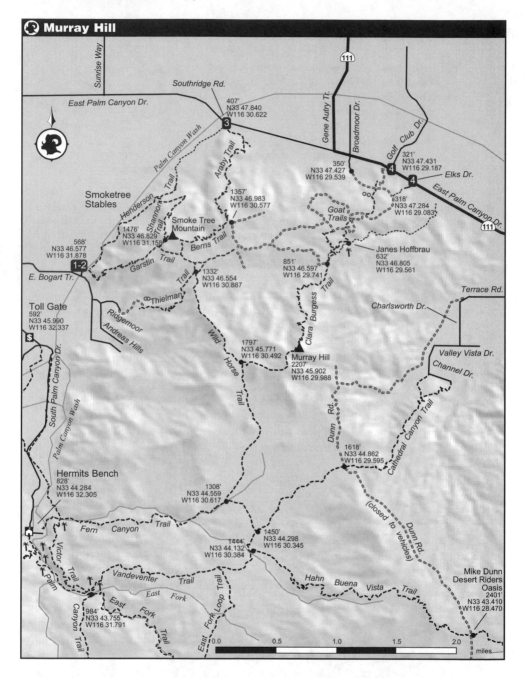

Murray Hill

Sunrise Way

Southridge Rd.

111

East Palm Canyon Dr.

407'
N33 47.840
W116 30.622

3

Gene Autry Tr.

Broadmoor Dr.

Golf Club Dr.

321'
N33 47.431
W116 29.187

Araby Trail

350'
N33 47.427
W116 29.539

4

Elks Dr.

4

318'
N33 47.284
W116 29.083

East Palm Canyon Dr.

111

Palm Canyon Wash

Smoketree Stables

Henderson Trail

Shannon Trail

1357'
N33 46.983
W116 30.577

Smoke Tree Mountain

Goat Trails

1476'
N33 46.829
W116 31.158

568'
N33 46.577
W116 31.878

1-2

Berns Trail

Garstin Trail

1332'
N33 46.554
W116 30.887

851'
N33 46.597
W116 29.741

Janes Hoffbrau
632'
N33 46.805
W116 29.561

Trail

Clara Burgess Trail

E. Bogart Tr.

Thielman

Charlsworth Dr.

Terrace Rd.

Toll Gate
592'
N33 45.990
W116 32.337

$

Ridgemoor

Andreas Hills

Wild Horse Trail

1797'
N33 45.771
W116 30.492

Murray Hill
2207'
N33 45.902
W116 29.988

Valley Vista Dr.

Channel Dr.

South Palm Canyon Dr.

Palm Canyon Wash

Dunn Rd.

Cathedral Canyon Trail

Hermits Bench
828'
N33 44.284
W116 32.305

1618'
N33 44.862
W116 29.595

1308'
N33 44.559
W116 30.617

(closed to vehicles)

Dunn Rd.

Fern   Canyon   Trail

1450'
N33 44.298
W116 30.345

1444'
N33 44.132
W116 30.384

Mike Dunn Desert Riders Oasis
2401'
N33 43.410
W116 28.470

Victor Trail

Vandeventer   Trail

East Fork Loop Trail

Hahn   Buena   Vista   Trail

East Fork

984'
N33 43.755
W116 31.791

Palm Canyon Trail

East Fork Trail

0.0   0.5   1.0   1.5   2.0

miles

ALTERNATIVE FINISHES

Hikers desiring a somewhat longer walk have two options.

(1) Continue straight 0.1 mile on the Berns Trail to another intersection with the Shannon Trail, then 0.1 mile farther to a high point on Smoke Tree Mtn. that offers outstanding 360-degree views. From here, either return the way you came or descend the Shannon Trail (0.9 mile), then turn left and follow the Henderson Trail 1.0 mile back to the start.

(2) Turn right and follow the Garstin Trail 0.5 mile to its end, passing two unmarked connector trails to the left along the way. There is a large sign for the Garstin Trail at the four-way junction at the end. Turn right and follow the unmarked Thielman Trail 1.0 mile southwest down to a dirt road near two water tanks. Turn right on the road and continue 0.3 mile down to a gate at the end of the paved Ridgemore Dr. in the posh Andreas Hills neighborhood. Follow this road down to its end, then make a right on Andreas Hills and another right on Bogart. Shortly before the bridge, turn right on Barona to regain the trailhead. This variation involves 0.6 mile of walking through the neighborhood.

---

trip 12.2 Murray Hill

Distance	7 miles (out-and-back)
Hiking Time	5 hours
Elevation Gain	1700'
Difficulty	Strenuous
Trail Use	Equestrians
Best Times	October–March
Agency	Santa Rosa and San Jacinto Mountains National Monument
Recommended Map	Santa Rosa and San Jacinto Mountains National Monument or Palm Springs, Cathedral City 7.5' (trail not marked)

see map on p. 252

DIRECTIONS From Interstate 10, take Highway 111 south into Palm Springs. The road changes name to North Palm Canyon Dr., then South Palm Canyon Dr. Most lanes turn left to become East Palm Canyon, but stay right (straight) and continue on South Palm Canyon Dr. for 1.9 miles. Turn left on E. Bogart Trail and follow it 0.9 mile over the bridge across Palm Canyon Wash, then immediately turn left on Barona Rd. and park at the end.

Prominent from many directions, the pyramid-shaped Murray Hill offers panoramic views across the southern Santa Rosa Mountains. It is best climbed on a clear, cool day. Its rather diminutive name belies the fact that Murray Hill is a steep and strenuous peak that challenges and rewards the intrepid explorer. Murray Hill is named for the Scottish rancher, Welwood Murray, who founded the Palm Springs Hotel in 1887 and drew attention to the area as a spa and resort. Murray Hill can be approached from the west, north, or south. This trip describes the western approach via the Garstin and Wild Horse Trails, but one can make an enjoyable longer loop or one-way trip in combination with the other routes.

The trail starts at an unmarked post at the end of Barona and leads east. In 150 yards, it reaches a signed fork. The Henderson Trail veers left and heads northeast along the toe of the ridge, but turn right and follow the Garstin Trail up steep switchbacks hewn from the hillside. Your efforts are rewarded by steadily widening views to the west.

Shortly before reaching the top of the hill, the trail forks. Both paths run parallel and rejoin in 0.1 mile; the right fork follows the ridgeline and is recommended for its views. Soon after, 1.2 miles from the start, come to a junction with the Berns Trail on top of the ridge.

From here, Murray Hill is clearly visible looming to the southeast. Your goal is to reach the Wild Horse Trail, which climbs the western ridge of the peak. Unfortunately, this area contains a maze of poorly marked trails. Turn right and head toward

Murray Hill. In 0.3 mile, stay right at a fork. Just beyond, at a four-way junction with the Thielman Trail, go straight onto the Wild Horse Trail.

Follow the Wild Horse Trail 1.2 miles up the ridge to a junction. The right fork drops down to Fern Canyon, but this trip stays left onto the Clara Burgess Trail, which follows the spectacular ridgeline 0.8 mile to the summit of Murray Hill. Return the way you came.

ALTERNATIVE FINISHES

Alternatively, descend to the north or south. The Clara Burgess Trail leads 1.4 miles north to a large metal sign marking its start near a wash. From here, you can turn left and follow a system of dirt roads back to the Garstin Trail, or can continue down the wash to Jane's Hoffbrau Oasis and the confusing network of Goat Trails (see Trip 12.4). If, instead, you return to the Wild Horse Trail (sometimes faint) and go south for 1.6 miles, you can reach the Fern Can-

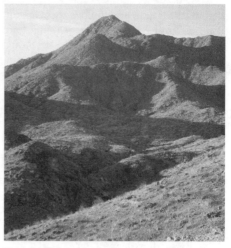

Murray Hill from the north

yon Trail (see Trip 11.11). The Fern Canyon Trail leads back to Hermits Bench. If you don't have a ride waiting there, you can slog about 3 miles down the sandy Palm Canyon Wash back to the Garstin Trailhead.

---

trip 12.3 Araby Trail

Distance	3.2 miles (out-and-back), or 4.6 miles (loop)
Hiking Time	2–3 hours
Elevation Gain	1000' to 1400'
Difficulty	Moderate
Trail Use	Equestrians
Best Times	October–April, daylight hours only
Agency	Santa Rosa and San Jacinto Mountains National Monument
Optional Map	*Santa Rosa and San Jacinto Mountains National Monument* or *Palm Springs* 7.5' (trail not marked)

see map on p. 252

DIRECTIONS From Interstate 10, take Highway 111 south into Palm Springs. The road changes name to North Palm Canyon Dr., then South Palm Canyon Dr. It then veers left and changes name to East Palm Canyon Dr. Drive 2.2 miles on East Palm Canyon Dr., cross a bridge over the wide Palm Canyon Wash, and turn right at a sign labeled Rimcrest/Southridge Rd. Make an immediate right and park in a dirt lot. Do not continue driving up the private road.

The Araby Trail climbs the canyon overlooking the modernistic Bob Hope estate on the southern edge of Palm Springs and offers close-up views of the comedian's sprawling ridge top compound. Actor Steven McQueen later owned the home until

his death in 1980. The Palm Springs International Airport is close by and you are likely to see the private jets of the rich and famous landing and departing as you hike. The hike also offers an accessible taste of the Santa Rosa Mountains with their rocky canyons, steep slopes, and fragile vegetation. The Araby Trail is a popular exercise hike for locals because it is short, steep, and close to town. The area is also a favorite of equestrians, especially the Desert Riders, who built many of the trails. The Santa Rosa Mountains are a bighorn sheep sanctuary, so dogs are not allowed. The trail is closed from dusk to dawn.

From the car, walk 100 feet up the private road to the signed Araby Trailhead on the left. The first part of the trail leads above a trailer park and below a row of homes. Respect the owners and do not stray from the trail. After passing above a pool area in the trailer park, the trail forks. The left fork descends to the trailer park. Take the marked right fork, which switchbacks up. It passes near a bend in the private road; then, a faint trail leads left 150 feet to a small hill with great views over Palm Springs and up to the Bob Hope estate and the mountains above. The main trail continues up the west slope of the canyon toward the estate, then cuts across the floor of the canyon over to the east slope. It climbs steeply up to gain the ridge at the head of the canyon, where large signs mark the junction with the Berns Trail. Climb the small hills to your left or right for a grand view. The homes, trees, and golf courses of Palm Springs sprawl across the valley to the north. The steep slopes of San Jacinto tower into the

sky to the west. And the pointy desert summit of Murray Hill draws your eye as you look southward into the Santa Rosa Mountains. At this point, you have hiked 1.6 miles and climbed 1000 feet. Enjoy the scenery and retrace your steps to the car.

ALTERNATIVE FINISH

For a 1.5-mile longer loop, turn right and walk 100 feet to a large metal sign indicating the start of the Berns Trail. At the sign, a short trail to the right leads up a hill with a good view, but the main Berns Trail stays left, switchbacks westward down into a canyon, and then switchbacks up the hill on the other side. The trail continues westward atop a low ridge with views southwest into the Indian Canyons. Pass an unmarked junction leading south to the Wild Horse Trail and climb another small hill (Smoke Tree Mtn.) marked with a huge cairn, 0.9 mile and 400 feet up from the end of the Araby Trail. This portion of the trail is notable for its assortment of barrel and cholla cacti. Beyond the hill is another signed junction. Turn right (north) on the Shannon Trail; the Garstin Trail leads down to the southwest (see Trip 12.1).

The Shannon Trail descends northward along the ridge just west of the Bob Hope estate and provides more views of the elaborate compound. It then switchbacks down the west slope of the ridge to a junction

Bob Hope's estate from the Araby Trail

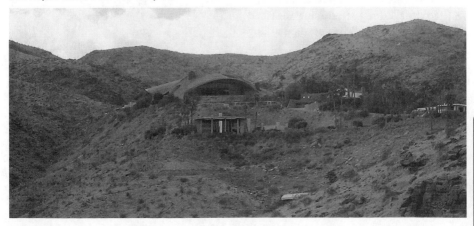

with the Henderson Trail (1 mile). Turn right (northeast) again and follow the Henderson Trail 0.5 mile past a house down to the valley floor. Cross a paved road to reach the huge Palm Canyon Wash (dry most of the year). Turn right and walk 0.6 mile northeast along the sandy floor of the wash toward the bridge where East Palm Canyon Rd. crosses the wash. Immediately before reaching the bridge, exit the right side of the wash and climb up to your car.

trip 12.4 Jane's Hoffbrau Oasis

Distance	2 miles (out-and-back)
Hiking Time	1 hour
Elevation Gain	700'
Difficulty	Moderate
Best Times	October–March
Agency	Santa Rosa and San Jacinto Mountains National Monument
Optional Map	*Santa Rosa and San Jacinto Mountains National Monument* or *Cathedral City* 7.5' (trail not marked)

see map on p. 252

DIRECTIONS There are two nearby trailheads for this hike. Both are located off East Palm Canyon Dr. (Highway 111) in Palm Springs 0.8 mile east of Gene Autry Trail. The recommended start is to turn south into a dirt clearing next to a restaurant at the traffic light opposite Golf Club Dr. Park in the dirt near the huge concrete storm drain. This area may be closed by future development. If so, continue east one short block and turn south on Elks Dr. Park behind the Elks Lodge by the gully leading south into the hills.

Tucked away in the sheer-walled Eagle Canyon scarcely a stone's throw from Palm Springs, Jane's Hoffbrau Oasis is certain to surprise and delight. It is named for Jane Lykken Hoff, a former president of the Desert Riders equestrian group. The oasis is located near the unmarked tangle of roads and bike paths called the Goat Trails, so it requires some navigational skills to locate.

If you are starting opposite Golf Club Dr., look for a dirt road leading west and then south up the hill behind the parking area. In 0.3 mile, the road switchbacks and ends part way up the hill. Look for a trail continuing south. It soon crosses another dirt road near some water tanks, then climbs 0.3 mile to a saddle where it meets dirt roads leading in three directions.

If you are starting behind the Elks Lodge, the unmarked and inauspicious route leads up the steep boulder and trash-strewn gully south of the parking lot. In 0.1 mile, reach a jeep road at the top of the gully. Turn left and follow the road south, then west 0.5

Jane's Hoffbrau Oasis

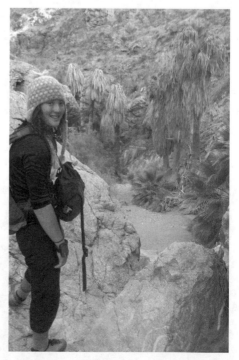

mile to the road junction on the saddle mentioned in the previous paragraph.

There are good views toward San Jacinto from the saddle. Take the dirt road leading south around a hill. In 0.1 mile, reach a T-junction near the top of a ravine. Look for a narrow trail on the far side of the junction shortcutting southwest around the right side of a hill. Follow it 0.1 mile to where it rejoins the road. Just west of this point, look for another trail leading south down into the dramatic Eagle Canyon. Follow this trail 0.2 mile to a point immediately overlooking Jane's Hoffbrau Oasis. Turn left and switchback down to the oasis on the canyon floor. You can't order a pastrami sandwich here, but you can enjoy your own snacks beneath the palms or beside a dry waterfall. Return the way you came.

ALTERNATIVE FINISHES

It is fun to explore Eagle Canyon or some of the Goat Trails. Those desiring a longer hike can continue up Murray Hill (see Trip 12.2). The Clara Burgess Trail to Murray Hill starts farther up Eagle Canyon. You can return to the trail just above the oasis and follow it southwest. If you enjoy scrambling, you can head directly up the canyon floor. This involves third-class climbing up a dry waterfall above the oasis, followed by easier scrambling up short dry falls farther up the canyon.

trip 12.5 Bump and Grind Trail

Distance	3 miles
Hiking Time	2 hours
Elevation Gain	800′
Difficulty	Moderate
Trail Use	Equestrians, cyclists
Best Times	Year-round, hot in summer
Agency	Santa Rosa and San Jacinto Mountains National Monument
Optional Map	*Santa Rosa and San Jacinto Mountains National Monument* or *Rancho Mirage 7.5′* (trail not marked)

see map on p. 258

DIRECTIONS From Highway 111 in Palm Desert between Bob Hope Dr. and Fred Waring Dr., turn south onto Painters Path. Proceed 0.5 mile to the trailhead and park on the side of the road behind Desert Crossing Shopping Center, taking care to observe the parking restrictions.

The Bump and Grind Trail, also known as the Desert Mirage Trail, is an extremely popular trail because it is so conveniently located in town and offers a vigorous workout over a short distance. On a pleasant weekend, you are likely to meet hundreds of hikers and joggers getting their exercise on the trail, which climbs the northern flank of Shadow Mtn. The trail has been rerouted from its former start in Rancho Mirage because of private property issues. The upper portion crosses the Magnesia Spring Ecological Reserve, and dogs are not allowed, even though you may see this rule being flagrantly violated. Some portions of the trail are quite steep, so shoes with good tread are recommended.

The rerouted loop begins at the Mike Schuler Trailhead. To make a counterclockwise loop, take the right fork. Climbing beneath the impressive varnished granite outcrops, the trail travels up well-built switchbacks to a notch on a ridge. Creosote bushes and brittlebushes cling to the sunbaked and sparsely vegetated hills. Continue across the next canyon above a nursery to reach the next ridge, 0.9 mile from the start.

Palm Desert Trails

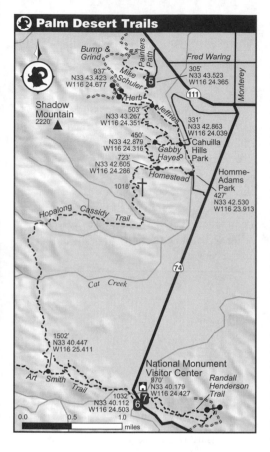

Here, you meet a dirt road, whose cut forms a deep scar on the slope.

The road rises up from the former trailhead in Rancho Mirage. This portion was named Bump and Grind by the cyclists who toil up the hill. Several side trails shortcut bends in the road. On a clear day, you will have splendid views over the Coachella Valley. San Jacinto and San Gorgonio to the west are capped with snow in the winter and spring. The Little San Bernardino Mountains to the north form a wall on the edge of Joshua Tree National Park. Countless bright green golf courses dot the arid Palm Springs region. In another 0.9 mile, the road turns hard right and reaches a gate. This is as far as visitors are allowed into the Ecological Reserve.

Turn left onto the unmarked Herb Jeffries Trail, named for the African-American star of Western films. The trail reaches a ridge, where you can admire the extensive network of trails covering the hills like a spider web. The rocky hills above the Art Smith Trail are clearly visible to the south, with Toro Peak and Martinez Mtn. in the background. The trail switchbacks down the steep ridge. In 0.6 mile, reach a four-way junction.

Rocks and palms from the Bump and Grind Trail above Rancho Mirage

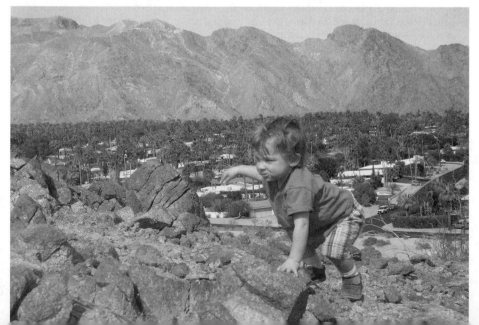

VARIATIONS————————————————

The right-most branch is the Hopalong Cassidy Trail. It leads along the hillside for 8 miles to join the Art Smith Trail (see Trip 12.6). Along the way, it passes the Gabby Hayes Trail, which leads down to Cahuilla Hills Park, and the Homestead Trail, which leads down to Homme-Adams Park. It then passes the Stone Eagle Golf Course and a large lighted cross before detouring around the Bighorn development. None of these trails are marked yet, and a variety of confusing social trails are starting to develop. Navigating this area requires a map and good sense of direction.

The center branch is a continuation of the Herb Jeffries Trail, which leads 0.7 mile down to the dirt Wash Rd., alongside the drainage canal. Turn left and walk back to Painters Path, or right to reach Cahuilla Hills Park.

————————————————————

Take the left-most branch, which is the bottom end of the Hopalong Cassidy Trail, named for one of American's best-known movie and television cowboy heroes. Cassidy and Jeffries were both once Palm Desert residents. The trail leads 0.6 mile back to the trailhead where you started.

trip 12.6 Art Smith Trail

Distance	6–16 miles (out-and-back)
Hiking Time	3–8 hours
Elevation Gain	1300'–3300'
Difficulty	Moderate–Strenuous
Trail Use	Equestrians, cyclists
Best Times	October–March, closed June 15–September 30
Agency	Santa Rosa and San Jacinto Mountains National Monument
Recommended Map	*Santa Rosa and San Jacinto Mountains National Monument* or *Rancho Mirage* 7.5' (trail not marked)
Permit	See below

see maps on pp. 248 & 258

DIRECTIONS The Art Smith Trailhead is on Highway 74, south of Palm Desert. It can be reached by exiting Interstate 10 at Monterey and driving south across Highway 111, where the road becomes Highway 74. It can also be reached directly from Highway 111, or by driving through the Garner Valley from Hemet. In any case, the trailhead is 4 miles south of Highway 111 on the west side of the road, directly across from the Santa Rosa and San Jacinto Mountains National Monument Visitor Center.

The Art Smith Trail, named in 1977 for the late long-time Trail Boss of the Desert Riders who was responsible for the development of numerous routes in these mountains, is the gem of the northern Santa Rosas, offering a grand tour through the heart of the wilderness. The trail features outrageous cacti, outlandish rock formations, several small palm oases, and a chance to commune with the desert. Despite its length and the rugged terrain, the trail gains less elevation than might be expected. Those looking for a quick jaunt can hike 3 miles out past palm oases to a vista point, then return. For a longer hike, go all 8 miles to the end at Dunn Rd., then return. Or better yet, connect to the Hahn Buena Vista Trail and follow it down to Fern and Palm Canyons.

This area is frequented by the endangered peninsular bighorn sheep. Dogs are prohibited at all times. The Art Smith Trail is closed from June 15 to September 30 west of its intersection with the Hopalong Cassidy Trail to protect bighorn sheep during the hot season. The trail once started up

Dead Indian Canyon, but this area has been closed and the trail rerouted to protect a water source for the sheep. The trails in this area are undergoing rapid development, so trail markings (and even trails) may have changed by the time you arrive; bring a map and good navigation skills.

The National Monument plans to require free self-issued wilderness permits for hikers on the Art Smith Trail west of its intersection with the Hopalong Cassidy Trail. When this permit requirement goes into effect, the permits will be available at a kiosk alongside the trail.

The signed Art Smith Trail begins at the north end of the parking lot. Follow it north along the levee 0.2 mile to a fence line. Turn left and walk another 0.2 mile until you reach the first of many BLM signposts marking the route. Switchback up the hill for 0.2 mile to the top.

Your goal is to follow the Art Smith Trail west. Unfortunately, unauthorized social trails make a maze of this area. Some trails are slated to be closed and obliterated in the near future, so any specific list of junctions will likely become incorrect soon. With

luck the trail will be better marked by the time you visit. When in doubt, pick a route leading west rather than dropping into the housing development to the north. In 0.7 mile, you should reach a signed junction where the Hopalong Cassidy Trail forks off north to Homme-Adams Park and the Art Smith Trail continues west.

Continue west up a hill through desert agaves and barrel cacti. The trail levels out amidst granite boulders varnished brown by centuries of exposure to the desert. In 0.6 mile, it reaches the first palm oasis in Cat Creek (usually dry). In another 0.6 mile, it passes several more small oases and contours northwest along the flank of flat-topped Haystack Mtn. 0.4 mile beyond, it crests a small hill from which you can see the Salton Sea glittering beyond the ridge to the east. You have now traveled 3 miles; this is a good turnaround point if you are looking for a short jaunt through the most scenic sections of the trail. Just past this overlook, you may see a sign marking the Schey Trail to the right, although this trail is slated to close in the near future.

Oasis along the Art Smith Trail

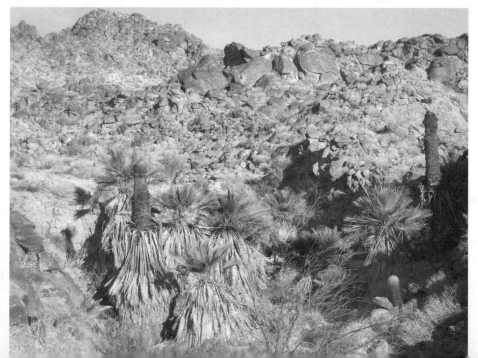

Continue west on the Art Smith Trail, reaching more palms in a wash in about 2 miles. You are in the heart of the Santa Rosa Mountains, out of sight of civilization, of the teeming hordes, the malls, golf courses, and galleries that sprawl across the Coachella Valley. In another 2 miles, enter a long sandy wash and pass through a narrow canyon, then exit the wash on the right. Follow the trail to the crest of a small ridge, where you are treated to panoramic views to the west. Look for Dunn Rd., a wide swath cut across the mountain range from north to south. Descend 0.2 mile through vast fields of agaves to reach the Mike Dunn Desert Riders Oasis, a grandiose name for a motley collection of weathered picnic tables and a broken-down bulldozer. Dunn used the bulldozer in the 1960s and 1970s to tear this road through the Santa Rosa Mountains. This marks the end of the Art Smith Trail, 8.2 miles from the start. Return the way you came.

ALTERNATIVE FINISHES

With a car shuttle or a pricey taxi ride, you can link up with other trails for an outstanding one-way hike.

Proceed straight onto the scenic Hahn Buena Vista Trail and explore the magnificent network of trails near Palm Canyon (see Trip 11.11). Depending on your route, this involves at least 6 miles of hiking, mostly downhill. Be sure to reach Hermits Bench before Palm Canyon closes at 5 P.M.

Another option is to turn right and follow Dunn Rd. and the Cathedral Canyon Trail down to Cathedral City (see the Murray Hill map on p. 252). To reach this trailhead from Highway 111 in Cathedral City, turn south on Cathedral Canyon Dr. At a T-junction in 0.5 mile, turn right on Terrace Rd. Then turn left on Paradise Way in 0.5 mile, right on Valley Vista in another 0.5 mile, and left on Channel Dr. in 0.3 mile. Meet a vehicle at the end of Channel Dr.

trip 12.7 Randall Henderson Loop

Distance	1.8–2.2 miles (loop)
Hiking Time	1–1.5 hours
Elevation Gain	300′–450′
Difficulty	Easy
Trail Use	Good for children
Best Times	All year, hot in the summer
Agency	Santa Rosa and San Jacinto Mountains National Monument
Recommended Map	Santa Rosa and San Jacinto Mountains National Monument

see map on p. 258

DIRECTIONS The Randall Henderson Loop starts at the Santa Rosa and San Jacinto Mountains National Monument Visitor Center on Highway 74 south of Palm Desert. Parking is available at the visitor center 9 A.M.–4 P.M. The trailhead can be reached by exiting Interstate 10 at Monterey and driving south across Highway 111, where the road becomes Highway 74. It can also be reached directly from Highway 111, or by driving through the Garner Valley from Hemet. In any case, the visitor center is 4 miles south of Highway 111 on the east side of the road. Park in the large lot. If the visitor center is closed, park across the highway at the Art Smith Trailhead.

The Randall Henderson Loop explores the valley above the Santa Rosa and San Jacinto Mountains National Monument Visitor Center. It is convenient for visitors looking for a short hike; it has fine views and a variety of interesting cacti. On a quiet day, you are likely to see rabbits, lizards, and other small desert animals. The visitor center periodically arranges naturalist-guided hikes in the cooler months; call ahead for a schedule. The trail was named for a long-time Palm Desert resident who published *The Desert Mountain* from the 1930s through the 1960s. Henderson's exploration, journalism, and vision were instrumental to the development of Palm Desert.

Walk back up the access road from the visitor center toward Highway 74 to the signed Randall Henderson Trail. The trail splits in 150 yards. Take the right fork. This is a good area in which to enjoy the desert plants. Smoke trees grow in the washes and creosote bushes are common. Different species of cacti prefer different altitudes and soils. Watch for silver, pencil, and teddy bear chollas in the lower elevations, and beavertail and barrel cacti higher up.

The trail leads up a wash and then gains a ridge. In 0.8 mile, reach a junction near a dirt road. To make the short loop (recommended), turn left and walk 100 yards to a second junction, then turn left again and walk 0.9 back down to the trailhead. There are some views across the highway to a palm oasis in Dead Indian Canyon (closed to protect the peninsular bighorn sheep) and Haystack Mtn. beyond. Much of this part of the trail follows the sandy wash, including a stretch through some narrows and then around a short dry waterfall.

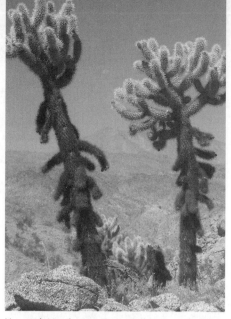

Haystack Mtn. between two Teddy Bear Chollas, from the Randall Henderson Trail

VARIATION

It is also possible to make a half-mile longer loop. At the junction in 0.8 mile, turn right and pass a field of desert agaves. Reach a dirt road and turn left, following the road across the head of the valley. Follow the road to a gate where the road is closed. Turn left on another trail that returns to the loop trail where you make your descent to the right through the wash.

trip 12.8 Living Desert Zoo and Gardens

Distance	5 miles (loop)
Hiking Time	2.5 hours
Elevation Gain	800'
Difficulty	Easy
Trail Use	Good for children
Best Times	October–April
Agency	Living Desert
Recommended Map	*Living Desert* (free at entrance)

see map on p. 248

DIRECTIONS From Interstate 10, exit south on Monterey and go 6 miles to Highway 111 in Palm Desert. Turn left (east) and proceed 1 mile to Portola Ave. Turn right (south) and go 1.5 miles to the signed entrance of the Living Desert Zoo and Gardens.

The Living Desert is a combination zoo and botanical garden in Palm Desert. Besides the zoo and garden, hikers will enjoy the wilderness trail system that leads east from the Living Desert grounds up onto the flank of Eisenhower Mtn. This trip

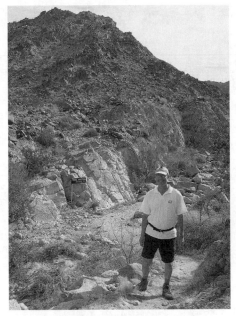

Hiker on the Living Desert Wilderness Trail

features good views of the Coachella Valley and surrounding mountains.

At the time of this writing, the Living Desert is open 9 A.M.—5 P.M., September 1–June 15. Summer hours are reduced to 8 A.M.–1:30 P.M.; this time of the year is too hot for enjoyable hiking. Admission is

$12.50, with discounts for seniors, military, and children. Ask for a brochure at the entrance showing the trails.

From the Living Desert entrance, walk east past the gift shop and model train display, then north past the bighorn sheep hill to the signed start of the wilderness trail system. The trail features numerous interpretive signs, including an exhibit marking the San Andreas Fault line. In 0.1 mile, pass the short Inner Loop Trail on the left that circles back to the start. In another 0.4 mile, pass the Middle Loop Trail on the left.

Soon after, the trail enters a rocky wash. In 0.8 mile, watch for a sign indicating where the trail exits the canyon bottom on the left.

Eventually, climb onto the side of Eisenhower Mtn., turn north, and reach a sheltered picnic ground at the halfway point. On a clear winter day, there are spectacular views of the snow-capped San Jacinto and San Gorgonio Mountains above the golf courses and sprawling development in the Coachella Valley.

The trail turns west and descends back to the Living Desert grounds. Be sure to enjoy the other attractions of the Living Desert before you depart.

trip 12.9 Bear Creek Oasis

Distance	9 miles (out-and-back)
Hiking Time	5 hours
Elevation Gain	2400'
Difficulty	Strenuous
Trail Use	Equestrians
Best Times	October–March, closed June 15–September 30
Agency	Santa Rosa and San Jacinto Mountains National Monument
Recommended Map	*Santa Rosa and San Jacinto Mountains National Monument* or *La Quinta, Martinez Mountain* 7.5' (trail not marked)
Permit	See below

see map on p. 264

DIRECTIONS From Interstate 10, exit south on Washington St. and drive south into La Quinta past Highway 111. Alternatively, from Highway 111, turn south on Washington. Proceed 1.3 miles south of 111, then turn right on Eisenhower. Follow it as it curves to the left and eventually ends in 3.7 miles at Avenida Bermudas. Turn right; Avenida Bermudas veers west and becomes Calle Tecate. Continue 0.5 mile to the end where Calle Tecate meets Avenida Madero and park on the street.

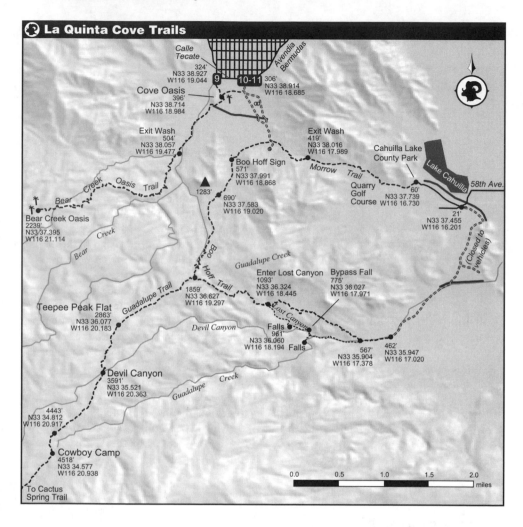

La Quinta Cove Trails

Calle Tecate
324'
N33 38.927
W116 19.044

9   10-11   306'
N33 38.914
W116 18.685

Avendia Bermudas

Cove Oasis
396'
N33 38.714
W116 18.984

Exit Wash
504'
N33 38.057
W116 19.477

Exit Wash
419'
N33 38.016
W116 17.989

Cahuilla Lake
County Park

Lake Cahuilla

58th Ave.

Boo Hoff Sign
571'
N33 37.991
W116 18.868

Morrow Trail

Quarry
Golf
Course

60'
N33 37.739
W116 16.730

Creek   Oasis   Trail

1283'

690'
N33 37.583
W116 19.020

21'
N33 37.455
W116 16.201

Bear

Bear Creek Oasis
2239'
N33 37.395
W116 21.114

Creek

Bear

(Closed to vehicles)

Boo Hoff Trail

Guadalupe Creek

Enter Lost Canyon
1093'
N33 36.324
W116 18.445

Bypass Fall
775'
N33 36.027
W116 17.971

1859'
N33 36.627
W116 19.297

Guadalupe Trail

Teepee Peak Flat
2863'
N33 36.077
W116 20.183

Devil Canyon

Lost Canyon

Falls
961'
N33 36.060
W116 18.194 Falls

462'
N33 35.947
W116 17.020

567'
N33 35.904
W116 17.378

Devil Canyon
3591'
N33 35.521
W116 20.363

Guadalupe   Creek

4443'
N33 34.812
W116 20.917

Cowboy Camp
4518'
N33 34.577
W116 20.938

To Cactus
Spring Trail

0.0   0.5   1.0   1.5   2.0
miles

Nestled among the canyons of the parched Santa Rosa Mountains, lush oases form where underground water is forced to the surface. The Bear Creek Oasis is hidden high on the slopes above the La Quinta Cove. This hike passes through a sandy wash and up the ridge along the dramatic Bear Creek Canyon through veritable gardens of cacti before abruptly rounding a corner and ending at the oasis. This trail is closed from June 15–September 30 to protect the bighorn sheep's access to water during the hot season.

The National Monument plans to require free self-issued wilderness permits for hik-ers on the Bear Creek Oasis Trail where it leaves Bear Creek Canyon. When this permit requirement goes into effect, the permits will be available at a kiosk along-side the trail.

A signed trailhead for Cove Oasis is located on the south side of the road. Hike south on the broad dirt path, reaching the Cove Oasis in 0.2 mile. The date palms at this park were a private gift to the city cel-ebrating the Coachella Valley date industry. Ninety percent of the US date supply comes from Coachella Valley. Look for the three-dimensional metal map of the area amidst the exhibits.

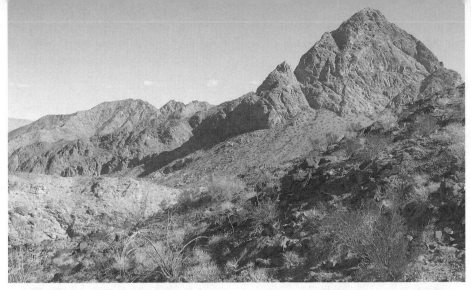

Peak 1283' from Bear Creek Canyon Ridge

Identify the prominent rocky hill (Peak 1283´) directly south of Cove Oasis. Your first goal is to hike up the Bear Creek wash right (west) of this peak. Pass around the south side of a hill adjacent to the oasis and then around the west end of a levee to drop into Bear Creek. Follow the sandy dry wash south until you reach a clear trail exiting on the west side and climbing onto Bear Creek Ridge. There are several use paths that veer off too soon; the correct trail is heavily used and departs the wash near the mouth of a major side canyon near trail signs. Hikers also enjoy continuing up the wash, so don't be distracted by the footprints and miss the turnoff. By the time you do this hike, better trail markings may be in place.

The trail parallels the wash, then crosses a minor canyon before gaining a ridge with dramatic views into Bear Creek Canyon. This region of the Santa Rosa Mountains supports diverse species of cacti, including pencil cholla, teddy bear cholla, barrel cactus and beavertail cactus. As you ascend, the Salton Sea and Joshua Tree National Park come into view. Eventually, veer north away from Bear Creek Canyon and continue up the ridge to cross the upper reaches of a tributary creek. Soon after, arrive at the densely vegetated Bear Creek Oasis tucked away in a small canyon high on the mountainside, 4.5 miles from the start.

After exploring the area, return the way you came.

Bear Creek Oasis, hidden among the cholla-covered hills

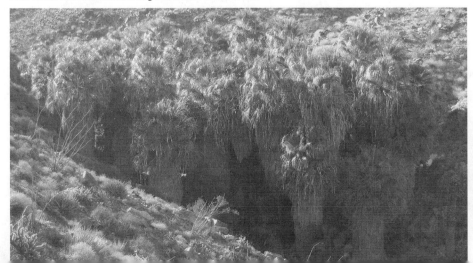

trip 12.10 Boo Hoff Loop

Distance	12 miles (loop)
Hiking Time	8 hours
Elevation Gain	2200′
Difficulty	Strenuous
Trail Use	Equestrians
Best Times	October–March
Agency	Santa Rosa and San Jacinto Mountains National Monument
Required Map	*Santa Rosa and San Jacinto Mountains National Monument,* or *La Quinta, Martinez Mountain* 7.5′ (trail not marked)
Permit	See below

see map on p. 264

DIRECTIONS From Interstate 10, exit south on Washington St. and drive south into La Quinta past Highway 111. Alternatively, from Highway 111, turn south on Washington. Proceed 1.3 miles south of 111, then turn right on Eisenhower. Eisenhower curves to the left and eventually ends in 3.7 miles at Avenida Bermudas. Turn right; in 0.2 mile, Avenida Bermudas turns right again (west) and becomes Calle Tecate. Park in the Top of Cove dirt lot near this corner.

The view south from the La Quinta Cove resembles an alien landscape. A maze of twisting canyons cut through the serrated ridges. Ocotillos and cacti dot the hillsides. The Boo Hoff Trail, named in 1979 for a long-time member of the Desert Riders, follows a historic Indian footpath through this curious wilderness. This hike makes a remarkable loop: It starts in the La Quinta Cove, climbs onto the north slopes of towering Martinez Mtn., then turns east and descends beside Devil Canyon. As an optional variation, you can descend to the canyon itself. The path then leads to Cahuilla Lake before returning to the Cove on the Morrow Trail.

The National Monument plans to require free self-issued wilderness permits for some segments of the Boo Hoff Trail. When this permit requirement goes into effect, the permits will be available at a kiosk alongside the trail.

From the trailhead, look south and identify Peak 1283′ standing alone 1.5 miles distant. Your first goal is to pass left of this peak. Unfortunately, there is a maze of trails and roads in the area, but no direct trail leads to this point. Begin walking south from the parking area on a dirt road. In 0.2 mile, it forks in 3 directions. The trail to the right leads to Cove Oasis, but you choose the road in the middle, passing on the west (right) side of two water tanks. In another 0.4 mile, reach the top of a levee. Ignore the no trespassing signs here; hikers have right-of-way to the Santa Rosa Wilderness.

The most direct path from here is to hike cross-country across the desert to gain the wash on the east side of Peak 1283′, reaching signposts marking the start of the Boo Hoff Trail in 0.6 mile. If you prefer to stay on trails, follow the dirt road as it descends past the levee and heads toward a water tank on the hill to the south-southeast. In 0.4 mile, just before the road begins climbing the hill, look for an unmarked footpath leading right (west) across the desert. Follow it 0.5 mile to the aforementioned signposts.

From here, there are several paths braiding up the wash; the one on the lip of the west bank is less sandy and may be easiest. Eventually, the steep walls of Peak 1283′ force you back into the bottom of the wash. Continue 0.6 mile up the wash, staying to the right following along the southeast slope of the peak and ignoring paths that might tempt you out, until you reach another large metal sign for the Boo Hoff Trail.

The Boo Hoff Trail leaves the wash and abruptly begins climbing a shallow ridge overlooking the east fork of Bear Creek (usually dry). The slopes are dotted with ocotillos and chollas. Occasionally, you will see traces of an old jeep road that once led up here, but stay on the established trail. As you gain elevation, the dominant cactus species visibly change. Pass the wilderness boundary in 1.5 miles. In another 0.1 mile, reach an unmarked trail junction that is critical but easy to miss. The right fork follows the Guadalupe Trail up into the remote wilds of Santa Rosa Wilderness (see Trip 12.11), but this trip veers left and begins descending eastward.

There are impressive views of the Salton Sea framed by the mountains as you hike down the ridge. In 0.8 mile, the trail dips into a wash, then promptly climbs out the other side. Do not miss the exit and continue down the wash. Soon, you can look down into Lost Canyon on the right (south). It is not named on the USGS *Martinez Mountain* 7.5′ map, but is the northwestern tributary of Devil Canyon. In another 0.4 mile, the trail dips again into a small wash that feeds into Lost Canyon.

Here, you have two options. You can cross the wash and continue following the trail 1.6 miles down to the desert floor where another large metal Boo Hoff sign marks the end of the trail, or you can hike cross-country down Lost Canyon.

VARIATION

Lost Canyon leads 1.5 miles down to rejoin the trail on the desert floor; this is a substantially more time-consuming and adventurous option. This cross-country route is only open from October–December. Note: never travel in canyons if there is the possibility of thunderstorms because of flash floods dangers.

If you take Lost Canyon, you will soon reach a short dry waterfall, which can be bypassed on the right, or climbed down directly (easy third class). 0.2 mile beyond, come to the top of a 150-foot drop. Here are impressive views of the Salton Sea framed by the steep walls of the canyon. The drop looks intimidating at first, but it is fairly easy to pick a path down to about halfway. When the cliffs become too steep to go farther, look for a trail on the left leading across the dirt slopes and down to

Lost Canyon

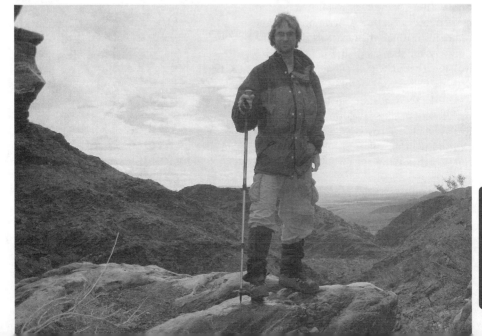

the canyon floor. Just beyond, Lost Canyon merges with Devil Canyon. Continue heading southeast and in another 0.2 mile, you may notice a few cairns and a trail leading out of the wash on the right. If you miss it and go around the bend, you will arrive at the top of a 30-foot overhanging dry waterfall. Go back 100 yards and look for the trail. The short bypass trail rejoins the bottom of the wash at the confluence of Devil Canyon and Guadalupe Creek. Consider taking a 0.1 mile side trip up Guadalupe Creek to another impressive waterfall (dry most of the year) with sheer polished granite walls and returning back to the confluence. You have now completed the slow part of the Lost Canyon descent; the remaining 0.7 mile are a simple matter of hiking down the boulder-strewn sandy wash until you reach its mouth and find the Boo Hoff sign on your left where the trail descends from the hill.

Hike down the wide wash for 0.3 mile to the wilderness boundary, marked with a sign and a former parking area. A jeep road leads northeast from here; it is now closed to motorized vehicles but open for horses and hikers. In 1.0 mile, stay left at a junction with a second jeep road. Just beyond, cross a levee. There is a maze of trails and old roads through the next part of the hike, but stay on the main dirt road, which is usually marked with trail signs. Your goal is to pass the dramatic hills ahead on their west side, then, at their north end, squeeze between a housing development and a levee until you reach a paved road at a Y-junction (1.2 miles). Then take Cahuilla Park Rd. 0.7 mile northwest to Lake Cahuilla Recreation Area.

The Morrow Trail begins at the northwest corner of the park at the base of the mountains. Look for a sign reading DOGS PROHIBITED; cross the dike and hike west to another sign reading MORROW TRAIL. This trail leads west for 1.6 miles, hugging the base of the hills north of The Quarry at La Quinta Golf Course. It sometimes stays in the wash and sometimes climbs up the toe of the ridge; there are several ways to go, all of which rejoin. When possible, choose the trail on the ridge rather than in the wash. As the wash enters a narrow canyon, be alert for a cairn and trail leading out on the left (south) side. If you reach the dead end of the canyon in a steep bowl, you have gone 0.2 mile too far. The trail climbs out of the canyon and reaches an improbable saddle. Then it descends 0.3 mile to a dirt road below a water tank (where you may have started if you stayed on trail at the beginning of the hike). Turn right (north) and follow the road 1.0 mile back to the trailhead.

Ocotillo and barrel cactus

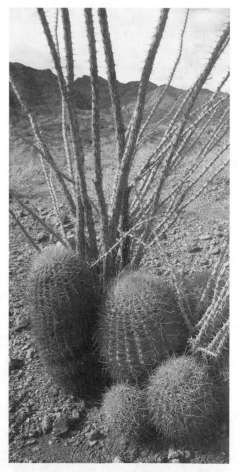

trip 12.11 Guadalupe Trail

Distance	14 miles (one-way)
Hiking Time	8 hours
Elevation Gain	5100′
Difficulty	Strenuous
Trail Use	Suitable for backpacking
Best Times	October–December
Agency	Santa Rosa and San Jacinto Mountains National Monument
Required Map	*Santa Rosa and San Jacinto Mountains National Monument* or *La Quinta, Martinez Mountain, Toro Peak* 7.5′ (trail not marked)
Permit	See below

see maps on pp. 248, 264 & 270

DIRECTIONS The Guadalupe Trail is a one-way hike from the La Quinta Cove to the Sawmill Trailhead in Pinyon Pines. Position a getaway vehicle at the Cactus Spring/Sawmill Trailhead. This is reached from Highway 74 at mile marker 74 RIV 80.50, by turning south onto Pinon Flats Trans Station Rd. (7S09). Go 0.3 mile to the vast Sawmill Trail parking area on the left. To reach the starting point, drive 15 miles north on Highway 74 to Highway 111, then turn right and drive 6 miles east on Highway 111. Turn right on Washington and proceed 1.3 miles south, then turn right on Eisenhower. Eisenhower curves to the left and eventually ends in 3.7 miles at Avenida Bermudas. Turn right; in 0.2 mile, Avenida Bermudas turns right again (west) and becomes Calle Tecate. Park in the dirt Top of Cove dirt lot near this corner.

The Guadalupe "Trail" is a cross-country route following an old Indian path through the heart of the Santa Rosa Mountains from the desert to the pines. The first part follows the Boo Hoff Trail, but the middle travels up a faint Indian footpath past Devil Canyon and Guadalupe Creek before rejoining the Cactus Spring Trail on the west side of Martinez Mtn. The Guadalupe Trail is strenuous and demands advanced route-finding skills, but also offers tremendous rewards to experienced hikers who undertake its challenge. Many desert plant species, ranging from ocotillo and cactus, to agave and yucca, to pinyon pine are represented. Each of these species favors a specific band of elevation. The route passes an old cowboy camp and sharp-eyed hikers may note old Indian artifacts along the way. Please leave what you find for the enjoyment of future hikers. It is helpful to wear gaiters to protect yourself from occasional brush and to carry pliers in case of an unfortunate encounter with a cholla cactus. The best way to do this hike is with a friend or group who knows the way; failing that, a GPS or exceptional map reading skills are necessary.

The National Monument plans to require free self-issued wilderness permits for hikers of the Guadalupe Trail. When this permit requirement goes into effect, the permits will be available at a kiosk alongside the trail.

From the trailhead, look south and identify Peak 1283′ standing alone 1.5 miles ahead. Your first goal is to pass left of this peak. Unfortunately, there is a maze of trails and roads in the area, but no direct trail to this point. Begin walking south from the parking area on a dirt road. In 0.2 mile, it forks in 3 directions. The trail to the right leads to Cove Oasis, but you take the road in the middle, passing on the west (right) side of two water tanks. In another 0.4 mile, cross the top of a levee. Ignore the no trespassing signs here; hikers have right-of-way to Santa Rosa Wilderness.

The most direct path from here is to hike cross-country across the desert to gain the wash on the east side of Peak 1283′, reaching signposts marking the start of the Boo Hoff Trail in 0.6 mile. If you prefer to stay

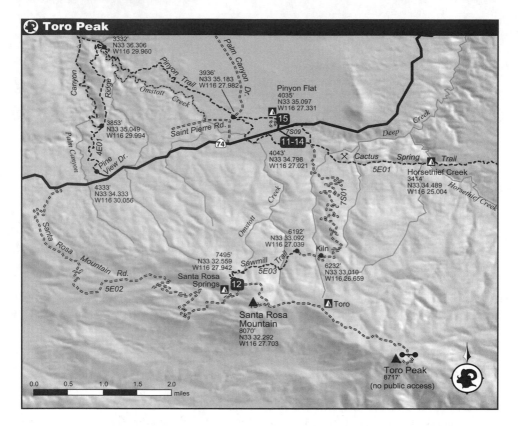

Toro Peak

3332'
N33 36.306
W116 29.960

3936'
N33 35.183
W116 27.982

Pinyon Flat
4035'
N33 35.097
W116 27.331

Canyon

Ridge

Omstott Creek

Pinyon Trail

Palm Canyon Dr.

Saint Pierre Rd.

3853'
N33 35.049
W116 29.994

4E01

Pine View Dr.

Palm Canyon

74

4043'
N33 34.798
W116 27.021

7S09

11-14

15

4333'
N33 34.333
W116 30.056

Santa Rosa Mountain Rd.

5E02

Omstott Creek

7S01

6192'
N33 33.092
W116 27.039

7495'
N33 32.559
W116 27.942

Sawmill Trail

5E03

Santa Rosa Springs

12

Santa Rosa Mountain
8070'
N33 32.292
W116 27.703

Kiln

6232'
N33 33.010
W116.26.659

Toro

Cactus Spring Trail

5E01

Deep Creek

Horsethief Creek
3414'
N33 34.489
W116 25.004

Horsethief Creek

Toro Peak
8717'
(no public access)

0.0 0.5 1.0 1.5 2.0
miles

on trails, follow the dirt road as it descends past the levee and heads toward a water tank on the hill to the south-southeast. In 0.4 mile, just before the road begins climbing the hill, look for an unmarked footpath leading right (west) across the desert. Follow it 0.5 mile to the aforementioned signposts.

From here, there are several paths braiding up the wash; the one on the lip of the west bank is less sandy and may be easiest. Eventually, the steep walls of Peak 1283' force you back into the bottom of the wash. Continue 0.6 mile up the wash, staying right along the southeast slope of the peak and ignoring paths that might tempt you out, until you reach another large metal sign for the Boo Hoff Trail.

Again, survey the territory in front of you. The biggest mountain ahead is Martinez Mtn., which is prominent from much of the eastern Santa Rosas. To the right is a

spire on the skyline locally known as "Teepee Peak." Your next goal is to follow the trail to the base of Teepee Peak.

The Boo Hoff Trail leaves the wash and abruptly begins climbing a shallow ridge overlooking the east fork of Bear Creek (usually dry). The slopes are dotted with ocotillos and chollas. Occasionally, you will see traces of an old jeep road that once led up here, but stay on the established trail. As you gain elevation, the dominant cactus species visibly change. Pass the wilderness boundary in 1.5 miles. In another 0.1 mile, reach an unmarked trail junction that is critical but easy to miss. The left fork continues on the Boo Hoff Trail descending east toward the Salton Sea (see Trip 12.10), but this trip veers right on the Guadalupe Trail and continues climbing.

Teddy bear chollas soon become the dominant cactus. Soon after, hike through a canyon full of agaves and come to a flat site at the base of Teepee Peak, 1.2 miles from the junction. This site was once popular with the Cahuilla Indians who lived in the area; it is a good place to take a break and explore.

In another half mile, reach a brush-choked canyon. Follow a faint path along the rocks on the right side until you can cross on a good trail and switchback up the far side. It is well worth your effort to find the trail. In 0.8 mile, reach a small plateau with a rocky point at the east end of the shelf. This was once another Indian camp. The trail becomes hard to follow here. Work your way south across the brushy bottom of Devil Canyon, then regain a faint ducked trail on the far side. Continue up a ridge, aiming for the saddle to the right of the pinyon-clad Martinez Mtn. Hike southwest up a shallow ridge on the right side of the Guadalupe Creek Canyon. Soon the trail becomes indistinct again; enter the Guadalupe Creek drainage and head for the saddle. Shortly below the saddle, arrive at Cowboy Camp, marked with a rusted cast iron stove

and assorted detritus. About 200 feet above the camp, you may sometimes be able to obtain murky water from a small spring. Continue 0.6 mile up the canyon and along a sandy wash to reach the saddle, 7.6 miles from the trailhead.

Look southwest and identify Toro Peak, the antenna-studded high point of the Santa Rosa Mountains. Hike toward Toro Peak until you enter a wash; follow the wash southwest and then west until you reach a wooden post marking the intersection with the Cactus Spring Trail in 1.3 miles. This intersection is easy to overlook, but very important.

Turn right and follow the Cactus Spring Trail west. Pass Cactus Spring (a grassy spot north of the trail where water rarely flows now), and in 2.4 miles reach the cottonwood-shaded camp at Horsethief Creek, the only reliable water source on the trip. Continue west past some historic mining operations and in another 2.2 miles reach a dirt road. Continue west 0.2 mile to the Sawmill Trailhead.

Martinez Mtn. and Teepee Peak from the Guadalupe Trail

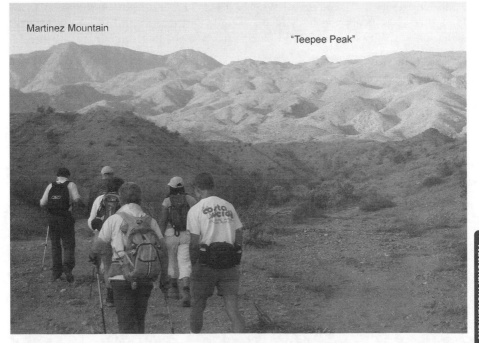

trip 12.12 Sawmill Trail

Distance	16 miles (out-and-back)
Hiking Time	8 hours
Elevation Gain	3900'
Difficulty	Strenuous
Trail Use	Suitable for backpacking
Best Times	October–November, March–April
Agency	Santa Rosa and San Jacinto Mountains National Monument
Recommended Map	Santa Rosa and San Jacinto Mountains National Monument or Toro Peak 7.5'

see map on p. 270

DIRECTIONS From Highway 74 at mile marker 74 RIV 80.50, turn south onto Pinon Flats Trans Station Rd (7S09). Go 0.3 mile to the Sawmill Trail parking area on the left. Optionally, arrange a second vehicle or bicycle at the top of the trail to do a one-way hike (or do the hike downhill). To reach the top, continue west on Highway 74 to the fair dirt Santa Rosa Mtn. Rd. near mile marker 74 RIV 77.00. Follow the mountain road 8.7 miles to the signed start of trail 5E03 near a bend and a side road. This is 0.5 mile above the turnoff for the Santa Rosa Springs Campground. There is parking for 2–3 vehicles near the trailhead.

From the Sawmill Trail parking area walk east along a dirt road, staying right at an immediate fork. In 0.2 mile at a signed junction with the Cactus Spring Trail, stay right on the Sawmill Rd. (7S01). Follow this road for 5.4 miles as it switchbacks unforgivingly up a chaparral-covered ridge.

Ribbonwoods and cacti give way to manzanitas and scrub oaks as you ascend. Watch for Steller's jays, quail, and birds of prey along the way. Views of the pinyon pines

community, Deep Creek's convoluted canyon, Sugarloaf and Asbestos Mountains, and the Desert Divide and San Jacinto become more expansive as you climb. The rough road is usually passable by high-clearance vehicles.

At the top of the Sawmill Rd. is an old charcoal kiln. Two faint roads continue. The left one reaches a reliable spring in 0.1 mile, but this trip follows the jeep tracks to the right that contour for another 0.4

Charcoal kiln at top of Sawmill Rd.

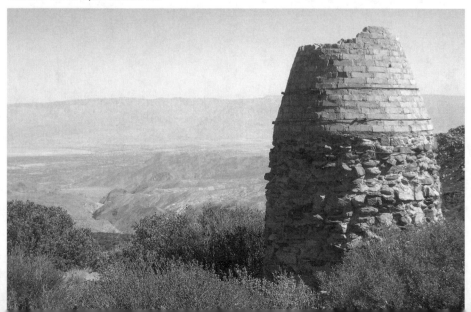

mile. Where they peter out, look for a signed trail marker for the recently constructed 5E03 trail. This trail crosses the headwaters of Omstott Creek, which flows down the mountainside much of the year from the Stump Spring area. Vegetation becomes momentarily lush along the banks of the creek, then fades to chaparral again before entering a band of black oaks. Not far beyond, climb into the mature forest of Jeffrey pines, white firs, and incense cedars that crowns the upper reaches of the Santa Rosa Mountains. The trail makes final switchbacks before reaching the Santa Rosa Mtn. Rd., 2.4 miles from the end of the jeep tracks.

From here, you can return the way you came. Alternatively, if a vehicle is parked at the top, your work is complete. The purist may choose to continue up to the summit of Santa Rosa Mtn. (8070´). This adds 500 feet of elevation gain. Either follow the dirt road to the top, or pick a cross-country route directly up the steep forested ridge.

trip 12.13 Horsethief Creek

Distance	5 miles (out-and-back)
Hiking Time	2.5 hours
Elevation Gain	900´
Difficulty	Moderate
Trail Use	Suitable for backpacking
Best Times	October–March
Agency	Santa Rosa and San Jacinto Mountains National Monument
Recommended Map	*Santa Rosa and San Jacinto Mountains National Monument* or *Toro Peak 7.5'*

see map on p. 270

DIRECTIONS From Highway 74 at mile marker 74 RIV 80.50, turn south onto Pinon Flats Trans Station Rd (7S09). Go 0.3 mile to the Sawmill Trail parking area on the left.

Between Highway 74 and Toro Peak is a high bench covered in chaparral and sliced by rugged canyons. Horsethief Creek flows through one of these canyons throughout the wet season. Alongside the creek is a small campsite shaded by cottonwoods. The trip to the creek is one of the few moderate hikes in this remote region of the Santa Rosa Mountains. According to legend, rustlers made their hideout here in the 19th Century as they preyed upon honest folk in San Diego and San Bernardino.

The signed Cactus Spring Trail (5E01) starts at the east end of the parking lot. Walk along the dirt path, staying right at an immediate fork. In 0.2 mile, turn left at the signed Cactus Spring Trail. Sign in at the wilderness box. Hike through fields of prickly pear cactus, agave, manzanita, and ribbonwood, and pass some old dolomite

Horsethief Creek

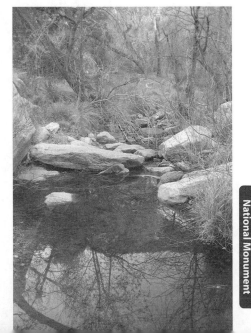

mining structures. An ominous sign warns you to BE PREPARED FOR HAZARDOUS CONDITIONS BEYOND THIS POINT. In 0.9 mile, you will reach the wilderness boundary. The trail descends through colorful hills and canyons. In another 1.2 miles, the trail drops down into the canyon of Horsethief Creek.

You can enjoy a picnic or spend a night here. It is possible to explore up or down the rough canyon alongside the creek. Return the way you came.

trip 12.14 Cactus Spring Trail

Distance	22 miles (one-way)
Hiking Time	11 hours
Elevation Gain	3000'/7000' loss
Difficulty	Very strenuous
Trail Use	Suitable for backpacking
Best Times	October–March
Agency	Santa Rosa and San Jacinto Mountains National Monument
Required Map	*Santa Rosa and San Jacinto Mountains National Monument* or *Toro Peak, Martinez Mountain, Clark Lake NE, Valerie* 7.5'

see maps on pp. 248, 270 & 279

DIRECTIONS This is a long one-way hike requiring a car shuttle. Position one vehicle at the corner of Van Buren and Avenue 66 amid the date palm groves northwest of the Salton Sea. This trailhead can be reached from Highway 111 in Indio by driving 10 miles south on Jackson, then 1 mile east on 66th Ave. Drive the second vehicle back to Highway 111, then 10.5 miles west to Highway 74, then 15 miles south to mile marker 74 RIV 80.50. Opposite the Pinyon Flats Campground road, turn left (south) onto Pinon Flats Trans Station Rd (7S09). Go 0.3 mile to the Sawmill Trail parking area on the left. This shuttle takes approximately 1 hour.

The Cactus Spring "Trail" is one of the wildest routes in the Santa Rosa Mountains, following an old Indian path from the forested heights around Martinez Mtn. down rugged Martinez Canyon to the date palm groves near the Salton Sea. The first half follows an established but sometimes faint trail; the second requires cross-country navigation skills. Long pants and gaiters are recommended because of the brush in Martinez Canyon and the perpetual cactus hazards.

The signed Cactus Spring Trail (5E01) starts at the east end of the Sawmill Trail parking lot. Walk along the dirt road, staying right at an immediate fork. In 0.2 mile, turn left at the signed Cactus Spring Trail. Sign in at the wilderness box. Hike through fields of prickly pear cacti, agaves, manzanitas, and ribbonwoods, and pass some mining structures. In 0.9 mile, reach the wilderness boundary. The trail

descends through colorful hills and canyons. In another 1.2 miles, reach Horsethief Creek, where a campsite is shaded with cottonwoods. Beyond this point, the trail is less used and sometimes requires attention to follow. Climb out of the canyon and in 0.6 mile enter a sandy wash. Watch for posts marking the entrance and exit of washes. In another 1.9 miles, look for Cactus Spring on the left (north) side of the trail. The spring is easy to miss; it is now just a grassy area that occasionally offers a trickle of water. This is one of the most sacred areas for the Cahuilla Indians who live in this area. Observant explorers may find bedrock mortars for grinding food, smooth rock dance floors, and pictographs and petroglyphs.

The trail continues southeast toward the looming Martinez Mtn. In 0.7 mile pass a post where the Guadalupe Trail veers off to the left side of Martinez Mtn. (see Trip

12.11). The Guadalupe Trail is a cross-country route and you are likely to miss it unless you are familiar with the area. The Cactus Spring Trail curves around the right side of Martinez Mtn. through a pinyon pine forest, passing over a 5168-foot saddle that marks the high point of the route, 6.9 miles from the start.

Beyond this point, the trail becomes even less distinct, but it is marked with cairns and is worth your while to find. Be especially alert when crossing washes in order to locate the trail on the far side. In 2.5 miles, the trail reaches the signed Agua Alta Spring campsite on the south side of Martinez Mtn. The campsite, complete with hitching post, is a few hundred feet up the canyon north of the trail. The spring is in the dense grass above the campsite and is not dependable.

VARIATION

From Agua Alta Spring, some hikers prefer to descend Agua Alta Canyon to rejoin Martinez Canyon near the bottom. This is also a very difficult journey.

Beyond the spring, the path traverses southeast across Pinyon Alta Flat and drops into Martinez Canyon. It is marked with the occasional cairn but is so seldom used that few traces remain. The best way to navigate is to look for the prominent rocky Peak 4345' to the southeast. The trail passes just right of the peak before following a steep ridge that drops down to the junction of Martinez and Tahquitz Canyons, 2.8 miles from Agua Alta Spring.

VARIATION

Intrepid explorers can walk up Martinez Canyon 1.2 miles to the two-room Jack Miller Cabin, built of stone in the 1930s. The miner's cabin, also called the Martinez Canyon Rockhouse, was placed on the National Register of Historic Places in 1999.

Your navigation problems are over, but the hiking is no easier. A trail once descended Martinez Canyon, but it is no longer maintained and few traces are left. Boulder hop eastward for 5 miles. Where springs flow, the narrow canyon is choked with reeds that are difficult to push through. Eventually, the canyon widens and Agua Alta Canyon joins in from the northeast. Finally, reach the wilderness boundary, where jeep tracks lead 5.5 miles out of the canyon and north past fields to your vehicle.

Cactus Spring Trail

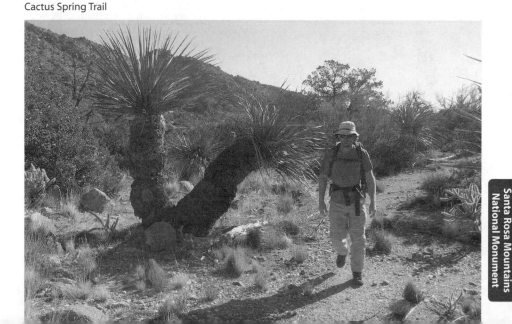

trip 12.15 Pinyon Trail

Distance	8.5 miles (out-and-back, or a cross-country loop)
Hiking Time	5 hours
Elevation Gain	1400'
Difficulty	Moderate
Trail Use	Equestrians, cyclists
Best Times	October–March
Agency	Santa Rosa and San Jacinto Mountains National Monument
Required Map	*Santa Rosa and San Jacinto Mountains National Monument* or *Toro Peak 7.5'*

see map on p. 270

DIRECTIONS From Highway 74 at mile marker 74 RIV 80.50, turn north onto Pinon Rd. In 0.1 mile, reach the entrance to the Pinyon Flats Campground. Unless you are staying at the campground, park on the shoulder of Pinon Rd.

The Pinyon Trail (5E02) is an alternative route into Palm Canyon originating from Highway 74. It was constructed by the Coachella Valley Trails Council in the 1990s. Starting at the Pinyon Flats Campground, it leads across a magnificent plateau covered with ribbonwoods, cacti, yuccas, and, of course, pinyon pines. It features great views of Santa Rosa Mtn. and the southern Desert Divide. It is easy to get lost in this part of the desert, so this trip is not recommended for beginning navigators. Adventurous hikers may make a loop, returning by the Palm Canyon Trail or Omstott Creek. For those wanting a truly wild backpacking trip from the Salton Sea to Palm Springs, the Pinyon Trail makes the critical link between the Cactus Springs Trail and Palm Canyon.

The trail starts next to the Pinyon Flats Campground sign and leads north along the west side of Pinon Rd. for 0.1 mile, then turns left and heads west. It generally follows the fence line marking the boundary between Forest Service and private land, and in another 0.6 mile reaches a pair of trail markers where the trail crosses the dirt Palm Canyon Dr. (private). This is a critical junction; be sure to depart this junction to the northwest on a signed trail rather than accidentally taking one of the power line roads or other dirt roads.

Pinyon pine at dawn on the Pinyon Trail

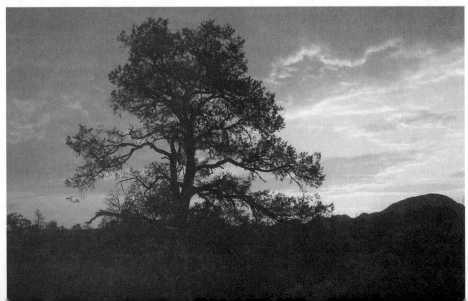

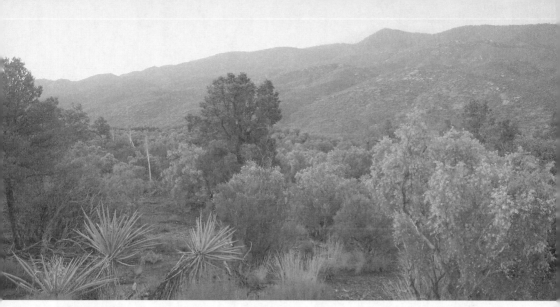

Ribbonwood, pinyon pines, and Mojave yucca along the Pinyon Trail, with Santa Rosa Mtn. in the background.

ALTERNATIVE START

An alternative start for this trip begins at the Sawmill Trailhead (see Trip 12.12), but it is difficult to follow. Hike west from the Sawmill parking area across the road to the signed Ribbonwood Equestrian Campground Rd. In 0.1 mile, where the campground road veers left, continue straight onto a trail at an unlabeled trail post. The equestrian trail braids repeatedly. In 1.0 mile, reach an equestrian tunnel passing beneath Highway 74. On the far side, the trail again braids countless times. If all goes well, you will arrive in 0.6 mile at a trail marker where the Pinyon Trail crosses the good dirt Palm Canyon Dr. Neither path is named at this intersection. If all does not go well, you will nevertheless eventually intersect Palm Canyon Dr. by hiking northwest.

The Pinyon Trail leads into the badlands of the Santa Rosa Mountains. Erosion has gouged the plateau with gullies that progressively deepen to canyons as you head north. The unusual ribbonwood trees are the dominant vegetation, but a wealth of sharp and pointy desert flora are sprinkled amidst the ribbonwoods.

In 1.1 miles, reach a cairn where an unmarked footpath comes in from the right, but stay straight on the main trail.

The trail begins to wind in and out of minor canyons, and then makes a steep series of switchbacks to drop into Omstott Creek. It climbs back up onto the hill beyond, then drops back into Omstott Creek at an unmarked junction with the Palm Canyon Trail. The junction is on the bottom of the canyon directly opposite the point where the Palm Canyon Trail begins switchbacking out of the canyon. This point is 3.6 miles from Palm Canyon Dr. The junction is hidden by bushes, so locating the Pinyon Trail from below would be difficult unless you know to look for it where the Palm Canyon Trail leaves the canyon floor. Return the way you came.

ALTERNATIVE FINISH

You can make a loop returning up the Palm Canyon Trail or Omstott Creek.

The Palm Canyon Trail switchbacks up onto a ridge and in 3.5 miles reaches Pine View Dr. by Highway 74, 2.7 miles west of Pinon Rd. (See Trip 11.12) This is an enjoyable hike, especially if you have arranged a vehicle at Pine View Dr. so that you don't have to trudge back along the highway.

The Omstott Creek route is shown on the National Monument map but is only for hardy cross-country travelers. It follows the canyon floor, roughly parallel to the Pinyon

Trail. While most of the hike is on an easy sandy creek bed, some sections are seriously overgrown and require pushing through dense brush. Watch out for rattlesnakes and for bees that are drawn to the damp creek bed. The lower part of the canyon features some magnificent pancake prickly pear cacti tenaciously rooted in the rock walls. In 3.3 miles, exit the canyon where it splits in two directions, and becomes hope-lessly choked with brush. Walk south across the desert to reach the dirt Saint Pierre Rd. near some houses. Turn left (east) and follow the road 0.4 mile to Palm Canyon Dr. Turn left (northeast) and continue 0.1 mile to the signed junction where the Pinyon Trail crosses the road. Turn right on the Pinyon Trail and return to Pinyon Flats Campground.

---

trip 12.16 Rabbit Peak from the Salton Sea

Distance	16 miles (out-and-back)
Hiking Time	12–14 hours
Elevation Gain	6800′
Difficulty	Very strenuous
Trail Use	Suitable for backpacking
Best Times	October–December (closed during the rest of the year)
Agency	Santa Rosa and San Jacinto Mountains National Monument
Required Map	*Rabbit Peak* 7.5′

see map on p. 279

DIRECTIONS From Interstate 10 in Indio, turn south on the 86S Expressway. Drive south, then turn right (west) on Highway 195 (also known as 66th Ave.) Stay on Highway 195. In 1.1 miles it turns left (south) and is also known as Pierce. In 4 miles, turn right (west) on 74th Ave. In 1 mile, cross Harrison and make an immediate left (south) on Filmore. Follow Filmore 2.3 miles to its end near some citrus groves. Park on the side of the street.

Rabbit Peak (6640+′) is the toughest mountain in Southern California to climb even when ascending by the easiest route. Anchoring the south end of the Santa Rosa Mtn. crest, it requires climbing more than 6000 feet of rugged trailless terrain from any direction. The rewards include fine views of the Salton Sea and Santa Rosa Mountains, close interaction with the full gamut of desert vegetation, and a great physical workout. The three most common routes on the mountain are this one from near the Salton Sea, an ascent of similar difficulty from Clark Dry Lake to the west (see Trip 12.18), and a tremendously long climb up the south ridge over Villager Peak (see Trip 12.17). These routes can be done as two-day backpacking trips, but you must haul all your water so it is questionable whether the difficulty is reduced. A few

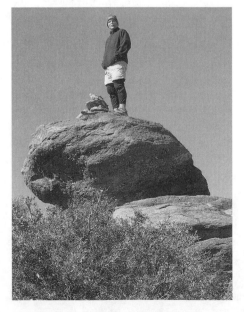

Rabbit Peak Summit Rocks

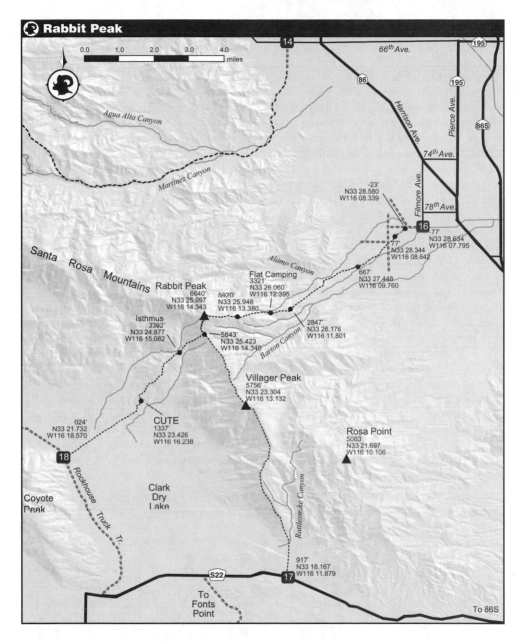

Rabbit Peak

0.0   1.0   2.0   3.0   4.0
miles

66th Ave.

Agua Alta Canyon

Harrison Ave.

Pierce Ave.

74th Ave.

Martinez Canyon

-23'
N33 28.580
W116 08.339

78th Ave.

77'
N33 28.634
W116 07.795

Santa   Rosa   Mountains

Alamo Canyon

77'
N33 28.344
W116 08.642

Rabbit Peak
6640'
N33 25.997
W116 14.343

Flat Camping
3321'
N33 26.060
W116 12.395

5920'
N33 25.948
W116 13.380

667'
N33 27.448
W116 09.760

Isthmus
3392'
N33 24.877
W116 15.082

5843'
N33 25.423
W116 14.340

Barton Canyon

2847'
N33 26.176
W116 11.801

024'
N33 21.732
W116 18.570

Villager Peak
5756'
N33 23.304
W116 13.132

CUTE
1337'
N33 23.426
W116 16.238

Rosa Point
5003'
N33 21.697
W116 10.106

Coyote
Peak

Rockhouse Truck Tr.

Clark
Dry
Lake

Rattlesnake Canyon

917'
N33 18.167
W116 11.879

To
Fonts
Point

To 86S

hardy souls have traversed the entire spine of the Santa Rosa Mountains from Toro Peak to Rabbit and on down over Villager Peak; this route is reportedly 31 arduous cross-country miles and involves 11,000 feet of elevation gain despite running the ridge in the net downhill direction.

The system of roads, levees, and ranches around the start of this trailhead has changed since the USGS map was printed and the navigation across the desert floor in the dark can be the crux of the route-finding challenge. Indeed, this area is developing rapidly and the network of roads may

Santa Rosa Mountains
National Monument

change again by the time you read this. Your first goal is to identify the long ridge between Alamo and Barton Canyons leading up Rabbit Peak. This is easiest to do in the daylight. The ridge is at a bearing of 230 degrees from the trailhead. A GPS receiver and extra batteries are helpful to record the route in the event that you retrace it after dark. Headlamps are indispensable for any route on Rabbit Peak.

From your vehicle, walk south past a gate at the end of Filmore, then immediately turn right (west) and follow a road on a levee between two citrus groves. In 0.4 mile, the levee veers right where two washes converge. Follow the left wash as it continues west. In 0.1 mile, turn left (south) at the west end of a grove. Follow the wash a few yards, then scramble up the west side into the desert, where you will find faint traces of an old dirt road leading toward Rabbit Peak. Follow it southwest.

Soon, you will begin seeing white cairns along the path. (The white rocks show up well by headlamp on a nighttime descent, but this section is nevertheless challenging and tedious to follow in the dark.) In 0.4 mile, cross a wash and arrive at a metal post. The road ends here, but the trail continues, marked by more cairns. In another 2.8

miles, the trail switchbacks and climbs onto the south side of the base of the ridge. It gradually climbs along the side of the ridge to the ocotillo-studded crest. From here on, cairns are found sporadically but are difficult to consistently follow. Your goal is simply to go up along the path of least resistance. Pay attention to the route so you can locate the correct ridges on the descent.

The ridge climbs to a small saddle at 2500 feet, ascends steeply, and then levels out into a jumbled field of boulders and agaves. Just west of Point 3235′, there are several clearings; these mark the half way point and offer fine but exposed dry camping for those backpacking the mountain.

Farther west, cross a narrow isthmus between two canyons and begin climbing in earnest, gaining 2600 feet in the next 1.1 miles. Pick your way around the innumerable cacti and agaves. Just before reaching the top, climb some class two slabs and traverse an easy knife-edge rock ridge to reach the long hogsback of Rabbit Peak. Continue another 1.1 miles west through juniper and scrub oak country to the summit boulders at the extreme west end of the ridge.

Return the way you came, or, with a car shuttle, descend to Clark Dry Lake. (See Trip 12.18.)

Rabbit Peak between Alamo and Barton Canyons. Note the lower approach ridge pointing down toward the trailhead.

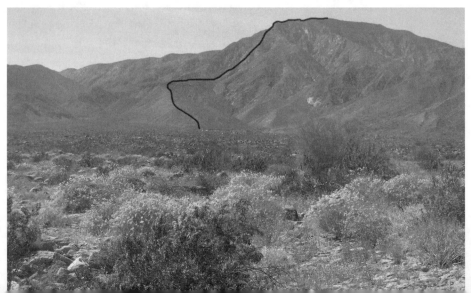

trip 12.17 Rabbit and Villager Peaks

Distance	21 miles (out-and-back)
Hiking Time	14 hours
Elevation Gain	7900'
Difficulty	Very strenuous
Trail Use	Suitable for backpacking
Best Times	October–December (closed during the rest of the year)
Agency	Santa Rosa and San Jacinto Mountains National Monument
Required Map	*Fonts Point, Rabbit Peak* 7.5'

see map on p. 279

DIRECTIONS From Interstate 10 in Indio, turn south on the 86S Expressway. Drive 35 miles, then turn right (west) on the Borrego Salton Seaway (S22). Proceed 14 miles, then park in a turnout on the north side of the road adjacent to call box S22-319; this point is 0.1 mile west of mile marker 32 and directly opposite the Thimble jeep trail.

This is the most strenuous of the routes on Rabbit Peak described in this book, but it also involves the simplest route-finding in the dark. It leads up the long crest of the Santa Rosa Mountains from the southern toe near the Borrego Salton Seaway, passing over Villager Peak en route to Rabbit. Bring headlamps and plenty of water; 6 quarts are merited on a cool day, more on a warm one.

From the parking area, identify the ridge to the north on the left (west) side of Rattlesnake Canyon. The Clark Fault has raised the interesting Lute scarp between the parking and the ridge. The scarp climbs gradually from the south but drops off precipitously on the north side. Hike across the desert toward the ridge, veering slightly right to remain east of the scarp. You may find ducks marking a path.

In 1.2 miles, gain the toe of the ridge. Look for switchbacks and a good use trail climbing unrelentingly. Watch for a spectacular display of cacti, ocotillos, and agaves. After 5.8 miles, the use trail reaches the summit of Villager Peak (5756').

If you have time and energy remaining, continue north 3.6 miles to Rabbit Peak. The undulating ridge involves 2000 feet of ascent and 1100 feet of descent that must be regained on the return. The use trail can generally be followed through the pinyon pines and scrub oaks to the summit of Rab-

bit, but if you lose the trail, simply pick the path of least resistance along the ridge.

Return the way you came. 1.8 miles south of Villager Peak, at an elevation of 4400 feet, the ridge forks. Be sure to stay right; the tempting left ridge lures hikers into the steep upper reaches of Rattlesnake Canyon. Once you reach the desert, finding your way back through the washes and boulders can be somewhat tricky at night. If you don't have a GPS, head south. The lights of passing vehicles show where the road lies, and the trailhead is near the closest point on the road.

Aerial view of Rabbit and Villager Peaks from the south

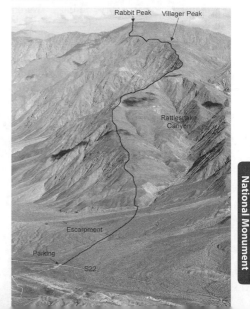

SIDE TRIP

If you have extra time before or after the trip, consider taking a drive to Fonts Point for a fantastic view over the colorful Borrego Badlands. The Fonts Point Rd. begins 2.4 miles west of the Villager Peak trailhead (0.5 mile west of mile marker 30) on S22. It follows a sandy wash and a 4WD vehicle is helpful, but ordinary passenger cars can usually navigate the wash with careful driving. Follow the wash 4 miles to the overlook.

trip 12.18 Rabbit Peak from Clark Dry Lake

Distance	15 miles (out-and-back)
Hiking Time	12–14 hours
Elevation Gain	6100′
Difficulty	Very strenuous
Best Times	October–December (closed during the rest of the year)
Agency	Santa Rosa and San Jacinto Mountains National Monument
Required Map	*Clark Lake, Lark Lake NE, Rabbit Peak* 7.5′

see map on p. 279

DIRECTIONS From Interstate 10 in Indio, turn south on the 86S Expressway. Drive 35 miles, then turn right (west) on the Borrego Salton Seaway (S22). Proceed 20 miles, then turn right (north) at the signed junction onto the Rockhouse Truck Trail; this point is 0.7 mile west of mile marker 27. Follow the good dirt road 5.4 miles to a large turnout on the west side of the road. This point is unmarked on the Clark Lake Map but is just southeast of the Noll benchmark.

The western approach to Rabbit Peak from a point just north of Clark Lake is shorter but even steeper than the others. It crosses the Anza Borrego Desert, which is justly famous for its remarkable cacti. Of all the trips in this book, this one offers the greatest opportunity to see all things sharp and pointy. Each plant occupies a distinctive habitat, and it is fascinating to watch the flora change as you climb.

This trip is entirely cross-country, and not even cairns mark the trail. Carefully study your maps. Note the landmarks where you started near Coyote Mtn. to assist your return, especially if it is after dark. A headlamp, GPS receiver, and spare batteries are helpful to find your way back to your vehicle at night.

From the parking area, look northeast and identify the major landmarks. Rabbit Peak is the highest point on the horizon. The long backbone of the Santa Rosa Mountains leads up from the south. The southernmost distinct high point is Villager Peak. Take a compass bearing of 50 degrees and identify a high point immediately north of Villager Peak. Walking on this bearing takes you to the south side of a ridge extending into the Clark Valley.

Follow the 50-degree bearing across the sandy desert floor past creosote bushes and pencil chollas. In 2.2 miles, reach the edge of the bajada, where walking becomes steeper and more difficult because of boulders and washes. Ocotillos, barrel cacti, and brittlebushes become common. Gain the toe of the ridge and pass the CUTE benchmark (1337′) in another 0.8 mile. Follow this poorly-defined ridge up to Point 2719′. As you climb, look for teddy bear and valley chollas, beavertail cacti, small fishhook cacti, dense stands of desert agaves, and, eventually junipers.

Continue northeastward up the ridge, which eventually narrows as it passes between two deep canyons. On this narrow isthmus are two small bivouac clearings with spectacular views. At this point, you have covered most of the distance but only half of the elevation gain. Follow the ridge

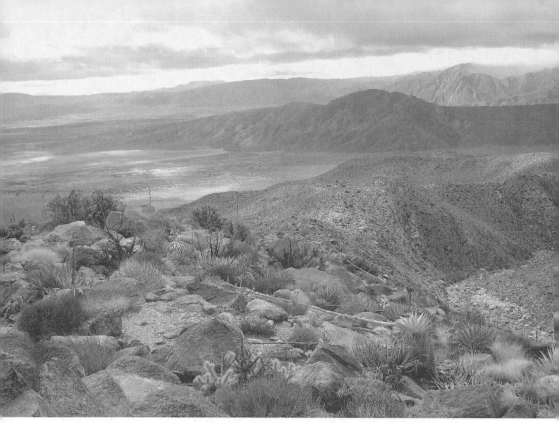

Clark Valley

photo by Tony Condon

northeastward toward the crest, gaining 2300 feet in the next 0.8 mile. There is one short band of rock to negotiate, but most of the climbing is simply walking up steep dirt and easy talus. As you climb, reach zones of prickly pear cacti, Mojave yuccas, and nolinas.

Upon reaching the crest of the Santa Rosa Mountains at 5800 feet, turn left (north). You may find a use trail, occasionally marked with cairns, on the east side of the crest. Pass over a small saddle, then make the final 800-foot ascent up slopes covered with pinyon pines and scrub oaks. Level out abruptly just south of the summit boulders.

Return the way you came or, with a car shuttle, take one of the other routes down. (See Trips 12.16 and 12.17.) There are several clearings where people have camped on the hogsback east of the summit.

chapter 13

Mecca Hills Wilderness

Fifteen miles southeast of Indio near the north shore of the Salton Sea, the dusty town of Mecca sits amid lush fields of carrots, peppers, and artichokes; thick groves of oranges, pecans, and date palms; and row upon row of rich grape vines. The earliest people to inhabit Mecca were the Cahuilla Indians. Because they lived so far inland, these Desert Cahuilla had little contact with the colonizing Spanish who established missions in San Gabriel and San Diego.

Although the Desert Cahuilla had dug an extensive network of wells to support agriculture in the Coachella Valley, it wasn't until the late 19th Century that Anglo-Americans considered developing the area for agriculture. In Mecca Hills' arid climate, it was the presence of water that led to the development of a railroad stop named Walters along the Yuma-Los Angeles rail line. Mecca's founder—R. Holtby Meyers—at the urging of his wife, changed the town's name from Walters to Mecca because the desert climate and burgeoning date palm industry so closely resembled the famed holy city. Developers capitalized upon this image and used the exotic images of Arabian oases to draw people to Mecca. It

Hikers in Ladder Canyon

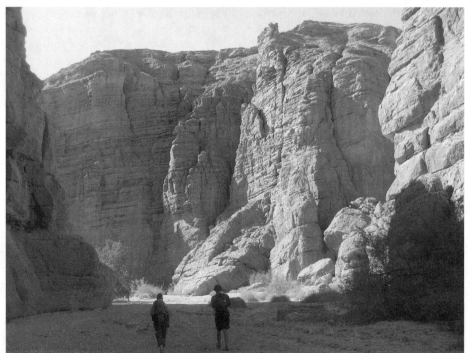

clearly worked; the area began to attract numerous family farmers. The completion of the Coachella Branch of the All-American Canal in 1948 transformed small family farms into sprawling commercial fields.

Agriculture is not only the lure in Mecca; the town lies beside a section of the San Andreas Fault zone that draws both professional and amateur seismologists. The seismic activity of the fault has thrust up a range of hills cut by a labyrinth of winding, narrow canyons, sandy washes, and caves, known locally as grottos. The violent upheavals that create the beautifully colored canyons of Mecca Hills Wilderness are the result of friction between the North American and Pacific plates along a spur of the San Andreas Fault. Much of

the rock, which has been upturned and exposed by centuries of earthquakes, is over 600 million years old. These rocks provide geologists and seismologists with valuable clues about the effects of temblors on the earth's crust. Because of its unique geological formations, the United States Congress designated the Mecca Hills as a federally protected wilderness area in 1994.

Mecca Hills Wilderness area is replete with flora and fauna that have adapted to the hostile desert environment. Yellowbloomed palo verde trees densely populate the deep washes in the area. The Mecca aster, a violet-tinted flower resembling a daisy, grows only in this area and in Baja Mexico. Majestic ocotillos stand sentry on the tops of mesas and on the gentler slopes.

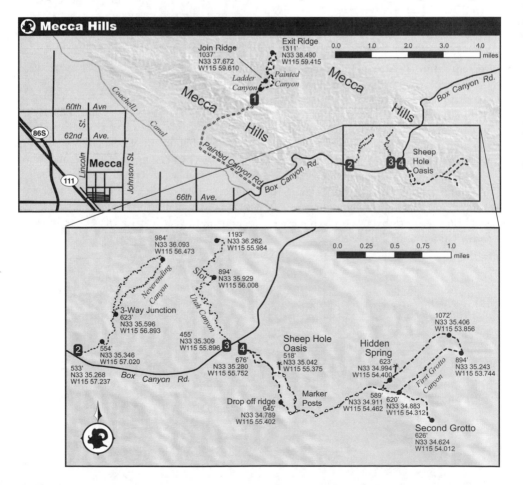

Their braches typically burst forth in a flurry of vermilion blooms in late spring, adding yet another layer of rich color to the painted canyons in the area. The rare spotted bat, famous for having the largest ears of any North American bat, lives in Mecca Hills Wilderness. Desert tortoises and prairie falcons also call the area home. Bighorn sheep cross into Mecca Hills from the Oracopia Mountains looking for reliable sources of water at Sheep Hole Oasis and Hidden Spring Canyon.

There are only a handful of established trails in Mecca Hills. This chapter describes the two most popular, Ladder Canyon and the Grottos, along with two cross-country routes exploring other spectacular canyons. However, inquisitive canyoneers will enjoy exploring the maze-like washes snaking through the colorful hills. Philip Ferranti's book, *140 Great Hikes in and near Palm Springs*, is a handy reference for more canyon adventures in Mecca Hills.

The 1994 California Desert Protection Act designated much of the Mecca Hills as Wilderness. No wilderness permit is required, but bicycles and motorized equipment are not allowed. Camping is allowed, with a maximum 14-day stay.

The pleasures of hiking in Mecca Hills include beautiful views of the Salton Sea. The Salton Sea lies in a basin more than 200 feet below sea level that was once connected to the Gulf of California until accumulated silt from the Colorado River cut the basin off and allowed the water to evaporate. The basin has refilled with water on many occasions. In 700 AD, the Colorado River turned north and formed Lake Cahuilla, which lasted a thousand years, until the Colorado River changed direction once again, leaving the lake to evaporate over time. Subsequent outpourings of the river have occasionally created small salt lakes. In 1901, the California Development Company built a system of irrigation canals to divert the Colorado River to farm the Imperial Valley. A flood breached the canals, sending the river pouring into the basin for a year and a half. By the time the canals were repaired, the present Salton Sea had formed. It now covers 376 square miles and is the largest lake in California. The water evaporates rapidly but is replenished by agricultural runoff. This causes the salinity to steadily increase, imperiling the fish that live in the lake and the migrating birds that depend on the fish. On the other hand, if the lake were to completely dry up, it would leave a basin full of carcinogenic dust that would be whipped about the Coachella Valley by the strong desert winds. The Salton Sea clearly presents substantial environmental and economic challenges, but it is also a source of fascination and wonder. Consider detouring to visit it if you have extra time on a Mecca Hills trip.

trip 13.1 Ladder and Big Painted Canyons

Distance	5 miles (loop)
Hiking Time	3 hours
Elevation Gain	750'
Difficulty	Moderate
Trail Use	Good for children
Best Times	October–April
Agency	BLM (Palm Springs Field Office)
Recommended Map	*Mortimar, Cottonwood Basin 7.5'*

see map on p. 285

DIRECTIONS From Interstate 10 in Indio, exit south on 86S and drive 10 miles to 62nd Ave. near the town of Mecca. Drive east 2 miles to its end at Johnson St., then turn right, proceed another 2 miles, then turn left on 66th Ave. The road changes name to Box Canyon Rd. and passes a signed turnoff for Painted Canyon Rd. Turn left on Painted Canyon Rd. A sign indicates 4WD vehicles only, but unless there have been heavy rains, the road is usually easily passable by low-clearance cars. Proceed 4.7 miles to the parking area in Painted Canyon.

Ladder Canyon and Big Painted Canyon are highlights of the Mecca Hills. The path snakes through a steep-walled canyon, up several ladders, and through a narrow slot canyon. The ladders are usually maintained by volunteers, but assess the conditions for yourself before trusting your footing. Once you leave Ladder Canyon, you will hike along the ridge, and find yourself surrounded by great views of Mecca Hills and the Salton Sea. After the ridge you will descend into the aptly named Big Painted Canyon for your hike back.

From the parking area, begin hiking northeast up the wide canyon behind the BLM sign. Look for healthy palo verde trees, smoke trees, and cat's claw acacia growing in the bottom of the wash. In 0.5 mile you will come to a trail marker on the right side of the canyon that points left toward the yawning boulder-strewn mouth of Ladder Canyon. Scramble into the side canyon and climb the ladders, then continue through the long narrow slot. After the canyon begins to open, stay right at a fork, 0.9 mile from the start. In less than 0.1 mile, look for the first easy way to walk up the right slope of the canyon. Follow a use trail up the wall of the canyon; you will need to negotiate a short but steep dirt wall part way up before reaching the ridge crest, 1 mile from the start.

Descending Ladder Canyon · *photo by Cidney Scanlon*

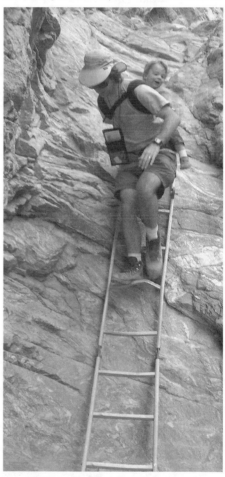

Turn left at the top of the ridge and hike north. Enjoy the views into the canyons on both sides, but don't get too close to the edge because the sandy slopes drop off abruptly over tall cliffs. Soon you will be able to see radio towers in the distance, follow the ridge toward these towers. In 1.1 miles, reach a saddle at the north end of the trail. To the left, you can see a dry waterfall near the head of Little Painted Canyon. The main trail turns right and drops into Big Painted Canyon.

Big Painted Canyon is a geologist's delight. Head down the canyon, staying right (downhill) at a junction. In 1.5 miles, climb down another pair of ladders where the canyon narrows and drops. Reach the trail junction 0.5 mile farther where you originally entered Ladder Canyon.

trip 13.2 Never Ending Canyon

Distance	3.5 miles (loop)
Hiking Time	2 hours
Elevation Gain	500'
Difficulty	Easy
Trail Use	Dogs
Best Times	October–April
Agency	BLM (Palm Springs Field Office)
Recommended Map	*Mortimar 7.5'*

see map on p. 285

DIRECTIONS From Interstate 10 in Indio, exit south on 86S and drive 10 miles to 62nd Ave. near the town of Mecca. Drive east 2 miles to its end at Johnson St., then turn right, proceed another 2 miles, then turn left on 66th Ave. The road changes name to Box Canyon Rd. and passes a signed turnoff for Painted Canyon Rd. Reset your odometer here. Drive on Box Canyon for 3.4 miles past the Painted Canyon sign, and pull off onto a dirt road on the left. The beginning of the trail is marked by a line of large rocks blocking the dirt road.

Never Ending Canyon is a gorgeous hike between the colorful walls of the Mecca Hills. The hike leads you through two separate canyons, the second of which rejoins the first, leading you back to your car. You are rewarded by a breath-taking view when you reach the crest at the head of the canyons. Most of the hike follows trailless washes so cross-country navigation skills are necessary. Do not attempt this hike when rain threatens because the slot canyons are at risk of flash floods.

From your car, dirt roads lead east and north. Walk east down the larger road, passing the line of boulders. Follow the wash as it bends to the left near a damaged signpost, and enter the first canyon. Stay in the main wash when you encounter small side canyons. The trail will soon fork into two distinct trails on either side of a large formation near a rusty old icebox; continue into the left canyon. Follow this canyon and admire its unique sand and mud walls imprinted with fascinating water patterns. Soon you will see an old rusted car wreck. Avoid the smaller trail on the left, staying in the main canyon, and soon come to a three-way junction. Do not take the first smaller canyon on the far right. Instead continue your path in the middle canyon, winding around the right side of a prominent round-topped formation with interesting strata. (You will return via the far left canyon.)

Stay in the larger canyon, avoiding smaller trails that branch off. Soon the canyon will narrow. Some fallen rocks and landslides may block your meandering path, but they are fun and easy to negotiate. Eventually the canyon opens up. At the head of the canyon ascend the rock field to the crest, and follow a path on the ridge crest outlined by rocks. The path leads to the left for a short distance to a cairn marking the high point. Take in the amazing view in all directions from the ridge.

Once you are finished enjoying the view, descend via the steep trail on the north-western slope into the second canyon. The slope is easy enough to handle and free from imminent dangers, but it consists of loose dirt so take care not to slip. Follow the main wash downhill for the rest of your journey, taking time to admire the amazing walls that make Mecca Hills such a beautiful place to hike. You will rejoin your previous trail at the three-way junction. From there retrace your steps back to your car.

Never Ending Canyon

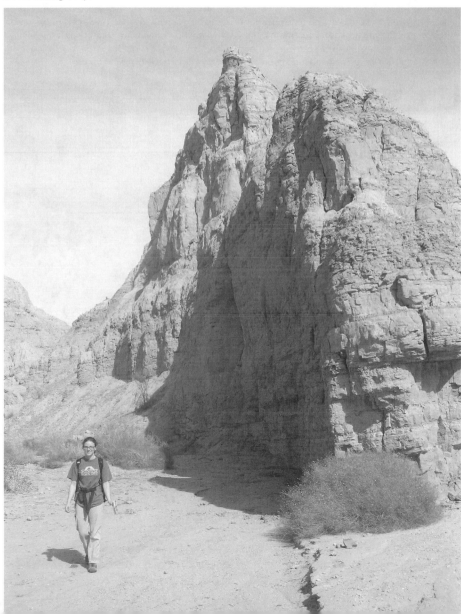

trip 13.3 Utah Canyon

Distance	4 miles (out-and-back)
Hiking Time	2 hours
Elevation Gain	500'
Difficulty	Easy
Trail Use	Dogs
Best Times	October–April
Agency	BLM (Palm Springs Field Office)
Recommended Map	*Mortimar 7.5'*

see map on p. 285

DIRECTIONS From Interstate 10 in Indio, exit south on 86S and drive 10 miles to 62nd Ave. near the town of Mecca. Drive east 2 miles to its end at Johnson St., then turn right, proceed another 2 miles, then turn left on 66th Ave. The road changes name to Box Canyon Rd. and passes a signed turnoff for Painted Canyon Rd. Reset your odometer here. Drive on Box Canyon for 4.9 miles past the Painted Canyon sign to the mouth of a canyon on the north, and park on the shoulder of the road. If you reach the Sheep Hole Oasis Trailhead marker on the south, you have gone 0.1 mile too far.

U tah Canyon, named for its resemblance to the colorful canyons of Southern Utah, features brilliant rocks and narrow winding passages. This hike is best done in the early morning or late afternoon when the sun highlights the intense reds, pinks, oranges, and mauves of the canyon walls.

Hike north up a wide, sandy wash lined with sprawling mesquite and palo verde trees. The wash promptly branches; stay to the left. As you hike up the wash, the canyon narrows considerably. Creosote bushes spread their lanky branches lazily through the wash, often blocking the trail. Negotiate around them as you journey up the canyon, enjoying the twists and turns of the trail.

In 0.5 mile, the trail curves around an impressive mudfall (like rockfall, but made of dried mud). In another 0.7 mile, the canyon forks again. Bear left into a canyon that soon becomes a slot just wide enough for two to walk abreast. Beyond the narrows, the canyon reopens. Spindly stands of ocotillo grace the rocky slopes. Stay in the main wash as you pass several side canyons. In 0.4 mile, veer left at a major fork. The canyon soon ends in a small valley. Follow the slopes up to the ridge for a birds-eye view of the multihued canyon systems winding down to the Salton Sea.

Return the way you came.

The Narrows in Utah Canyon

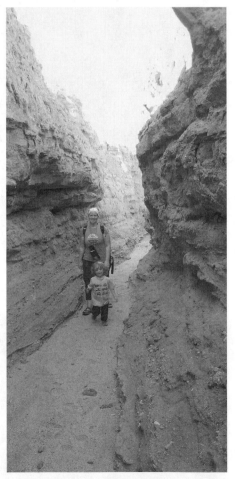

trip 13.4 The Grottos

Distance	7 miles (semi-loop)
Hiking Time	5 hours
Elevation Gain	1500′
Difficulty	Moderate
Trail Use	Dogs
Best Times	October–April
Agency	BLM (Palm Springs Field Office)
Required Map	*Mortimar 7.5′*

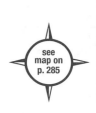

see map on p. 285

DIRECTIONS From Interstate 10 in Indio, exit south on 86S and drive 10 miles to 62nd Ave. near the town of Mecca. Drive east 2 miles to its end at Johnson St., then turn right, proceed another 2 miles, then turn left on 66th Ave. The road changes name to Box Canyon Rd. and passes a signed turnoff for Painted Canyon Rd. Reset your odometer here. Continue 5.0 miles to the signed Sheep Hole Oasis Trailhead on the right.

The Grottos are two slot canyons nestled in the outlandishly colorful Mecca Hills. They have filled with giant boulders to form remarkable cave systems. Two palm oases bring further wonder to this unusual trip. If your time is limited, you can shorten the trip by visiting only one of the Grottos. Be sure to bring a flashlight; a helmet is also helpful. The terrain is complicated and is crisscrossed with a warren of trails, so a map and good navigational skills are essential. The main trail is almost always well-used, so if the path becomes faint, you are probably on the wrong trail.

From the parking area, the Hidden Spring Trail leads into the canyon. You

Hidden Spring Canyon below Second Grotto

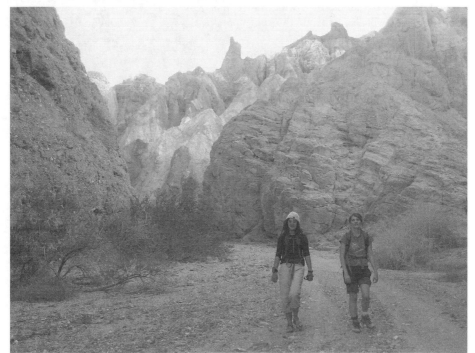

will soon reach a fork; stay left, then follow the trail straight up the ridge to reach a hilltop with panoramic views of the Mecca Hills, the Salton Sea, and the Santa Rosa Mountains, 0.25 mile from the start. Turn left and follow the crest of the ridge. You will see the Sheep Hole Oasis below on your left, but pass the side trail leading down and continue south along the ridge until the main trail drops eastward into the canyon, 0.8 mile from the start. Cross the wash to a post, then continue east up a small side canyon to the top of a rise with another trail junction. Descend east into the large Hidden Spring Canyon. A series of posts marks the route northeastward up the sandy canyon floor. The canyon narrows and the walls become vertical, then they change into exotic purple, brown, and tan colors. The first canyon on your left after entering the narrows is home to Hidden Spring and is marked with a post. You will later come down the canyon leading from Hidden Spring and return to this spot. The second canyon on the left is the entrance to the First Grotto, marked by a 6-foot-tall tree stump. You will also return to this spot, so be sure that you can recognize it.

Continue east and then south up the main canyon to the very end passing spires and battlements of green, pink, purple, red, and yellow sedimentary rock. Then turn left and enter a narrow slot canyon that is home to the Second Grotto. Explore the cave system until it ends at a 15-foot wall. Climbers will enjoy scrambling up the fourth-class conglomerate rock to the top, but our hike returns the way you came. Retrace your steps to the First Grotto Canyon.

Ascend First Grotto Canyon 0.4 mile until it becomes choked with boulders. Climb into their maw and pick your way through the cave system. Cross over to the left side of the canyon, walk a wooden plank, and descend into the tunnel. If the scrambling becomes difficult, you are off route. After navigating through three stretches of caves, reach the upper portion of the can-

yon. Look for a steep jeep road cut through the canyon wall on the left. Ascend on the road until it levels out at a four-way junction, then turn left and follow the jeep trail as it crosses a wash and climbs another very steep hill. Beyond the hill, leave the jeep road at a faint trail leading left at a cairn. The trail heads west, then traverses a ridge southwest until the Hidden Spring Oasis comes into view on the left. As the ridge narrows to a knife-edge, follow a steep trail down to the oasis. After enjoying the palms, work your way down the narrow canyon back to the main Hidden Spring Canyon Trail at the post that you passed earlier.

Turn right and retrace your steps out of the canyon, down the wide wash, and over the small rise. You may continue back up the ridge the way you came, or you may follow posts to Sheep Hole Oasis. At the oasis, beyond the topmost palm, a steep path climbs up the left wall of the canyon to the ridge top and rejoins the main trail.

Second Grotto is not for the claustrophobic.

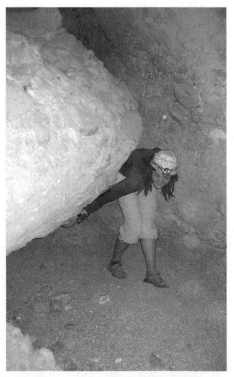

chapter 14

Desert and Mountain Preserves

In recent years, the population explosion in Southern California has led to tremendous development in once quiet communities near Banning Pass. Development has threatened to partition the desert and mountains into "islands" that disrupt traditional patterns of wildlife movement. The natural wind-blown movement of sand has also been disturbed by construction and off-road vehicles, threatening the fragile sand dune habitats. In response to these problems, a number of homegrown and national conservation groups have teamed with government agencies to purchase and preserve critical habitat. The groups have also built several fine trail systems so that hikers can enjoy these special places. This chapter describes trips in several of these preserves.

The Wildlands Conservancy

The Wildlands Conservancy, founded in 1995, has developed a grand vision of the Sand-to-Snow Preserve System; the group has been remarkably effective at carrying it out. They have identified strategic blocks of land at the periphery of the San Bernardino National Forest, Joshua Tree National Park, and other preserves in the area, and have raised funds to create the largest non-profit preserve system in Southern California. This 37,000-acre system includes the

Whitewater Canyon Ranger Station

photo courtesy of The Wildlands Conservancy Staff

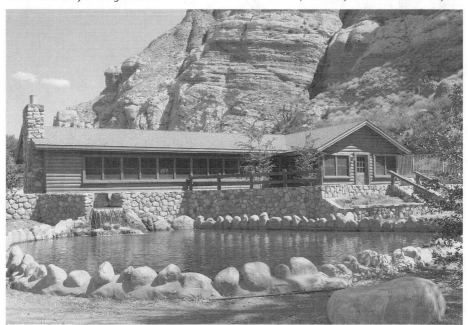

Pioneertown Mountains Preserve, the Oak Glen Preserve, the Mission Creek Preserve, and the Whitewater Preserve. Several hikes in this system are described in this chapter.

Coachella Valley Preserve

The 17,000-acre Coachella Valley Preserve, located northeast of Palm Springs and south of Joshua Tree, was established in 1986 to protect the sand dune habitat of the endangered Coachella Valley fringe-toed lizard. The preserve is managed by the non-profit Center for Natural Lands Management in partnership with the public agencies that own land on the Preserve. The Preserve's visitor center is located on the San Andreas Fault. The crushed rock and clay in the fault is nearly impermeable to groundwater, directing the water to the surface and resulting in a series of springs that support spectacular palm oases in the midst of the parched desert. Unlike some other local palm oases that are fed by creeks, the 12 oases on the Coachella Valley Preserve are fed only from these earthquake seeps.

Before pioneers arrived in the Palm Springs area, the Coachella Valley was covered with nearly 100 square miles of sand dunes. The Coachella Valley fringe-toed lizard is specially adapted to sand dune habitat, with snowshoe-like hind toes that give traction in the shifting sand. The lizard uses its shovel-like snout to burrow into the sand to avoid the extreme summer heat and to elude predators. In fact, the lizard has more adaptations than any other known species for survival in this extreme environment, where surface temperatures can reach 120–140°F in the heat of the summer. Development projects and off-road vehicles have wiped out 95% of the lizard's dune habitat. The Coachella Valley Preserve system contains the Thousand Palms Preserve, along with two smaller satellite preserves, Whitewater and Edom Hill/Willow Hole. The preserve system protects some of the remaining dunes as well as the precious "sand source" areas of the hills that replenish the sand in the dune systems.

Coachella Valley Preserve map

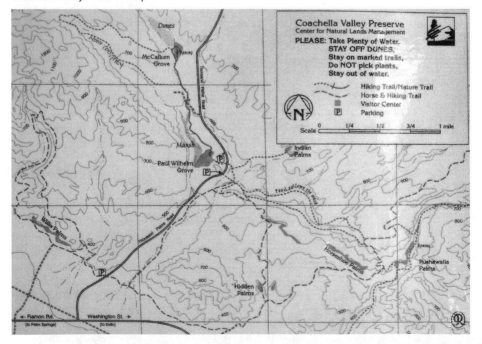

The Coachella Valley Preserve Visitor Center is located in the Palm House in the second largest grove of palms in the valley, known as the Thousand Palms or Wilhelm Grove. It was named for Paul Wilhelm, the writer, naturalist, and long-time resident of the oasis. At the center, you can pick up a free brochure with a reasonably good map of the area, and can get hiking advice from the volunteer staff. About 20 miles of hiking trails radiate through the desert to the other palm oases.

The preserve is open from sunrise to sunset during most of the year and from 5 A.M. to 10 A.M. in July and August. The visitor center is closed in the summer. To protect the habitat, pets, camping, and smoking are not permitted. The Preserve Management asks that you stay off the sand dunes and out of the water.

Big Morongo Canyon Preserve

Big Morongo Canyon, surrounded by cactus-studded desert, is the unlikely site of a lush wetland. Snowmelt from the San Bernardino Mountains flows underground through sandy soils until it encounters an earthquake fault in Big Morongo Canyon. The impermeable rock in the fault directs the water to the surface, creating an array of springs that support a marsh and grove of cottonwoods. Bighorn sheep and many other animals are drawn to the area for water and food, especially in the dry season. Birders from around the world flock to the preserve seeking rare species, especially during spring and fall migration. There are regularly scheduled bird walks; check www.bigmorongo.org for a calendar of events. The land around the preserve was seized from the Morongo band of the Serrano Indians in 1846, and was used for ranching until 1968, when 80 acres were acquired by the Nature Conservancy. Now it encompasses 31,000 acres and is administered by the Bureau of Land Management as an Area of Critical Environmental Concern.

Crafton Hills Open Space Conservancy

The Crafton Hills rise out of the valley south of the San Bernardino Mountains between Yucaipa and Mentone, and they offer commanding views in all directions. On a clear day, you can admire many of the prominent peaks surrounding the Los Angeles Basin including San Gorgonio, San Bernardino, San Jacinto, Santiago, Baldy, and Keller. Zanja Peak (3543′) is the high point of the Crafton Hills. The Spanish word *zanja* (big ditch), pronounced "zan-ha," commemorates the irrigation canal from Mill Creek to Mission San Gabriel's Asistencia outpost laboriously dug from 1820 to 1822 by Native Americans on behalf of the Spanish.

The Crafton Hills Open Space Conservancy was formed in 1992 to protect 4500 acres of chaparral and sage habitat. In collaboration with local governments, the conservancy is working to keep the hills open and to develop and maintain the trail network. By the time you visit, more trails may have been completed. Look for free trail maps at the trailheads, and visit their website at craftonconservancy.homestead.com for the latest information and for a calendar of organized hikes. The Crafton Hills are sun-scorched in the summer, so the cooler months are the best time to visit. The trails attract mountain bikers, equestrians, and birders as well as hikers. Springtime is especially attractive, with the wildflowers in bloom and panoramic views of high peaks clad in snow, but do watch out for rattlesnakes.

For more information about the area, consider a visit to the Yucaipa Valley Historical Society at the Mousely Museum on the corner of Panorama and Bryant in Yucaipa. At the time of this writing, the museum is open on Saturdays from 10 A.M. to 3 P.M. and Wednesdays from 5 P.M. to 8 P.M. The museum phone number is (909) 760-4685.

trip 14.1 McCallum Nature Trail

Distance	2 miles (out-and-back)
Hiking Time	1 hour
Elevation Gain	100'
Difficulty	Easy
Trail Use	Good for children
Best Times	October–March
Agency	Coachella Valley Preserve
Recommended Map	*Coachella Valley Preserve* map

DIRECTIONS From the 10 Freeway, exit on Ramon Rd. and drive east (on the north side of the freeway) for 4.5 miles. Turn left on Thousand Palms Rd. and proceed 2 miles to the visitor center parking area on the left.

This self-guided nature walk brings you through the Thousand Palms Oasis, across the San Andreas Fault, and reaches the McCallum Grove of palms where there is a pond and large sand dune. The trail departs from the Palm House Visitor Center in the midst of the Thousand Palms Oasis.

This oasis has one of the world's largest groves of California fan palms (*Washingtonia filifera*), the only palm native to California The palms grow to 60 feet and live for about 250 years. Their fruit, produced in the spring, is important to birds and other animals in the oasis.

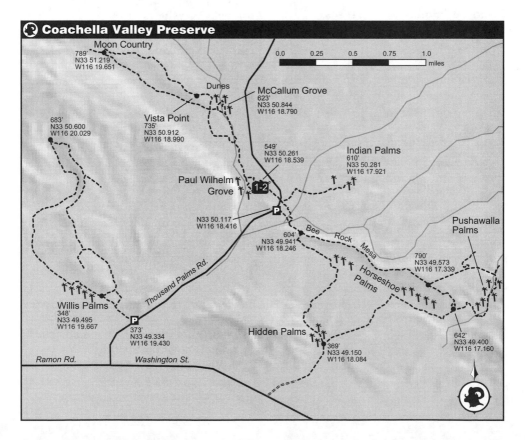

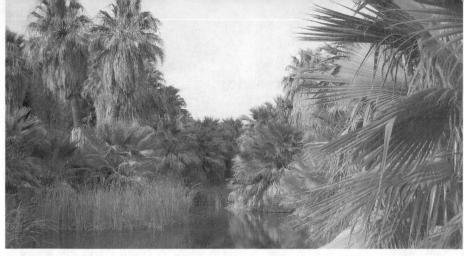

McCallum Grove Oasis

The brochure at the visitor center includes a map and guide to the sights along the way.

From the parking area, walk into the oasis and stop at the Palm House to pick up a map and check out the information on display. Continue through the grove to the beginning of the McCallum Trail, which crosses some wetlands on a boardwalk.

The trail then departs the north side of the grove and follows the edge of the wetlands through the desert. The Coachella Valley is shielded from moist air by the San Bernardino and San Jacinto mountains, so it normally receives only 4–5 inches of rain per year. However, the rainfall is irregular; some years have virtually none, while others have brief but intense rains that cause flash flooding. You will cross the San Andreas Fault, California's infamous earthquake fault. The fault is responsible for pushing up many of the bluffs and hills in this area. The unique geology of the fault zone keeps the water close to the surface, supporting numerous palm oases in the preserve.

In 0.2 mile from the start, a signed trail forks off to the right, leading directly back to the parking area. In another 0.3 mile, pass some private ranch houses. Stay on the trail, taking care not to disturb the residents. In another 0.3 mile, reach the south end of the McCallum Grove. The trail forks here and makes a loop. Take the right fork directly into the grove. Explore the palms, the pond, and the nearby sand dunes.

The oasis and pond are nourished by a spring. The pond is home to the desert pupfish, an endangered minnow-like fish adapted to shallow salty desert pools. The pupfish burrows into the bottom of the pool and lies dormant during the cold winter, then becomes active in the spring and mates in the summer. The pupfish's habitat has been nearly eliminated through development, pollution, and the introduction of exotic species. Keep an eye out for the fish in the spring, but do not feed or disturb it. The sand dunes north of the oasis are built by strong winds that carry grains of sand for long distances. As the wind patterns shift and subside, the grains are deposited to form large piles. This preserve has been established to protect the dunes and fringe-toed lizard, so walking on the dunes is prohibited.

At the far end of the McCallum Grove, the trail loops around to return along the west edge of the grove. In 0.1 mile, pass a signed turnoff for Moon Country and the Vista Point. This optional loop along a desolate ridge and back through a wash adds 2 miles to the hike and is recommended only on a cool day.

When you have finished exploring, return to the Thousand Palms Oasis. You can take a shortcut back to the parking area at the marked trail near interpretive post #5 shortly before reaching the oasis.

trip 14.2 Pushawalla, Horseshoe, and Hidden Palms Loop

Distance	6.5 miles (loop)
Hiking Time	4 hours
Elevation Gain	1000'
Difficulty	Moderate
Best Times	October–March
Agency	Coachella Valley Preserve
Recommended Map	*Coachella Valley Preserve* map

see map on p. 296

DIRECTIONS From the 10 Freeway, exit on Ramon Rd. and drive east (on the north side of the freeway) for 4.5 miles. Turn left on Thousand Palms Rd. and proceed 2.1 miles to the visitor center parking area on the left. If you don't plan to stop at the visitor center for a map, you can save a little walking by parking 0.3 mile back down Thousand Palms Canyon Rd. at a turnout on the east side.

This loop hike offers a tour of the southeastern part of the preserve featuring three separate palm groves and expansive views from a narrow ridge. The diversity of scenery makes this our favorite moderate hike in the preserve. The Pushawalla Oasis is in a narrow canyon, so avoid this trip on rare rainy days when flash flooding is a hazard.

If you haven't already been to Coachella Valley Preserve, stop by the Palm House in the oasis next to the parking area and pick up a pamphlet with a map. Docents at the Palm House can tell you about current conditions and wildlife.

A sign on the south side of the visitor center parking lot indicates the start of the trail to the Pushawalla, Horseshoe, and Hidden Palm Oases. The trail leads through the desert and crosses Thousand Palms Rd., then immediately reaches a signed junction. The left fork leads a half mile to the Indian Palms Grove, but this trip takes the right fork, following frequent signposts. Keep your eyes open for steps cut up a steep hill onto Bee Rock Mesa. When you reach a large wash, turn right, hike a short distance along the wash, and exit the other side where the trail leads up the steps to the mesa. A sign at the top of the hill points

Hikers on the ridge above Horseshoe Palms Grove

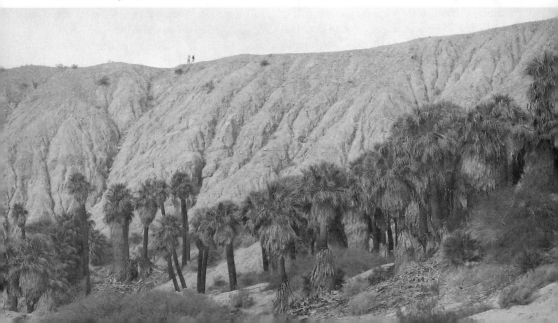

left along the top of the ridge to Pushawalla Palms and right to Hidden Palms. This hike leads to Pushawalla, then will return via Hidden Palms to form a loop.

The trail follows the narrow and exposed crest of the ridge eastward for a mile. Here you will find panoramic views of the desert, the mountains ringing the Coachella Valley, and the Horseshoe Palms to the south. At a signed trail junction at the end of the ridge, stay right and follow the trail down off the ridge to another junction. Stay left for Pushawalla Palms; you will return to this junction later to take the other fork going to Horseshoe and Hidden Palms. Descend a narrow gully and arrive at the oasis in Pushawalla Canyon. In the wet months, a trickle of water is often found in the canyon bottom, though it is not suitable for drinking. Turn left and explore up the canyon to find the two main palm groves, 2.7 miles from the trailhead.

VARIATIONS

From here, you have several options. You may return the way you came. You may continue up the canyon for 0.2 mile to reach a trail exiting the canyon to the left at the end of the oasis near an old car wreck.

This trail loops back to the junction on the end of the long ridge that you followed; it also offers the opportunity to walk back along the wash to the north of the ridge. But if time permits, make a loop to visit the Horseshoe and Hidden Palms. Retrace your steps through the Pushawalla Oasis and up the narrow gully to the signed junction that you passed earlier. Go west toward the Horseshoe Palms, nestled at the foot of the ridge. The maze of trails through the valley can be confusing; follow the trail markers that eventually lead you onto an old jeep track down the middle of the valley. After passing the Horseshoe Palms, come to a fork in the road at a hitching post. Take the right fork into the Hidden Palms Oasis. The road ends at a turnabout at the north end of the oasis and continues north as a trail, then eventually rejoins jeep tracks. The network of trails through the desert can be confusing here. A map and navigation skills are important. At another fork beneath the power lines near the toe of the main ridge, take the right fork and return to the signed junction on Bee Rock Mesa. Descend the stairs and retrace your steps to the trailhead.

trip 14.3 Big Morongo Canyon Preserve

Distance	0.6–10+ miles, depending on the route
Hiking Time	30 minutes–5 hours
Elevation Gain	negligible
Difficulty	Easy–Moderate
Trail Use	Good for children, some wheelchair access
Best Times	October–May
Agency	Big Morongo Canyon Preserve
Recommended Map	*Big Morongo Canyon Preserve* map

see map on p. 300

DIRECTIONS From Highway 62 in Morongo Valley, 11.3 miles north of Interstate 10, turn east on East Dr. at a sign for the Big Morongo Canyon Preserve. In 0.2 mile, turn left into the park entrance (11055 East Dr.).

Numerous trails lace this preserve and it is easy to choose as short or long a hike as you wish. There are benches and observation platforms along the way. All hikes start at the kiosk adjacent to the parking lot. Excellent maps are available here; take one and plan your excursion. The preserve is open from 7:30 A.M. to sunset.

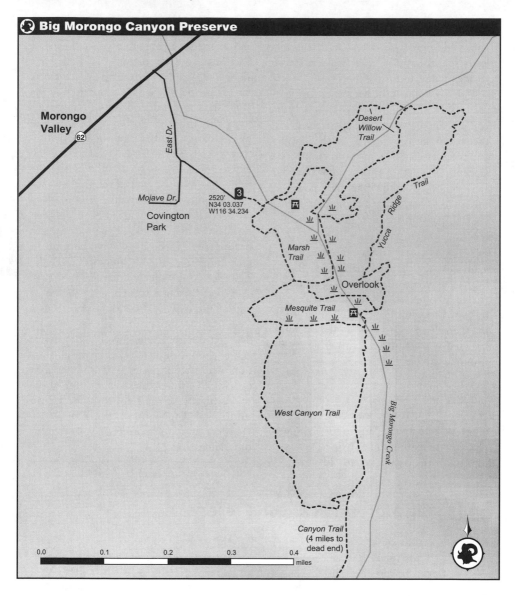

Big Morongo Canyon Preserve

Morongo
Valley
62

East Dr.

Desert
Willow
Trail

Yucca Ridge Trail

Mojave Dr.

2520'
N34 03.037
W116 34.234

3

Covington
Park

Marsh
Trail

Overlook

Mesquite Trail

West Canyon Trail

Big Morongo Creek

Canyon Trail
(4 miles to
dead end)

0.0   0.1   0.2   0.3   0.4
miles

The 0.6 mile Marsh Trail is not to be missed. Pick up a brochure at the kiosk describing 28 signed attractions along the wheelchair-accessible boardwalk. Hike the loop counterclockwise to follow the markers in order. Remarkably, this area burned in 1992, but large, fast-growing cotton-woods have already reached maturity and there are few signs of the destruction.

For a 1.7-mile hike offering views of more of the preserve, hike the north half of the Marsh Trail, then turn left on the Desert Willow Trail. This trail zigzags along a path cut through the enormous honey mesquite trees. The protein-rich bean pods once formed an important part of the diet of many Indian bands. Beware of the long thorns! In 0.3 mile, turn right on the Yucca

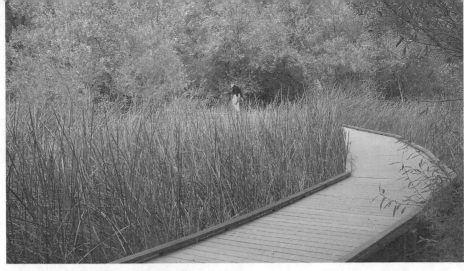

Morongo Preserve Marsh Trail boardwalk

Ridge Trail and climb up to the ridge. Unfortunately, this area was devastated in a June 2005 fire (started in a nearby private residence) that destroyed the splendid Mojave yuccas and cholla cacti that once dotted the hills. Recovery will not be nearly as fast as in the wetlands below. Enjoy the views of the preserve, along with more distant views to San Gorgonio and San Jacinto, covered in snow through the winter and spring. At the end of the ridge, turn right on the Mesquite Trail and follow it back down to the Marsh Trail.

VARIATION

For a longer workout, follow the Mesquite and West Canyon Trails to the Canyon Trail. The Canyon Trail leads south for 4 miles, often following the remains of an old jeep route. The trail ends near the mouth of the canyon overlooking the Coachella Valley at a private land boundary. Retrace your steps the way you came. Including the walk to the start of the canyon makes for an out-and-back hike of about 10 miles, or even more if you make a figure eight along some of the other trails.

trip 14.4 Pipes Canyon

Distance	5.6 miles (loop)
Hiking Time	3.5 hours
Elevation Gain	1100'
Difficulty	Moderate
Best Times	October–May, trail open 8:00 A.M.–5:00 P.M.
Agency	The Wildlands Conservancy
Recommended Map	Rimrock 7.5
Permit	See below'

see map on p. 302

DIRECTIONS From Highway 62 in Yucca Valley 0.5 mile east of mile marker 062 SBD 10.00, turn left on Pioneertown Rd. Drive through Pioneertown, which was built in 1946 as a set for western movies and now operates as a tourist attraction. In 7.6 miles, turn left on the good dirt Pipes Canyon Rd. In 0.7 mile, stay right at a fork and continue 0.2 mile to the parking area.

Pipes Canyon is located west of Yucca Valley in the transition zone between the Mojave Desert and the San Bernardino Mountains. Pipes Creek is one of the few dependable streams in the area, and its lush riparian habitat is a critical resource

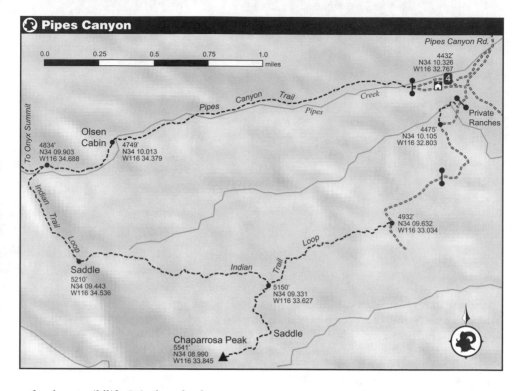

Pipes Canyon

Pipes Canyon Rd.

0.0   0.25   0.5   0.75   1.0
miles

4432'
N34 10.326
W116 32.767

4

Pipes Canyon Trail

Creek

Pipes

Private
Ranches

4475'
N34 10.105
W116 32.803

Olsen
Cabin

4749'
N34 10.013
W116 34.379

4834'
N34 09.903
W116 34.688

To Onyx Summit

Indian Trail Loop

4932'
N34 09.632
W116 33.034

Loop

Saddle

5210'
N34 09.443
W116 34.536

Indian Trail

5150'
N34 09.331
W116 33.627

Chaparrosa Peak

5541'
N34 08.990
W116 33.845

Saddle

for desert wildlife. It is thought the canyon was named after an attempt by an early rancher to pipe water from the stream. South of the canyon are weird and wonderful geological features, including basalt hills and the aptly-named Sawtooth Mountains. The land has been purchased by The Wildlands Conservancy to protect a corridor for wildlife to travel between the mountains, large conservation areas, and Joshua Tree National Park. The area is now part of the Conservancy's 20,000-acre Pipes Canyon Wilderness within the Pioneertown Mountains Preserve. The Indian Trail makes a scenic loop through the preserve, with an optional side trip to Chaparrosa Peak.

This area was devastated by the lightning-triggered Sawtooth Fire in July 2006, which also burned portions of Pioneertown. The original route was burned and washed out, and is being rebuilt at the time this book is going to press. It is now a good place to watch the process of regeneration. Unfortunately, most of the pinyon

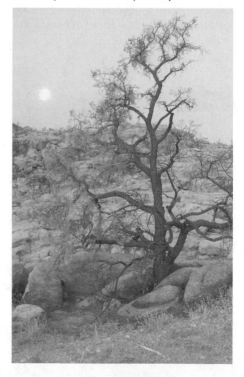

Burnt Pinyon Pine above Pipes Canyon

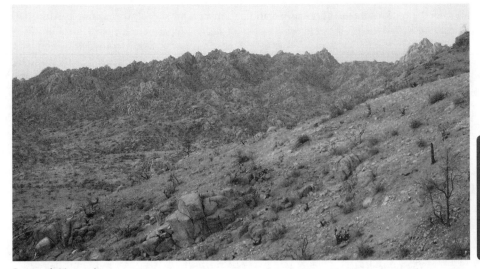

Sawtooth Mountains

pines and majestic Joshua trees were burnt beyond recovery, but many hardy nolinas are showing signs of new life and the scrub oak is rapidly returning. Call ahead at (760) 369-7105 to find out about current trail conditions and permit requirements.

From the ranger station near the parking area, hike west past a gate up a dirt road. In 0.2 mile, pass a second gate where the road narrows to a trail. The trail leads along a section of year-round wetlands, where cottonwoods and desert willows fill the streambed and animals come for food and water. In another 1.6 miles, look for the ruins of the stone Olsen Cabin on the northwest side of the creek. Swedish prospectors working the Onyx Mine during the Great Depression built this winter cabin.

Beyond the Olsen Cabin, reach a signed turn in 0.4 mile at the first tributary canyon on the left (south). Be certain to take this route, called the Indian Trail, rather than continuing up Pipes Canyon along traces of an old jeep road. On the Indian Trail hike up the steep draw through ghostly stands of juniper and scrub to a saddle in 0.7 mile. Turn left (east) and begin a long gradual descent. In 0.7 mile, a signpost marks the turnoff for Chaparrosa Peak.

VARIATION

If you have the time and energy, this 1.4-mile round trip to Chaparrosa Peak is well worth making and adds 500 feet of climbing. The trail leads south, curling around a volcanic hill to a saddle on the ridge. It then veers right (southwest) along the ridge to the 5541-foot summit. The peak's name contains the Spanish root chaparro, or scrub oak, which is a common species on these hills and is also the root of English word chaparral. From the summit, there are impressive views of the boulder-filled canyon to the south, San Jacinto, and the desert.

The main trail continues east from the Chaparrosa turnoff. There are excellent views along this stretch, including the volcanic mesas north of Pioneertown and the jagged Sawtooth Mountains to the south. In 0.8 mile, the trail ends at a jeep road. Turn left and follow the road down the ridge, passing around the right side of a locked gate. In another 0.8 mile, the road turns right and leads toward private ranches, but you can follow a trail that leads 0.2 mile across a dry wash to rejoin the road near a gate beyond the ranches. Continue north for another 0.2 mile near a former roadbed and gates to return to the trailhead parking.

SIDE TRIP

If time remains after your hike, movie buffs should consider stopping in Pioneertown. The town was built by the Hollywood movie industry after World War II as a set for Westerns starring the likes of Gene Autry and Roy Rogers. Actors lived in the houses and ate at the saloons. Although it is no longer actively used for film, Pioneertown was saved from demolition and is now a living community, with a motel, restaurants, and theaters. You might catch a shootout on Mane Street each Saturday and Sunday at 2:30.

trip 14.5 Oak Glen Preserve

Distance	2 miles (loop)
Hiking Time	1 hour
Elevation Gain	300'
Difficulty	Easy
Trail Use	Good for children, dogs
Best Times	Year-round, Saturday and Sunday 9:00 A.M.–4:30 P.M.
Agency	The Wildlands Conservancy
Optional Map	*Forest Falls* 7.5' (trail not shown)

see map on p. 305

DIRECTIONS The preserve can be reached from the west or from the south, or the two driving routes can be combined for a scenic tour through the foothills.

From Yucaipa to the west, exit Interstate 10 at Oak Glen Rd. and follow it northeast for 10 miles into Oak Glen. Pass Oak Tree Village (with pony rides, animals, and other family attractions) and continue 1.1 miles to Los Rios Rancho at 39611 Oak Glen Rd. Turn right, then right again into the parking area across a bridge from the restaurant.

Alternatively, from Beaumont to the south, exit Interstate 10 at Highway 79/Beaumont Ave. Follow Beaumont Ave., which later becomes Oak Glen Rd., 9.2 miles north to Los Rios Rancho at 39611 Oak Glen Rd. Turn left, then right into the parking area.

Oak Glen, tucked away in the foothills below Yucaipa Ridge, is famous for its apple orchards and New England scenery. The Wildlands Conservancy has established its headquarters at Los Rios Rancho. Here you will find a nature trail that leads through a historic orchard and evergreen forest to a pond and then along a creek. This family-friendly trail has special merits in the fall during apple-picking season, in the winter when the Yucaipa Ridge is blanketed in snow, and in the spring when the sweet scent of blooms draw butterflies to the orchards. The trail is open to the public on Saturdays and Sundays from 9:00 A.M. to 4:30 P.M. Bring a picnic or purchase lunch and a homemade apple pie at the adjacent restaurant. The first part of the trail to the

Wildflowers along the boardwalk attract bees and butterflies

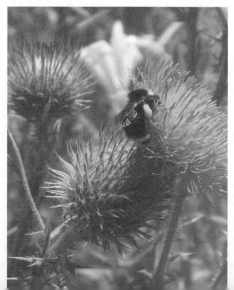

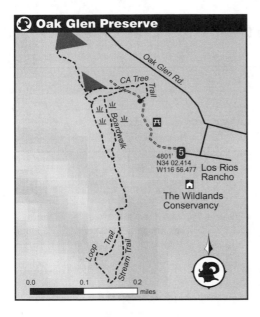

Oak Glen Preserve

Oak Glen Rd.

CA Tree Trail

Boardwalk

4801' **5**
N34 02.414
W116 56.477 Los Rios
Rancho

The Wildlands
Conservancy

Loop Trail

Stream Trail

0.0   0.1   0.2
                        miles

shady picnic area. Just beyond, a sign on the right indicates the California Tree Trail, which parallels the dirt road and leads through a grove of huge evergreens. When the Tree Trail rejoins the road, veer left across a small bridge to a pond, a quarter mile from the trailhead. Look for the floating dock in the pond, where you can get close-up views of the waterfowl and fish.

At the far end of the pond, the trail makes a T-junction. The right fork leads a short distance up to a second pond. The left fork leads down through a forest of black oaks, and along a creek overgrown with thickets of invasive but delicious Himalayan blackberries. Pass a boardwalk on the left leading through the wetlands. Signs identify some of the trees and bushes along the trail. Soon, reach a fork; the Stream Trail leads left, while the Loop Trail leads right. Take either one to the bottom of the preserve, where you can loop back on the other trail and return via the boardwalk through a delightful wetland full of wildflowers.

pond is easily passable with a large-wheeled stroller.

The signed trail starts at the northwest end of the parking lot. Follow a dirt road past the apple orchard and restrooms to a

Desert and Mountain Preserves

The Oak Glen Boardwalk

photo courtesy of The Wildlands Conservancy Staff

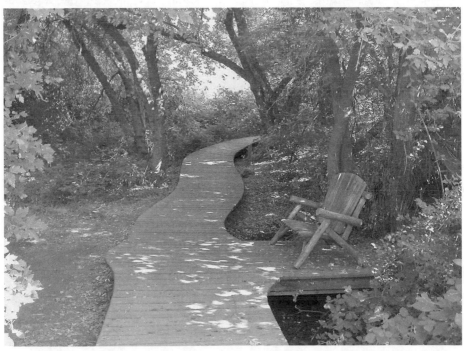

trip 14.6 Whitewater Preserve to Mission Creek Preserve

Distance	8 miles (one-way)
Hiking Time	4.5 hours
Elevation Gain	800'
Difficulty	Moderate
Trail Use	Dogs; equestrians enter via Mission Creek
Best Times	October–April, 8 A.M.–5 P.M.
Agency	The Wildlands Conservancy
Recommended Map	*Whitewater, Catclaw Flat, Morongo Valley* 7.5'

see map on p. 307

DIRECTIONS If you plan to make a one-way trip, you'll need to arrange a 15-mile car shuttle between Mission Creek Preserve and Whitewater Canyon Preserve.

First, position one vehicle at the Mission Creek Preserve Trailhead. From Interstate 10, exit north on Highway 62 and drive 5 miles to mile marker 062 RIV 05.00, then turn left onto Mission Creek Rd. The sign is easy to miss. Follow the good dirt road for 2.3 miles, staying left at a junction, to its end at a gate.

To reach Whitewater Canyon, return to Interstate 10 and drive one exit west to Whitewater Canyon Rd. Exit north. Follow a frontage road that veers east, then immediately turn left onto Whitewater Canyon Rd. and proceed 4.9 miles to the end of the road at the parking area for Whitewater Preserve.

This trip follows the Pacific Crest Trail (PCT) along two of the major waterways rushing down the southeast flank of San Gorgonio Wilderness. It offers outstanding mountain, river, and desert scenery. The best time to visit is in the spring after good rains when the wildflowers are in bloom. Animals large and small visit the canyons for the reliable water; this is a great place to watch for prints and scat. Consider bringing a pair of sandals for the river crossings because your feet are likely to get wet.

Whitewater Canyon Preserve and Mission Creek Preserve are both operated by The Wildlands Conservancy as part of their Sand-to-Snow Preserve system. They border a portion of the San Gorgonio Wilderness administered by the Bureau of Land Management and form critical corridors to protect wildlife and guarantee hikers access to the wilderness.

The Whitewater River is the biggest river between the Mojave and the Colorado. It pours out of the San Bernardino Mountains and flows through Palm Springs before emptying into the Salton Sea. The Whitewater Trout Farm had operated for

65 years in Whitewater Canyon. It was a popular fishing destination, but the farm did not permit hikers to cross their land and access the canyon upstream. When the trout farm closed, the land was slated for housing development. The Wildlands Conservancy obtained the land in 2006 through a partnership with the Friends of the Desert Mountains and the Coachella Valley Mountains Conservancy. The Whitewater Preserve opened to the public in April 2008. The gate to the parking area is open daily from 8 A.M. to 5 P.M. If you expect to exit later, ask at the ranger station for a combination to open the gate. There is a picnic area and a free campground (call

Bear tracks along Whitewater River

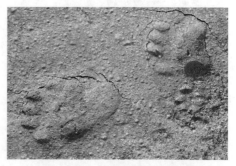

for a reservation). Gas stoves are permitted, but wood fires are not allowed. The trout ponds are now closed to the public, and are used for catch-and-release fishing programs for youths. The cliffs above the ranger station are made of fanglomerate, cemented remains of an old alluvial fan carried down from San Gorgonio. Raptors roost on these cliffs and bighorn sheep can be seen roaming the ledges.

Mission Creek is named for the Serrano band of Mission Indians who once roamed the San Bernardino Mountains. Many of the Serrano were forcibly relocated to Mission San Gabriel in 1834 by the Spanish missionaries. The American government again relocated the Serrano to a system of reservations in 1875, including one on Mission Creek. The land later passed into private hands before being purchased by the Nature Conservancy. It was later turned over to The Wildlands Conservancy

for management. The preserve includes a group camping area at the Stone House. With a week's advance notice, visitors can get a permit and gate code to drive up to the Stone House, shaving 1.6 miles off the end of this hike. Call the Desert Field Office for more information (see Appendix B).

This trip is worth the trouble of arranging a shuttle for a one-way hike. It is also possible to hike halfway or all the way and then return on foot. This trip follows part of the PCT, which continues all the way up to Big Bear Lake and beyond. The Whitewater River is a popular destination for families, who explore the first mile of the trail and play in the water (not recommended during times of peak runoff.) The Whitewater Preserve lacks horse facilities and the trail crosses some sensitive wetlands, so equestrians are asked to access the area from the Mission Creek Preserve.

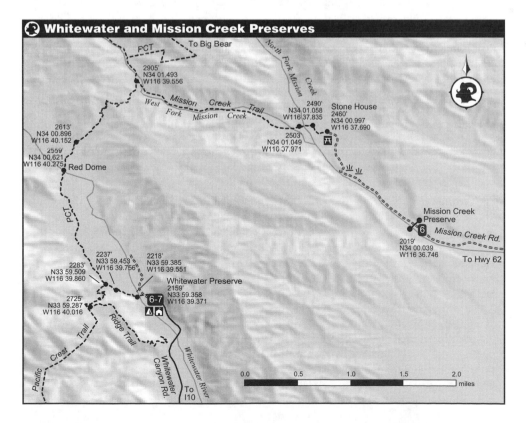

Whitewater and Mission Creek Preserves

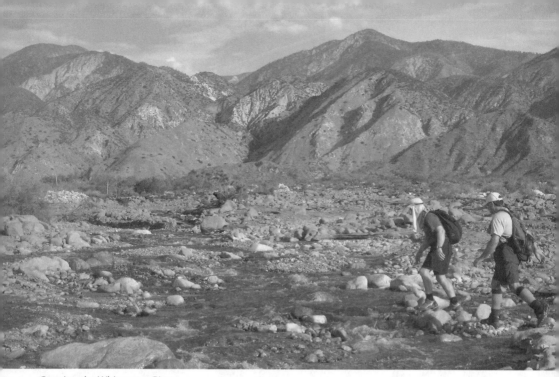

Crossing the Whitewater River

Before beginning this hike, inquire at the Whitewater Preserve Ranger Station about current trail conditions. The Whitewater River follows a broad wash and shifts its course after each major flood. Portions of the trail wash out from time to time. Crossing the river can be dangerous during times of peak runoff or during intense summer thunderstorms.

The trail starts on the north side of the parking area near a billboard with a map. The trail follows a rock-lined path between two palm trees. It then leads west, reaching the Whitewater wash in 0.2 mile. Along the way, it crosses an old jeep road leading north on the east side of the wash; don't be lured up this road. If the river hasn't flooded recently, you may find a marked trail across the wash. Reach a well-defined trail on the other side in 0.3 mile and follow it through a grove of desert willows for 0.1 mile to a junction with the PCT at the mouth of a tributary canyon.

Turn right and follow the PCT upstream (north). In 1.4 miles, reach a corner where the Whitewater River begins to turn left. On the right side of the trail is a small volcanic lump called Red Dome. The PCT crosses the wash here. It can be difficult to follow, but you can pick it up again at a post in 0.4 mile at the mouth of a broad side-canyon on the far side. The trail then climbs northeast, passing brittle bushes, cat's claw acacias, and Mojave yuccas, and makes a few switchbacks to reach a saddle at the head of the canyon in 0.7 mile. A fence across the ridgeline delimits the boundary of the historic Whitewater Cattle Allotment.

The PCT then descends 0.6 mile into the West Fork of Mission Creek. A jeep road once led up the canyon, but it was torn up by bulldozers fighting the 2006 Sawtooth Complex Fire, and is becoming indistinct. As soon as you reach the canyon floor, watch for a faint trail on the left. It may be marked by a small circle of rocks. If you start traveling upstream and reach a signed junction where the PCT crosses the jeep road and starts climbing north out of the canyon, you've gone 0.3 mile too far. The correct trail leads down the canyon, crossing the intermittent creek and joining the jeep trail for a while. It is poorly defined in places, but if you lose the trail, just pick your own path down the canyon. There are some beautiful green, purple, brown, and white formations in the sedimentary rocks overlooking the canyon. You may see coveys of quail running through the bushes.

In 1.9 miles, reach the junction with another canyon coming in from the left. A sign here indicates PCT 1.9 MILES. Hike east across the North Fork of Mission Creek. The trail becomes indistinct again in the wide wash but resumes in 0.2 mile at another trail marker. 0.2 mile beyond, reach the Stone House in Mission Creek Preserve. The building, picnic ground, and

campground are open to the public and have information about the preserve and The Wildlands Conservancy.

After refreshing yourself, follow the good dirt road down the canyon. Pass the Painted Hills Wetlands where wild grape vines fill the creek beneath a magnificent cottonwood tree. In 1.6 miles, pass the ruins of the T Cross K Ranch, once a working ranch, which also hosted Hollywood stars looking for a desert retreat. Just beyond the ruins, reach the gate and parking area where you may have pre-positioned another vehicle.

trip 14.7 Whitewater Canyon Ridge Loop

Distance	3.2 miles (loop)
Hiking Time	2 hours
Elevation Gain	600'
Difficulty	Easy
Trail Use	Dogs
Best Times	October–April
Agency	The Wildlands Conservancy
Optional Map	*Whitewater, Catclaw Flat, Morongo Valley* 7.5'

see
map on
p. 307

DIRECTIONS From Interstate 10 between Highway 111 and Highway 62, exit north on Whitewater Canyon Rd. Follow a frontage road that veers east, then immediately turn left onto Whitewater Canyon Rd. and proceed 4.9 miles to the end of the road at the parking area for Whitewater Preserve.

The Whitewater River is the biggest river between the Mojave and the Colorado. It pours out of the San Bernardino Mountains and flows through Palm Springs before emptying into the Salton Sea. The river cuts a spectacular canyon down the southeast side of San Gorgonio. This hike starts at The Wildlands Conservancy's Whitewater Preserve and follows the PCT up to a ridge where there are great views of the canyon. It then descends the ridge and returns along the river's wide wash.

The Whitewater Trout Farm had operated for 65 years in Whitewater Canyon. It was a popular fishing destination, but the farm did not permit hikers to cross their land and access the canyon upstream. When the trout farm closed, the land was slated

for housing development. The Wildlands Conservancy obtained the land in 2006 through a partnership with the Friends of the Desert Mountains and the Coachella Valley Mountains Conservancy. The Whitewater Preserve opened to the public in April 2008. The gate to the parking area is open daily from 8 A.M. to 5 P.M. If you expect to exit later, ask at the ranger station for a combination to the gate. There is a picnic area and a free campground (call for reservations). Gas stoves are permitted, but wood fires are not allowed. The trout ponds are now closed to the public, and are used for catch-and-release fishing programs for youths. The cliffs above the ranger station are made of fanglomerate, cemented remains of an old alluvial fan carried down

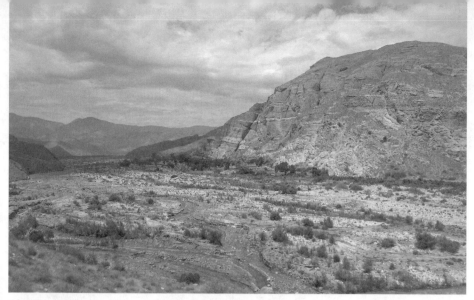
Whitewater River

from San Gorgonio. Raptors roost on these cliffs and bighorn sheep can be seen roaming the ledges.

Before beginning this hike, inquire at the Whitewater Preserve Ranger Station about current trail conditions. The Whitewater River follows a broad wash and shifts its course after each major flood. Portions of the trail wash out from time to time. Crossing the river can be dangerous during times of peak runoff or during intense summer thunderstorms. At the time of this writing, part of the trail was overgrown and the end was washed out, but the Whitewater Preserve expects to repair the path soon.

This area was once home to an incredible assortment of spectacular cactus, especially in the nearby Devil's Garden. By the 1920s, it became fashionable to collect cactus to decorate private gardens in Southern California. Poachers soon stole most of the cactus from this area; you will have to roam far from the beaten path to find the remaining stands. The problem was so severe that Minerva Hoyt of Pasadena organized a campaign that established Joshua Tree National Monument to protect a broad swath of desert vegetation. Collecting cactus from the wild is now illegal, but there is again a growing problem with cactus rustlers stealing cactus to sell on the black market.

The trail starts on the north side of the parking area near a billboard with a map. The trail follows a rock-lined path between two palm trees. It then leads west, reaching the Whitewater wash in 0.2 mile. Along the way, it crosses an old jeep road leading north on the east side of the wash; don't be lured up this road. If the river hasn't flooded recently, you may find a marked trail across the wash. Reach a well-defined trail on the other side in 0.3 mile and follow it through a grove of desert willows for 0.1 mile to a junction with the PCT at the mouth of a tributary canyon.

Turn left (south) and follow the PCT as it switchbacks up the south wall of the canyon. In 0.7 mile, reach the top of the ridge where views open up to the south. The PCT continues south, but this trip goes to the left on the Ridge Trail. The trail leads south, then southeast for 0.7 mile to the end of the ridge, then switchbacks 0.6 mile down the toe to the Whitewater River.

Turn left and follow the Whitewater River wash 0.5 mile back up to the parking area. This may involve some rock hopping and an interesting river crossing. If conditions do not look good, it is possible to turn right instead and reach Whitewater Canyon Rd., then turn left and follow the road over a bridge back to the trailhead.

trip 14.8 Wildwood Canyon State Park

Distance	2.6 miles (loop)
Hiking Time	1.5 hours
Elevation Gain	500'
Difficulty	Easy
Trail Use	Equestrians, cyclists
Best Times	All year, but hot in the summer (day use only)
Agency	California State Parks (in development)
Optional Map	*Forest Falls* 7.5' (trails not marked)

see map on p. 312

DIRECTIONS From Interstate 10, exit east on Yucaipa Blvd. and go 5 miles to Bryant St. Turn right (south) and go 1.2 miles to Wildwood Canyon Rd. Turn left (east) and go 1.8 miles to Canyon Dr., a narrow road that is the first left turn past Mesa Grande Dr. Go 0.1 mile and park in the large dirt equestrian staging area on the right side of Canyon Dr.

Wildwood Canyon, scarcely a stone's throw from Yucaipa's bustling center, invites you to hike along shady trails past historic ranches. It is enormously popular with local equestrians, but was until recently a well-kept secret outside of Yucaipa. A developer purchased the canyon in the 1980s and planned to build thousands of homes, but a fortuitous accidental fire and subsequent flooding delayed construction and ultimately the developer sold the land to the Yucaipa Valley Conservancy. The State of California purchased the 850-acre parcel to establish a new state park, dedicated in 2003. At the time of this writing, the master plan for the park has not yet been completed and the park is not officially open, but hikers, equestrians, and cyclists are welcome to use the trails during daylight hours. Look for updated information at www.wildwoodcanyonstatepark.com.

Wildwood Canyon is laced with trails on seemingly every ridge and canyon. Fast-growing brush periodically overtakes some of the trails until dedicated volunteers cut them clear. When the State Park opens, it is possible that some trails will change. By the time you visit, the map and trail description may no longer exactly match the situation. Take a careful look at the landmarks and remember that traveling downhill or southwest will generally lead you back toward the trailhead should you become disoriented. This trip describes a short loop through some of the most attractive parts of Wildwood Canyon, but part of the fun of the park is to roam the twisting maze and explore the rich trail network.

The Cahuilla and Serrano Indians used to come to Wildwood Canyon to gather acorns before continuing up to Yucaipa Ridge in search of pine nuts. Canyon Rd. follows one of their ancient trails, and shards of pottery can still be found. More recently, miners and ranchers have occupied the canyon, which was long known as Hog Canyon until a developer decided that "Wildwood" was more marketable. Feral pigs roamed the canyon into the 1990s. Animals and birds now visit the canyon in search of water and food. If you are fortunate, you may see deer, bears, or even shy mountain lions.

The East Canyon Trail starts beside the ruins of a 1920s lodge and leads east into the mysterious oak groves. Water once ran year-round in the creek, but Southern California's insatiable demand for water has lowered the water table and dried up the creek. In 0.5 mile, come to a four-way junction. Turn right and hike 0.2 mile to another junction in a ravine. Turn left here onto the Oak Canyon Trail and follow the cool canyon, which lights up with wildflowers in the spring. Watch out for poison oak

Desert and Mountain Preserves

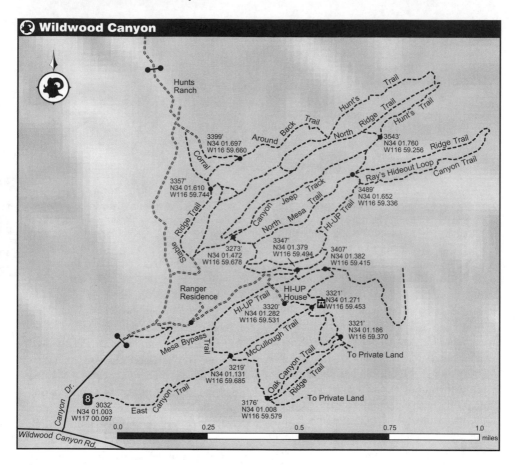

and look for the spiny and inedible wild cucumber growing on vines.

In 0.3 mile, come to a T-junction on a ridge. Turn left and promptly reach another junction. An unmaintained old wagon road veers right, but this trip curves left on the trail that cuts through the chamise. Enjoy the views; to the south is Black Mtn. and the Hidden Meadows subdivision, and to the southwest is Santiago Peak, the high point of Orange County. Pass the wagon road again on your right before reaching another four-way junction. The trail straight ahead leads to the Hi-Up House, and the Hi-Up Trail to the left returns to the trailhead, but this trip turns right toward a picnic bench and tie rail.

The trail curves around and reaches a T-junction with a wagon road in 0.2 mile. The

McCullough family cut this road decades ago to climb onto the hill to the right where they could watch glorious sunsets. This trip turns left down the road and passes fields of buckwheat. Veer right where the road becomes overgrown and pass a trail on the left leading down toward the house. Shortly after, reach another T-junction. The right path leads to the former site of Huebner's Ranch, but we turn left (west) and reach a graded dirt road.

Consider making a short excursion to the left (south) on the dirt road to see the Hi-Up House, well-situated to command an excellent view. The resourceful McCollough family built the house during the Great Depression using mostly recycled materials. The blocks are from an icehouse that burned down in Yucaipa. Surplus wood

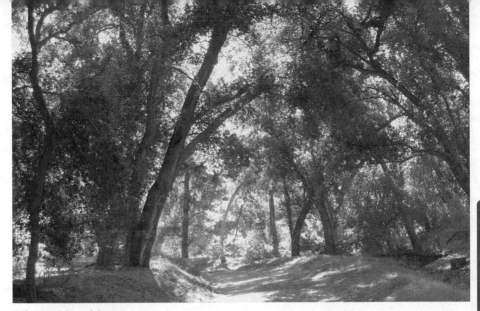
Oaks in Wildwood Canyon

came from a job site at March Airbase. Boulders were collected from Mill Creek.

Return along the dirt road, which turns west. Follow it down through a lovely grove of oaks that arch gracefully over the road. When you reach a T-junction with the main road, turn left and follow it down past a gate to the trailhead.

VARIATION

If you haven't had enough, you can explore more of the intricate web of trails that follow almost every ridge and valley in Wildwood Canyon. Beware that trail conditions are highly variable, but the fun is in the discovery. The chaparral provides shelter and food for numerous birds, lizards, and other small animals. It is not uncommon to hear the piercing cry of a hawk circling overhead in search of prey. Be particularly alert on these trails for poison oak bushes in the canyons and rattlesnakes prowling the tall grass looking for rodents.

trip 14.9 Crafton Hills: Park-to-Peak Loop

Distance	5 miles (loop)
Hiking Time	2.5 hours
Elevation Gain	1100′
Difficulty	Moderate
Trail Use	Dogs, cyclists
Best Times	October–April
Agency	Crafton Hills Open Space Conservancy, Yucaipa Regional Park
Optional Map	Yucaipa 7.5′

see map on p. 314

DIRECTIONS From Interstate 10 exit north/east on Yucaipa Blvd. Proceed 2.9 miles, and then veer left on Oak Glen Rd. In 1.0 mile, turn left into the Oak Glen Rd. Trailhead parking area opposite Shadow Hills Dr.

This loop is the shortest way to reach Zanja Peak and offers the greatest diversity of scenery. The steep climb provides a great workout. Gold Gulch, just west of the trail, was the site of California's first gold mining operations from 1820 to 1840.

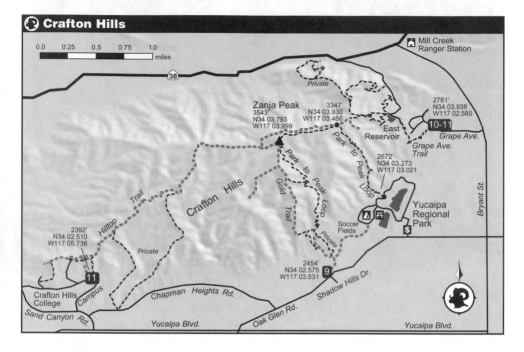

Crafton Hills

Dozens of adits (horizontal mineshafts), most tight enough to require crawling, were chopped into the hillside in search of the precious metal. The shafts are now unsafe for entry. The trip ends with a walk through Yucaipa Regional Park. Tent and RV camping is available at the regional park.

Crafton Hills

Starting from the message board/trail map, hike northeast up the paved road beyond a gate. In 0.2 mile, look for a trail marker pointing up a dirt road to the left. Take this dirt road 200 yards, and then look for a marked trail on the left. Follow the trail up to the junction with the Gold Trail.

From this junction, there are two routes to Zanja Peak: a trail to the right leading up the canyon and a road to the left leading to a steep fire break / road called the Gold Trail that follows the ridge. The easiest path is to turn right and follow the canyon trail, which switchbacks up above a steep narrow gorge. In 0.8 mile, reach another signed trail junction. A lightly used track leads left up to the Gold Trail on the ridge, but the main trail continues straight up the scenic canyon. In another 0.7 mile, reach the ridge. The trail turns right and climbs steeply for less than 100 yards to the top of Zanja Peak.

After enjoying the summit views, follow a trail to the right that leads northeast along the crest of the Crafton Hills. In 0.6 mile, the trail passes alongside a fire road that also runs along the crest. But stay right on the trail and descend 1.1 miles through another canyon to reach the paved road at a trailhead marker in Yucaipa Regional Park.

Families with young children may especially enjoy a detour to the fine playground on a peninsula in the lake below. Otherwise, turn right and follow the road, which crosses a ravine and then turns south. Pass a road leading right to the group tent camping area, then make a right just after and follow a road past the large group picnic shelters. Go around a yellow gate to some soccer fields and follow the road along the south side of the fenced earthworks back to the trail marker 0.2 mile north of the Oak Glen Rd. Trailhead, and 0.8 mile from the Yucaipa Regional Park Trailhead.

trip 14.10 Crafton Hills: Grape Avenue Trail

Distance	4 miles (loop)
Hiking Time	2 hours
Elevation Gain	1000'
Difficulty	Moderate
Trail Use	Dogs, equestrians, cyclists
Best Times	October–April
Agency	Crafton Hills Open Space Conservancy
Optional Map	*Yucaipa* 7.5'

see map on p. 314

DIRECTIONS From Interstate 10 exit north/east on Yucaipa Blvd. Proceed 2.9 miles, and then veer left on Oak Glen Rd. In 2.6 mile, turn left on Bryant St. In 1.1 miles, turn left on Grape Ave. In 0.5 mile, park on the residential street. The trailhead is marked with a small sign on the south side of the road just before reaching the house at 34889 Grape Ave.

This hike explores the east end of the Crafton Hills, with good views into Oak Glen and San Gorgonio Wilderness. The first part of the trail leads behind a neighborhood to East Reservoir. The trail then climbs up to the Crafton Hills backbone and loops around before returning.

From the trailhead, follow the narrow path southwest into the chaparral. Even though the trail backs up against a row of houses, the dense trees give you an immediate sense of entering the wilderness. In 0.3 mile, climb up to a ridge marked by a metal tower. Stay right at a fork and descend behind a house 0.2 mile to an access road below a dam. Follow the trail 0.3 mile up to the right (east) end of the dam, where you meet another paved dam-access road. Continue west on the trail overlooking East Reservoir for 0.1 mile to a three-way split. A well-maintained trail veers off to the left. A steep firebreak rises straight to the west (not recommended). And another marked trail veers off to the right. This loop ascends

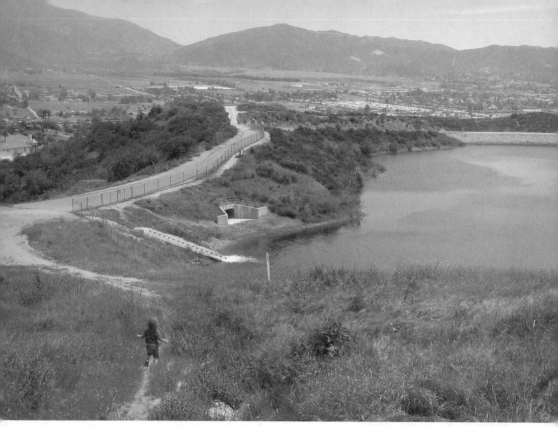

East Reservoir

the left trail and returns on the one to the right.

Follow the left trail 0.6 mile as it switchbacks up to a junction where it rejoins the firebreak. In another 200 feet, look for a fork on the right (northwest). From here, there is an option to continue west for a mile to Zanja Peak before returning; otherwise, head down the right fork on the north side of the hills. The first section has multiple paths, giving you the option of switchbacking or descending straight down

the ridge. In 0.2 mile, look for an unmarked fork. The steep bike trail to the left leads into unmarked private property. Veer right instead and hike across the head of a canyon, then down another ridge overlooking Mill Creek, then switchback into a canyon and arrive at a paved road in 0.9 mile. Turn right and hike up the road 0.2 mile until you can pick up another trail on the right that follows an old roadcut 0.4 mile back up to the junction above East Reservoir. Then return the way you started.

trip 14.11 Crafton Hills: Hilltop Trail

Distance	7 miles (out-and-back)
Hiking Time	3 hours
Elevation Gain	1200'
Difficulty	Moderate
Trail Use	Dogs, equestrians, cyclists
Best Times	October–April
Agency	Crafton Hills Open Space Conservancy
Optional Map	*Yucaipa 7.5'*

see map on p. 314

DIRECTIONS From Interstate 10 exit north/east on Yucaipa Blvd. Proceed 1.6 miles, and then turn left onto Sand Canyon Rd. In 0.2 mile, turn right at Campus into Crafton Hills College. In 0.5 mile where the road bends left, look for a large white trailhead sign on the right (north) side of the road. Parking is available on Campus opposite the trailhead, but a parking permit is required. At the time of this writing, the permit can be purchased for $1 from a machine in the main parking lot. On weekends, Parking Lot I is free for hikers.

This hike follows the crest of the Crafton Hills from their southwest terminus at Crafton Hills College to the high point at Zanja Peak (3543'). You can follow the gently graded fire road, or choose to hike the steep strenuous trail that undulates along the very tops of the hills.

From the trailhead sign, walk up the dirt road along the east side of the golf course. At a trail marker in 100 yards, turn sharply right and take a paved trail up to a bench. The trail then narrows and leads up a ridge to the hill overlooking the water tank, 0.3 mile from the start. Turn left to the water tank and follow its access road down to the fire road. Crafton Hills College is beginning a major construction project in 2008 and

the start of this trip may be rerouted, but the general idea is to park at the college and find your way onto the fire road along the ridge.

Turn right and follow the fire road northeast. At various junctures you have a choice of staying on the easy road or taking steeper but shorter trails directly along the ridge top. In about 3 miles, the trail runs alongside the road just below Zanja Peak. There are fine views along the ridge. Follow the trail 0.2 mile northeast to the summit, where you can take in the 360-degree panorama.

Return the way you came, or with a car or bicycle shuttle, explore more of the trail network lacing the Crafton Hills.

Crafton Hills Hilltop Trail

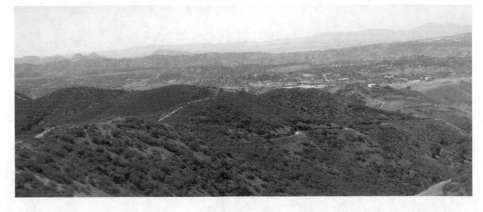

chapter 15

Joshua Tree National Park

Joshua Tree National Park draws visitors from around the world to see its famous yuccas and outlandish geology. It is an international rock climbing mecca and one of the authors spent years dashing from climb to climb before noticing the fantastic hiking possibilities. The park is full of trails leading up mountains, to old mines, and through maze-like canyons, and it features many of the most interesting family-friendly hikes in the Inland Empire.

The Joshua Tree region is primarily composed of ancient Pinto gneiss (pronounced *nice*) formed 1.6 billion years ago. About 100 million years ago, molten rock forced its way upward, then slowly cooled to form large blobs of monzogranite about 15 miles underground. Earthquakes and stress from cooling caused the granite to crack, forming systems of horizontal and vertical joints. In wetter times, groundwater flowed through these cracks, eroding the sharp-cornered blocks into rounded boulders. Mountain-building action has lifted the rock and removed the upper layers, exposing the granite boulders. The boulders often form giant piles called *inselbergs*. On many hikes, you can see the contrast of the white monzogranite against the brown gneiss. The monzogranite is most striking in the Wonderland of Rocks, where the boulders form a formidable barrier to passage. The

Joshua trees at sunset

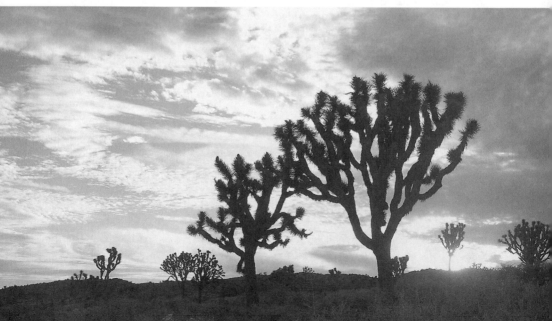

Geology Tour Rd. is another good place to explore these features. Trent and Hazlett's award-wining book *Joshua Tree National Park Geology* is a friendly introduction to the park's geological wonders.

The signature plant in the park is, of course, the Joshua tree. This many-armed yucca stands as tall as a house. The tree purportedly received its name from Mormon settlers who imagined the upstretched arms of Joshua leading the faithful to the Promised Land. John Frémont, the famous explorer and California's first Senator, dubbed the Joshua tree "the most repulsive tree in the vegetable Kingdom." Millions of visitors to the park would likely quarrel with his ungenerous assessment. In more recent times, the curious tree has inspired the band U2 and the art of Dr. Seuss. Joshua Tree is also an excellent place to find other spiky desert residents, especially the Mojave yucca and several species of cacti. In the spring of a good rain year, the whole desert bursts into glorious bloom.

Joshua Tree National Park lies at the border of two major ecosystems. The higher western end is part of the Mojave Desert, and tends to be slightly cooler and moister. The eastern end is part of the Colorado Desert, characterized by creosote bushes. Six palm oases are scattered about canyons where water comes to the surface. Both deserts are full of spectacular cacti that pose a barbed threat to the unwary hiker.

Centuries ago, the land received more rainfall and Native Americans lived and hunted in the region. Even in the late 1800s, cattle ranchers were lured by reliable water. Soon, drought drove the ranchers away, and gold lust brought a flood of miners in their stead. Tourists were attracted to the exotic scenery, but also to poach the cacti, and to ignite the Joshua Trees as giant torches. The park owes its formation largely to the efforts of Minerva Hoyt, who founded the International Deserts Conservation League and lobbied Franklin Roosevelt. In 1936, Roosevelt set aside 825,000 acres for Joshua Tree National Monument. Less than two decades later, mining interests chopped more than a quarter of the area out of the monument, but in 1994, Congress passed the Desert Protection Act that increased the area to 794,000 acres and changed Joshua Tree from a Monument to a National Park.

Joshua Tree offers the services you would expect in a National Park. There are visitor centers near the park entrances, staffed by knowledgeable rangers. There are numerous campgrounds across the park, and most are located near fascinating rock formations. Note that only Black Rock and Cottonwood Campgrounds have water, so plan to bring your own if going elsewhere. See www.nps.gov/jotr/ for information and www.recreation.gov for campground reservations. There are also a dozen self-guided nature walks scattered around the park; these are good ways to learn about the unique environment here. The park charges a $15 entrance fee, or you can purchase an annual pass. Campground fees run $10–$15. Dogs and bicycles are not allowed on trails in the park.

Many hikers discover that route-finding in the desert, and particularly in Joshua Tree, is more difficult than on more conventional mountain trails. The footpaths in Joshua Tree are often poorly marked. Many follow dry washes where it is impossible to maintain a conventional trail because of annual washouts. Locating proper exits from washes requires careful attention. A good map (especially the Trails Illustrated *Joshua Tree* map) and a compass or GPS are essential, even on many of the shorter hikes. Pay close attention to your surroundings and watch for footprints of previous hikers.

Hiking in Joshua Tree is most enjoyable in the fall, winter, and spring. From June to August, the temperatures normally exceed 100°F in the shade. In December and January, temperatures sometimes fall below freezing and the park occasionally receives spectacular snow. Some winter days are

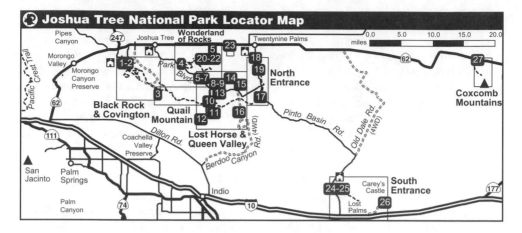

Joshua Tree National Park Locator Map

cold and windy, but the majority are ideal for a brisk walk.

If you venture far from a road, you are likely to enter a designated wilderness area. Wilderness permits are not required. However, if you will be out overnight, you must park and sign in at a backcountry registration board. Backcountry camping is free, but you must camp at least a mile from a road and 500 feet from any trail. Be sure to carry adequate water for your entire trip (typically a gallon per day in the cool seasons).

If you spend much time in the park, you will inevitably pass through burn areas. Wildfire has become a serious threat to Joshua Tree National Park. To some extent, wild fire is a normal and necessary part of the desert ecosystem. However, before 1965, lightning strikes tended to burn small patches of vegetation. Now, nonnative grasses are flourishing on the desert floor,

fertilized by the nitrogen-rich smog that creeps in from the Los Angeles Basin. By late summer, the dry grasses act as tinder for fearsome brush fires. Catastrophic fires that once occurred every other century now ravage the park twice a decade, threatening to eliminate some of the diverse and unusual plant life that makes Joshua Tree so attractive. As a result, wood fires are not allowed in the backcountry.

There are scores of fine hikes in Joshua Tree National Park. Although this chapter is the longest in the book, it only covers some of the most popular trails and cross-country routes. These trips include the park's major peaks, palm oases, a free-standing arch, the Wonderland of Rocks, and a miner's "castle" built under an overhanging rock. Patty Furbush's *On Foot in Joshua Tree National Park* is recommended for frequent park visitors who want to investigate even more possibilities.

Joshua Trees at dawn from Ryan Campground

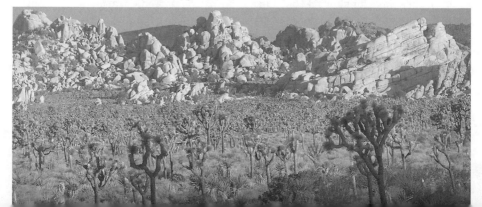

trip 15.1 Black Rock Canyon Panorama Loop

Distance	6 miles (semi-loop)
Hiking Time	4 hours
Elevation Gain	1200'
Difficulty	Moderate
Trail Use	Equestrians
Best Times	October–April
Agency	Joshua Tree National Park
Required Map	Trails Illustrated *Joshua Tree* or *Yucca Valley South* 7.5'

see map on p. 322

DIRECTIONS From Highway 62 in Yucca Valley, turn south on Joshua Lane at the sign for the Black Rock Campground (opposite where Highway 247 intersects 62, 0.4 mile east of mile marker 062 SBD 12.00). Follow Joshua Lane as it winds east then back south, and then reaches a T-junction in 4.4 miles. Turn right, then immediately left on Black Rock Canyon Rd., which leads into the campground. The trail begins at the top of the campground adjacent to site #30. There is parking northeast of the site where you will not block campsite users.

Black Rock Canyon is located near the western edge of Joshua Tree National Park and is connected to the main park only by way of a long and strenuous footpath. While it lacks the outlandish rock formations characteristic of the main park, Black Rock makes up for this with an exceptionally lush and beautiful assortment of prickly desert vegetation. An extensive but poorly marked trail network fans out from the Black Rock Campground. The trails are not shown on USGS topographic maps and can be difficult to follow at times, so you should have a good sense of direction if you venture out in this area. The Panorama Loop is our favorite moderate hike in this area. It explores a series of washes before climbing up to a ridgeline with a splendid view, then returns via another wash system.

Hike south up a dirt road for 0.2 mile to a water tank through a classic scene of junipers, Mojave yuccas, silver cholla cacti, and, of course, Joshua trees. Follow the road as it veers left, then, just beyond, take a signed trail on the right. In 0.1 mile, reach an unsigned junction. The right fork is the West Side Loop, which hugs the base of the hills before heading west over a pass (not shown on the map). This trip takes the left fork, which leads down to a system of washes in 0.2 mile. The area around the washes is confusing, with several poorly

marked variations that eventually reconverge. The best choice is to cross the first wash, then continue 0.1 mile to a signed junction at the confluence of two more washes. Take the right wash, signed PL + WP (Panorama Loop + Warren Point). In 0.3 mile, stay left at another fork, following the PL + WP sign.

Joshua Tree along Panorama Loop

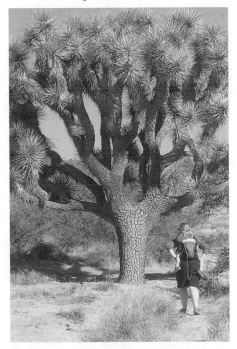

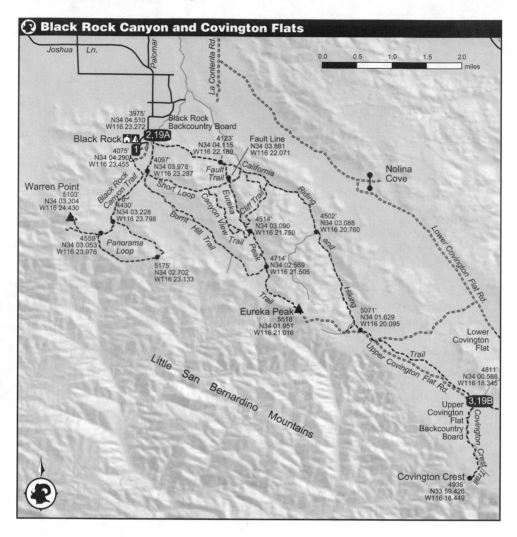

Black Rock Canyon and Covington Flats

Joshua Ln.

Palomar

La Contenta Rd.

0.0   0.5   1.0   1.5   2.0
miles

3975'
N34 04.510
W116 23.272

Black Rock
Backcountry Board

Black Rock

2, 19A

1

4075'
N34 04.290
W116 23.455

4097'
N34 03.978
W116 23.287

4123'
N34 04.115
W116 22.189

Fault Line
N34 03.881
W116 22.071

Fault
Trail

California

Warren Point
5103'
N34 03.304
W116 24.430

Black Rock Canyon Trail

Short Loop

4430'
N34 03.228
W116 23.798

Burnt Hill Trail

Canyon View Trail

Eureka

Cliff Trail

Peak

Riding

Nolina
Cove

4514'
N34 03.090
W116 21.750

4502'
N34 03.088
W116 20.760

Lower Covington Flat Rd.

4559'
N34 03.053
W116 23.976

Panorama
Loop

5175'
N34 02.702
W116 23.133

4714'
N34 02.569
W116 21.505

and

Trail

Hiking

5071'
N34 01.629
W116 20.095

Lower
Covington
Flat

Eureka Peak
5518'
N34 01.951
W116 21.016

Little San Bernardino Mountains

Upper Covington Flat Rd.

Trail

4811'
N34 00.588
W116 18.345

3, 19B

Upper
Covington
Flat
Backcountry
Board

Covington Crest Trail

Covington Crest
4935'
N33 59.426
W116 18.449

In 0.5 mile, the wash narrows and threads through a canyon between the hills. At the mouth of the canyon, the vegetation becomes lusher, including oaks, pinyon pines, mesquite bushes, and prickly pear cacti. You may notice the Black Rock Spring on the left side, but its tiny trickle is more of interest to desert animals and bees than to humans. In 0.2 mile, emerge at a major signed fork. This is where the Panorama Loop begins. This trip describes a counterclockwise loop, so turn right following the WP sign. Hike up the sandy wash for 0.3 mile to a signed junction. Warren Point lies to the right.

VARIATION

If you would like to make a detour to the summit, follow the trail west up the wash. Soon, you will see Warren Point ahead and to the right; it is the only rocky summit in the vicinity. In 0.3 mile, turn right at a signed fork and follow the trail up to the east ridge of Warren Point, reaching the summit in another 0.4 mile. There are great views of San Jacinto and San Gorgonio and the Little San Bernardino Mountains from the top. This enjoyable excursion adds 500 feet of elevation gain and 1.4 miles of hiking.

The Panorama Loop Trail continues south through a forest of Joshua trees, pinyon pines, and oaks; it is one of the most enjoyable wash hikes in the park. As you gradually climb, the path becomes a set of old jeep tracks. Just before reaching the crest, take the signed trail veering left off the jeep tracks, 1 mile from the last junction.

Follow a good trail east along the ridge for 0.3 mile, enjoying the fine views, to a truly panoramic vista at the high point. Then drop down a steep and sandy trail to the north. As you drop into a canyon, the trail becomes a wash and passes through a narrow section before returning to the signed fork in 1.4 miles. Turn right and return the way you came via Black Rock Spring.

`trip 15.2` Eureka Peak

Distance	5 miles (one-way), or 10 miles (loop)
Hiking Time	6 hours (loop)
Elevation Gain	1800'
Difficulty	Strenuous
Trail Use	Suitable for backpacking
Best Times	October–April
Agency	Joshua Tree National Park
Required Map	Trails Illustrated *Joshua Tree* or *Yucca Valley South, Joshua Tree South* 7.5'

see map on p. 322

DIRECTIONS From Highway 62 in Yucca Valley, turn south on Joshua Lane at the sign for the Black Rock Campground (opposite where Highway 247 intersects 62, 0.4 mile east of mile marker 062 SBD 12.00). Follow Joshua Lane as it winds east then back south, and then reaches a T-junction in 4.4 miles. Turn right, then immediately left on Black Rock Canyon Rd., which leads into the campground. The trailhead is on the east side of the road shortly past the entrance. The road is divided and the trail can be hard to see.

If you plan to do this as a one-way hike, arrange to be picked up at the top near Upper Covington Flat, which is accessed via a long dirt road. The road is usually, but not always, passable by low clearance passenger vehicles. From Highway 62 between Yucca Valley and Joshua Tree 0.2 mile east of mile marker 062 SBD 15.00, turn south on La Contenta. In 1 mile, the road becomes good dirt. In another 1.9 miles, veer left at a sign indicating Covington Flat. Cross the park boundary (no fee station) and through an area recovering from a catastrophic fire triggered by lightning in the summer of 2006. In 6 miles, stay right at a junction, then in 2.8 miles, turn right at another junction. Proceed 1.4 miles to the end of the road on a hilltop 0.1 mile south of Eureka Peak.

Eureka Peak (5518') is one of the major summits above 5000 feet in Joshua Tree National Park. It is accessed by a trail from Black Rock Campground and by a road from Upper Covington Flat. This trip can be done as a one-way hike with a shuttle, or as a loop trip from Black Rock Campground. The peak itself is unimpressive (save for its views of San Gorgonio), but the journey is rewarding. The trail explores beautiful washes and ridges lushly blanketed by yuccas and cacti. This trip is described in the uphill direction from Black Rock Campground, but it is also possible to hike downhill from the peak. There is a maze of other trails through this area. They are usually marked, but be sure to carry a map and navigation equipment.

From the backcountry board at the trailhead, hike east and then south up a wash for 0.2 mile through a forest of Joshua trees. Take a signed turnoff for the California Riding and Hiking Trail leading east out of the wash. Admire the diverse plant life, including silver cholla cacti, Mojave yuccas, and junipers amidst the Joshua trees. In another 1.1 miles, reach a second signed junction. Turn right (south) on the Fault

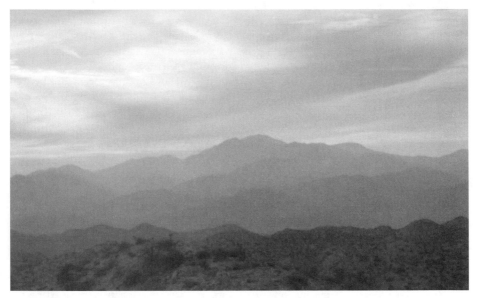

San Gorgonio Mtn. from Eureka Peak

Trail; the California Riding and Hiking Trail continues left.

The Fault Trail climbs gradually for 0.3 mile, and then steeply ascends a low ridge with views of a wide wash beyond. From this ridge, it is worth making a detour left (east) for 150 feet. Just before reaching a small hill, look for a foot-wide crevice between two rocks near a stand of nolinas. Geologists believe this crevice formed during the 1992 Landers earthquake, which tore the hill asunder. Most of the gap has been filled in by erosion, but the line may be faintly seen continuing down the hill.

Continue 0.1 mile down off the ridge to the end of the Fault Trail where there is a signed junction with the Short Loop Trail. Turn left and walk a few yards to a second sign indicating the Eureka Peak Trail leading south up a broad sandy wash.

Follow the Eureka Peak Trail all the way up the wash. The wash has some dramatic sections with sheer walls. Several signs point out other trails climbing out along the way. In 0.8 mile, the Cliff Trail exits up a narrow defile on the left. 0.2 mile beyond, the Canyon View Trail exits to the right. In another 0.1 mile, the wash forks and a confusing wooden marker seems to indicate "EP" in both directions. Stay right in the main wash. The left fork follows a very faint path through a system of washes to the Bigfoot Trail; few traces remain and the route is not recommended (although the trail is shown on the Trails Illustrated map). In another 0.6 mile, the Burnt Hill Trail exits to the right. The Eureka Peak Trail continues over a saddle at the head of the wash, reaching another junction in 0.9 mile with the south end of the Bigfoot Trail. Continue 0.2 mile up to the summit of Eureka Peak. If you left a vehicle near the summit, your trip is essentially finished.

ALTERNATIVE FINISH

There are many ways to return to Black Rock on foot. You can retrace your steps. You can descend the dirt road for 0.8 mile toward Upper Covington Flat, then join the California Riding and Hiking Trail (see Trip 15.19) and follow it back to Black Rock. Or you can return via any of the other trails that branch off the Eureka Peak Trail. The Burnt Hill Trail is especially recommended; the distance is scarcely longer and it traverses a beautiful valley full of Joshua trees.

trip 15.3 Covington Crest

Distance	3 miles (out-and-back)
Hiking Time	2 hours
Elevation Gain	100'
Difficulty	Easy
Trail Use	Equestrians
Best Times	October–April
Agency	Joshua Tree National Park
Recommended Map	Trails Illustrated *Joshua Tree* or *Joshua Tree South, East Deception Canyon* 7.5'

see
maps on
pp. 322
& 325

DIRECTIONS Covington Flat is accessed via a long dirt road. The road is usually, but not always, passable by low-clearance passenger vehicles. From Highway 62 between Yucca Valley and Joshua Tree 0.2 mile east of mile marker 062 SBD 15.00, turn south on La Contenta. In 1 mile, the road becomes good dirt. In another 1.9 miles, veer left at a sign indicating Covington Flat. Cross the park boundary (no fee station) and through an area recovering from a catastrophic fire triggered by lightning in the summer of 2006. In 6 miles, stay right at a junction, then in 2.8 miles; turn sharply left at another junction. Proceed 1.8 miles to the end of the road at Upper Covington Flat.

Covington Flat is a rarely visited gem in the crown of Joshua Tree National Park, offering seclusion among some of the park's largest Joshua trees. The short Covington Crest Trail leads past some of these trees to the lip of the Little San Bernardino Mountains, where unfathomable canyons twist down into the Coachella Valley below. This trip is especially enjoyable near sunset on a partially cloudy day, when you can watch the sky light up in rich red splendor as the sun retires behind San Jacinto.

Two trails depart from the Upper Covington Flat parking area. One trail is marked Covington Crest and leads south. The unmarked trail leads east along the California Riding and Hiking Trail (see Trip 15.19). It is worth taking a 0.1 mile jaunt

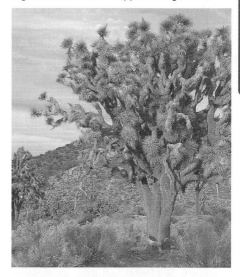
Gigantic Joshua Tree at Upper Covington Flat

Joshua Tree
National Park

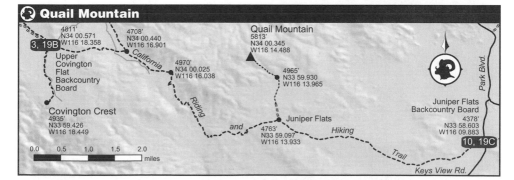

Quail Mountain

4811'
N34 00.571
W116 18.358

3, 19B

4708'
N34 00.440
W116 16.901

Upper
Covington
Flat
Backcountry
Board

California

4970'
N34 00.025
W116 16.038

Quail Mountain
5813'
N34 00.345
W116 14.488

4965'
N33 59.930
W116 13.965

Riding

Covington Crest
4935'
N33 59.426
W116 18.449

and

Juniper Flats

4763'
N33 59.097
W116 13.933

Juniper Flats
Backcountry Board
4378'
N33 58.603
W116 09.883

Hiking

Park Blvd.

10, 19C

Trail

Keys View Rd.

0.0   0.5   1.0   1.5   2.0
miles

along the eastern trail to see some of the park's largest Joshua trees up close. Along the way look for the remains of what once was the park's largest Joshua tree. Nearby is another gigantic multi-armed behemoth.

Return and take the signed Covington Crest Trail. The path is narrow but reasonably well defined. It leads 1.6 miles to an overlook at the edge of the valley. There are fantastic views of the Santa Rosa Mountains, San Jacinto, and the Little San Bernardinos. For an even better view, walk 0.3 mile northwest along the lip to a nearby hill with a single prominent tree. After enjoying the scenery, return to the parking area.

trip 15.4 Maze and Window Rock Loop

Distance	6.5 miles (loop)
Hiking Time	4 hours
Elevation Gain	1100'
Difficulty	Moderate
Best Times	October–April
Agency	Joshua Tree National Park
Recommended Map	Trails Illustrated *Joshua Tree* or *Indian Cove* 7.5' (the Trails Illustrated map is the only one showing this new trail)

see map on p. 327

DIRECTIONS From the West Entrance Station of Joshua Tree National Park, drive 1.8 miles into the park on Park Blvd. to an unsigned gravel parking area on the left (north) side of the road next to mile marker 24.

Visitors driving through the West Entrance of Joshua Tree are treated to views of outrageously jagged hills on the skyline. The Maze Loop explores some of these peaks and canyons, offering a taste of what makes Joshua Tree National Park famous. The hike travels through the Mojave Desert environment, presents some spectacular views, and passes the unusual Window Rock. This is a new trail and is not always well marked, especially in the Maze. When in doubt, look for cairns or footprints. Although the trip is relatively short, it is not recommended for inexperienced desert navigators at this time. A new parking lot and better trail signs may be in place by the time you do this hike.

The trailhead is a dirt path heading away from the road. After 40 yards there is a junction at a dip in the trail; turn left and

Window Rock

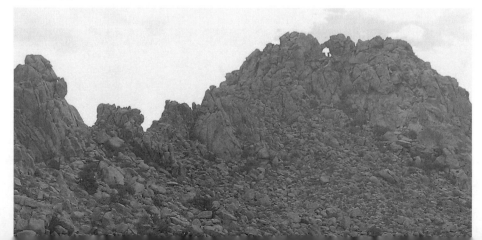

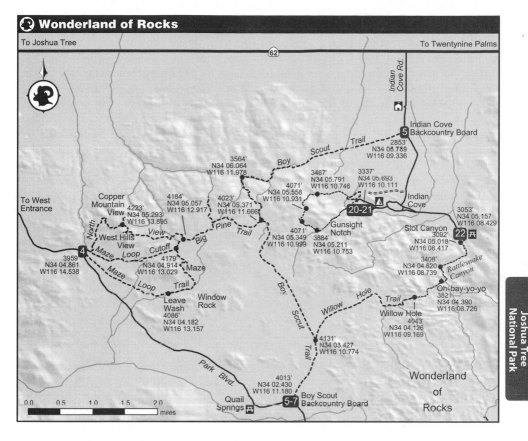

Wonderland of Rocks

To Joshua Tree

To Twentynine Palms

62

Indian Cove Rd.

Indian Cove
Backcountry Board 5

2853'
N34 06.789
W116 09.336

Scout Trail Boy

3467'
N34 05.791
W116 10.746

3337'
N34 05.693
W116 10.111

4071'
N34 05.558
W116 10.931

Indian
Cove

3564'
N34 06.064
W116 11.978

To West
Entrance

Copper
Mountain
View

4184'
N34 05.057
W116 12.917

4023'
N34 05.371
W116 11.666'

20-21

4223'
N34 05.293
W116 13.895

Pine Trail

Gunsight
Notch

Slot Canyon
3092'
N34 05.018
W116 08.417

3053'
N34 05.157
W116 08.429

22

View

Big

4071'
N34 05.349
W116 10.999

3884'
N34 05.211
W116 10.753

West Hills
View

4

Cutoff

Maze Loop

3959'
N34 04.861
W116 14.538

4179'
N34 04.914
W116 13.029

Maze

3408'
N34 04.620
W116 08.739

Rattlesnake
Canyon

Loop Trail

Maze

Boy

Oh-bay-yo-yo
3821'
N34 04.390
W116 08.726

Leave
Wash
4086'
N34 04.182
W116 13.157

Window
Rock

Scout

Willow Hole Trail

Willow Hole
4043'
N34 04.126
W116 09.169

Trail

4131'
N34 03.427
W116 10.774

Wonderland
of
Rocks

Park Blvd.

4013'
N34 02.430
W116 11.180

Quail
Springs

Boy Scout
Backcountry Board 5-7

0.0   0.5   1.0   1.5   2.0
miles

proceed for 70 yards. Here you will find a sign reading MAZE LOOP NORTH ACCESS (NO DOGS, NO FIRES) that marks the beginning of the trail. Turn right and follow the trail down the hill. You will return to this point from the other branch of the trail upon your return. Pass north of the gravel pit and, in 0.2 mile, reach another sign reading: NORTH VIEW TRAIL. The Maze Loop Cutoff continues straight up the wash, but this trip takes the North View Trail on the left, which leads through various washes past yuccas, junipers, and cat's claw acacias.

Continuing along the rocky mountainside, hike another 1.4 miles and climb up some switchbacks to reach a saddle. Here, the Copper Mtn. view sign marks the first of two optional side jaunts that lead to some of the best vistas on the trip. To take it, follow the indicated trail north for 0.2 mile until reaching the peak. Copper Mtn. is visi-

ble across the desert to the north. Follow the same trail back to continue the loop. After 0.3 mile more you reach the second side trail, marked with a sign reading WESTERN HILLS VIEW. To take in the view, turn right and travel west less than 0.1 mile to reach the viewpoint, from here you can see the parking area where you started. Follow the trail back to the sign to continue the loop.

The trail remains on the high slopes for some time, and then drops steeply into a sandy dry wash. Follow it downstream a short way, then, when reaching a junction with a second wash, turn right and proceed up the second wash. In 40 yards, stay left where the wash forks. Look for cairns or footprints marking this potentially confusing section of trail.

The sandy trail leads into a grove of Joshua trees and reaches a signed junction with the Big Pine Trail, 1.3 miles from the

Western Hills view turnoff. It is possible to turn left here and cross the desert 1.7 miles to the Boy Scout Trail (see Trip 15.5), but this trip veers right on the Maze Loop Trail. In another 0.1 mile, reach a wash at another sign for the Big Pine Trail. Stay left (on the trail) and head for the Maze, and Window Rock.

The trail enters a flat area after another 0.2 mile. At an unsigned junction, the Maze Loop Cutoff Trail leads to the right back to the trailhead. This trip stays in the wash to the left, heading towards the maze. The trail winds its way through the Maze, an area of large boulders and impressive rock formations. After exiting the Maze, the trail crosses some small ridges. 1.0 mile from the last junction, it enters a major wash at the base of Window Rock. Keep your eyes open for the window near the top. Turn right here and follow the wash for 0.5 mile. Watch carefully so that you do not miss the trail exiting the wash on the right. This trail leads across a plain dotted with Joshua trees, roughly paralleling the road. In 1.7 miles, near the gravel pit and parking area arrive at the last MAZE LOOP SOUTH ACCESS TRAIL sign.

trip 15.5 Boy Scout Trail

Distance	8 miles (one-way)
Hiking Time	4 hours
Elevation Gain	negligible; 1300' loss
Difficulty	Moderate
Trail Use	Suitable for backpacking
Best Times	October–April
Agency	Joshua Tree National Park
Recommended Map	Trails Illustrated *Joshua Tree* or *Indian Cove* 7.5' (note: the start and end of the trail have been rerouted since the 1995 edition of the map)

see map on p. 327

DIRECTIONS Arrange one vehicle at the Indian Cove backcountry board in Indian Cove and a second one at the Boy Scout backcountry board in the main park. The two trailheads are only 8 miles apart, yet involve a half-hour's drive because they are separated by the nearly impenetrable Wonderland of Rocks.

To reach Indian Cove from Highway 62, drive 8.8 miles east from Park Blvd. in the town of Joshua Tree, then turn south on Indian Cove Rd. (0.4 mile east of mile marker 062 SBD 27.00). Pass the entrance station in 1.1 miles, then park at the backcountry board on the right side of the road 0.5 mile beyond.

To reach the Boy Scout Trailhead, return to Park Blvd. in Joshua Tree and turn left (south). Pass the West Entrance Station and reset your odometer. In 6.4 miles, reach the large paved parking area for the Boy Scout backcountry board on the north side of the road (0.8 mile east of mile marker 20).

The popular Boy Scout Trail connects the main park to Indian Cove, following the western edge of the outlandish Wonderland of Rocks. It treats the hiker to Joshua tree forests, massive granite boulder piles, yuccas, cacti, and scenic washes. The hike is long enough that it is preferable to do one-way rather than out-and-back. Or better yet, combine the Boy Scout Trail with Willow Hole and Rattlesnake Canyon (see Trip 15.7) to make the best loop hike anywhere in the park. The Wonderland of Rocks is a day-use area, but camping is allowed on the west side of the Boy Scout Trail. There are excellent sites in the sandy wash about halfway down the trail, but beware of flash flooding anytime thunderstorms threaten the desert.

From the Boy Scout backcountry board, follow the broad trail north across the

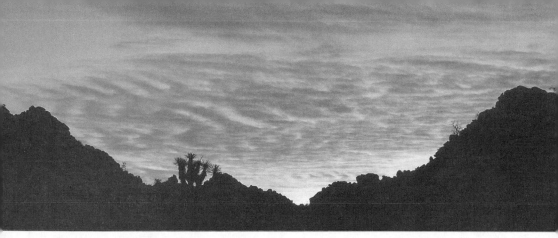
Dawn from the Boy Scout Trail

Joshua tree-studded desert toward the largest granite boulder pile on this side of the Wonderland (Peak 4602′). Beware of the impressive hedgehog cactus in the middle of the trail. In 1.2 miles, come to a junction on the far side of the boulder pile. The Willow Hole Trail leads right (see Trips 15.6 and 15.7), but the Boy Scout Trail continues to the left across the desert. After another 2.5 miles of easy walking, enter a dry wash and soon come to a signed fork. The Big Pine Trail leads west toward the Maze Loop (see Trip 15.4), but the Boy Scout Trail follows the wash downstream. There is good camping for small parties along this stretch of the wash.

In 0.2 mile, reach a sand-filled tank (a barrier across the wash once used by ranchers to create a small pond). In another 0.2 mile, the trail leaves the wash to the northwest before the wash drops into a steep boulder-filled ravine. Adventuresome travelers may try to navigate the ravine, but it is much easier to follow the trail as it crosses a low ridge and switchbacks down into a second dry wash. This soon turns right (east) and rejoins the original wash 1.3 miles from where you left it.

The trail continues in and alongside the wash for another 0.9 mile before the canyon opens up. It then leads 1.6 miles straight across the gently sloping desert to the Indian Cove backcountry board.

trip 15.6 Willow Hole

Distance	7 miles (out-and-back)
Hiking Time	4 hours
Elevation Gain	200′
Difficulty	Moderate
Best Times	October–April
Agency	Joshua Tree National Park
Recommended Map	Trails Illustrated *Joshua Tree* or *Indian Cove* 7.5′ (note: the start of the trail has been rerouted since the 1995 edition of the map)

see map on p. 327

DIRECTIONS From Highway 62 in Joshua Tree, turn south on Park Blvd. Pass the West Entrance Station and reset your odometer. In 6.4 miles, reach the large paved parking area for the Boy Scout backcountry board on the north side of the road (0.8 mile east of mile marker 20).

The Wonderland of Rocks is an intricate maze and obstacle course whose gigantic monzogranite boulder piles stymie most travelers. One of the few easy ways in is the Willow Hole Trail, which follows a broad sandy wash into this clearing tucked away

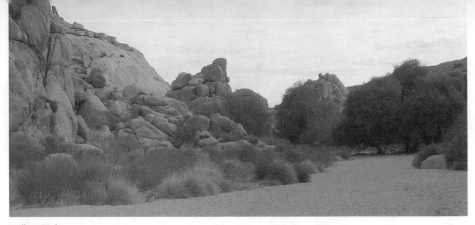

Willow Hole

in the heart of the Wonderland. There is no overnight camping in the Wonderland of Rocks, so make this a daytrip.

From the Boy Scout backcountry board, follow the broad trail north across the Joshua tree-studded desert toward the largest granite boulder pile on this side of the Wonderland (Peak 4602′). In 1.2 miles, come to a junction on the far side of the boulder pile. Turn right (northeast) and follow an old jeep road that eventually enters a wash in 1.6 miles. Follow the wash downstream, passing two washes coming in from the right. Stone walls begin to squeeze the wash into a narrow corridor. In another 0.7 mile arrive at Willow Hole.

In the wet season, deep pools of water may be found here. The vegetation is far lusher than elsewhere in this part of the Mojave Desert. This is a pleasant place to have lunch and explore the rock formations. When you have had enough, return the way you came. Alternatively, continue down the Boy Scout Trail to Indian Cove (see Trip 15.5) or continue down the wash through the Wonderland for 1.5 amazing but difficult boulder-strewn miles to Rattlesnake Canyon (see Trip 15.7).

trip 15.7 Wonderland Traverse

Distance	6 miles (one-way)
Hiking Time	6 hours
Elevation Gain	negligible; 1300′ loss
Difficulty	Strenuous
Best Times	October–April
Agency	Joshua Tree National Park
Required Map	Trails Illustrated *Joshua Tree* or *Indian Cove* 7.5′ (note: the start and end of the Boy Scout Trail have been rerouted since the 1995 edition of the map)

see map on p. 327

DIRECTIONS Unless you plan to do a loop hike, arrange one vehicle at the Rattlesnake Canyon Picnic Area in Indian Cove and a second one at the Boy Scout backcountry board in the main park. The shuttle arrangements involve a half-hour's drive even though the two trailheads are only a few miles apart because they are separated by the Wonderland of Rocks.

To reach Indian Cove from Highway 62, drive 8.8 miles east from Park Blvd. in the town of Joshua Tree, then turn south on Indian Cove Rd. (0.4 mile east of mile marker 062 SBD 27.00). Pass the entrance station in 1.1 miles, and the backcountry board in another 0.5 mile, and then continue 1.4 miles to the campground. Turn left (east) and pass through the campsites and on to reach the picnic area at Rattlesnake Canyon in another 1.3 miles.

To reach the Boy Scout Trailhead, return to Park Blvd. in Joshua Tree and turn left (south). Pass the West Entrance Station and reset your odometer. In 6.4 miles, reach the large paved parking area for the Boy Scout backcountry board on the north side of the road (0.8 mile east of mile marker 20).

Travel through the Wonderland of Rocks is arduous, involving constant up and down climbing on gigantic granite boulders. It is seldom possible to see more than 100 yards ahead of you and there are few landmarks, so simply describing a route in most parts of the Wonderland is nearly impossible. A rare exception is Wonderland Traverse, which follows a well-defined wash full of jumbo rocks between Willow Hole and Rattlesnake Canyon. Even though this stretch is only 1.5 miles long, it will take hours of challenging scrambling to get through. This is no place for inexperienced hikers, especially those traveling alone. An interesting attraction on this hike is the valley of Oh-bay-yo-yo, where locals have built and maintained a fascinating "fortress" beneath an overhanging boulder. The Wonderland of Rocks is a day-use area; no camping is allowed.

This trip can be done as a one-way hike, or as a loop in conjunction with the Boy Scout Trail (see the variation below).

The traverse is best done downhill because washes converge rather than diverge, making navigation much easier.

From the Boy Scout backcountry board, follow the Boy Scout Trail 1.2 miles to the Willow Hole junction, then hike 2.3 miles on an old dirt road and downstream through a wash until the wash seems to end at Willow Hole (see Trip 15.6).

At the big trees in Willow Hole, look ahead for the path. The easiest way is straight forward over a small rise and down the other side. The path to the left is choked with vegetation. The path into a narrow alcove to the right looks promising, but emerges atop a band of cliffs. If you find yourself scrambling on difficult boulders, you haven't found the right path. Beyond the rise, cross a clearing and drop down between two rock piles into a wash. From here on, all travel should be down hill. You may find occasional cairns marking the route.

Boulder-hop down the wash. It soon veers left (take care not to miss this turn

Aerial view of the Wonderland of Rocks

and start walking up hill), then back right. The next stretch is choked with huge boulders and is slow, complicated going. The wash opens up again at a grassy clearing 0.7 mile from Willow Hole, and shortly merges with another wash on the right (south). Oh-bay-yo-yo can be found in the clearing to the left beneath a huge boulder. Visitors sometimes stock the fortress with supplies. Please take good care of this special spot.

Beyond the confluence, the wash turns left (north) and abruptly descends 0.4 mile over huge boulders and dry waterfalls into the heart of Rattlesnake Canyon. This is one of the few weaknesses in the south wall of the canyon; farther east are sheer cliffs. Turn right (east-northeast) and follow the refreshingly easy path on the floor of Rattlesnake Canyon for 0.5 mile until it bends left. This is a fine place to admire the geology of the park. The light-colored White Tank monzogranite of the Wonderland abuts the brownish Pinto gneiss on the flank of Queen Mtn. making an interesting contrast.

Shortly beyond, reach a series of potholes marking the top of a rare slot canyon. It is worthwhile to peer over the top, but descending into the canyon here would involve a tricky rappel. Instead, backtrack to the sandy area above the potholes and look for a path to scramble up left to a notch. Descend through the notch past a number of oak trees, and then walk down slabs, taking care to stay left, until you reach easy terrain and can veer right back toward the base of the slot canyon. There are more interesting potholes at the base, some of which may be sheltering frogs or killer bees.

The final stretch involves some more boulder hopping. The wash veers right, then left again before reaching the broad flat bottom. On the way you pass granite boulders peppered with enormous pinkish feldspar crystals. Look for a path out of the wash to the left leading to the Rattlesnake Canyon Picnic Area.

VARIATION

This trip can be done as a challenging but magnificent loop starting at the Indian Cove backcountry board; this loop is our favorite trip in Joshua Tree National Park. This option is 14 miles with 1500 feet of elevation gain and takes about 10 hours. Start early because you will navigate the Wonderland at the end of the trip; this is not a place to get stranded after dark.

From the Indian Cove backcountry board, hike up the Boy Scout Trail 6.8 miles to the Willow Hole Trail (see Trip 15.5), then turn left and join the route described above. Unless you have left a second vehicle at the Rattlesnake Canyon Picnic Area, follow the paved road 1.3 miles back to the Indian Cove Campground, then turn right and walk 1.4 miles down Indian Cove Rd. to the backcountry board.

Oh-bay-yo-yo

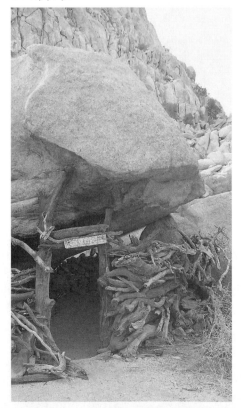

trip 15.8 Barker Dam Nature Trail

Distance	1.5 miles (loop)
Hiking Time	1 hour
Elevation Gain	100'
Difficulty	Easy
Trail Use	Good for children
Best Times	October–April
Agency	Joshua Tree National Park
Optional Map	Trails Illustrated *Joshua Tree* or *Indian Cove* 7.5'

see map on p. 334

DIRECTIONS From the main Park Blvd. through Joshua Tree National Park immediately east of the Hidden Valley Campground (and 0.2 mile east of mile marker 17), turn north onto a paved road, following signs for Barker Dam. Follow this road 1.6 miles to its end at the Barker Dam parking area.

It is also possible to walk to the trailhead from the Hidden Valley Campground. Look for a trailhead marker near campsite #36. The trail begins across the road about 50 yards beyond this marker. This adds 1.2 miles in each direction.

A century ago, the climate in Joshua Tree National Park was wet enough to support limited cattle ranching. Ranchers dug wells and built reservoirs to obtain vital water. Barker Dam is the largest of these efforts. Built by the Barker & Shay Cattle Company, it creates a substantial lake during the wet season. This nature trail past the dam at the edge of the Wonderland of Rocks offers some of the most varied and interesting scenery and vegetation of any short walk in the park. This trip can

Barker Dam

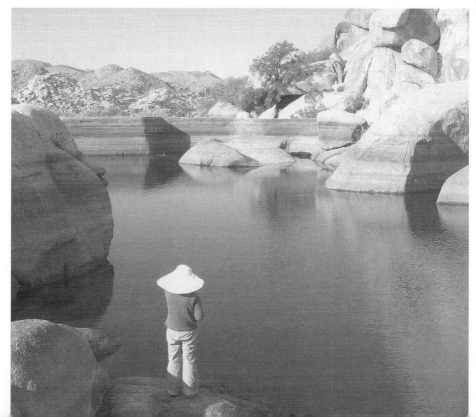

Joshua Tree National Park

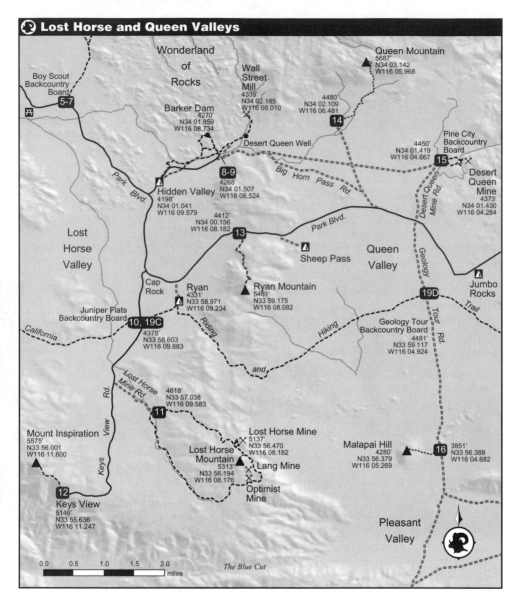

Lost Horse and Queen Valleys

Wonderland
of
Rocks

Queen Mountain
5687'
N34 03.142
W116 05.968

Boy Scout
Backcountry
Board
5-7

Wall
Street
Mill
4339'
N34 02.185
W116 08.010

4480'
N34 02.109
W116 06.481

14

Barker Dam
4270'
N34 01.859
W116 08.734

Pine City
Backcountry
Board
4450'
N34 01.419
W116 04.667

15

Desert Queen Well

Park Blvd.

Big Horn Pass Rd.

Desert
Queen
Mine
4373'
N34 01.430
W116 04.284

8-9
4268'
N34 01.507
W116 08.524

Hidden Valley
4198'
N34 01.041
W116 09.579

4412'
N34 00.156
W116 08.182

13

Park Blvd.

Sheep Pass

Queen
Valley

Lost
Horse
Valley

Cap
Rock

Ryan
4331'
N33 58.971
W116 09.234

Ryan Mountain
5461'
N33 59.175
W116 08.082

Geology Tour
Backcountry Board
4481'
N33 59.117
W116 04.924

19D

Jumbo
Rocks

Juniper Flats
Backcountry Board

10, 19C
4378'
N33 58.603
W116 09.883

California

Riding

Hiking

and

Lost Horse Mine Rd.

4618'
N33 57.038
W116 09.583

11

Mount Inspiration
5575'
N33 56.001
W116 11.600

Keys View Rd.

Lost Horse
Mountain
5313'
N33 56.194
W116 08.176

Lost Horse Mine
5137'
N33 56.470
W116 08.182

Lang Mine

Optimist
Mine

Malapai Hill
4280'
N33 56.379
W116 05.269

3851'
N33 56.388
W116 04.682

16

12
Keys View
5146'
N33 55.636
W116 11.247

Pleasant
Valley

0.0 0.5 1.0 1.5 2.0
miles

The Blue Cut

be combined with the adjacent Wall Street Mill (Trip 15.9) to make a pleasant half-day jaunt.

From the parking area, walk north on the broad trail. In 100 yards, stay left at a junction; the right fork goes to Wall Street Mill. In 0.1 mile, reach the start of the loop trail. Stay right to take the loop counterclockwise. There are numerous interpretive signs along the path identifying local flora

and explaining their struggle for survival under the harsh desert conditions.

The loop trail leads through a narrow corridor and opens into a valley. During the wet season, a good-sized lake forms behind Barker Dam, nestled beneath the dramatic cliffs of the Wonderland of Rocks. Do not try swimming here. The murky and uninviting water is a precious resource for park wildlife. Look for high water marks indicating the level to which the lake rises. Keep your eyes out for rock climbers who frequent the cliffs in this area.

The trail passes along the south side of the large dam, and then enters another valley full of Joshua trees and yuccas. Hike south to another junction. The path straight ahead is a shortcut back to Hidden Valley Campground. Follow it a few yards to a large rock on the left covered in petroglyphs. Unfortunately, most of the artwork has been vandalized. Return to the junction and turn east for a short jaunt back to the start of the loop.

trip 15.9 Wall Street Mill

Distance	2 miles (out-and-back)
Hiking Time	1 hour
Elevation Gain	100'
Difficulty	Easy
Trail Use	Good for children
Best Times	October–April
Agency	Joshua Tree National Park
Recommended Map	Trails Illustrated *Joshua Tree* or *Indian Cove* 7.5'

see map on p. 334

DIRECTIONS From the main Park Blvd. through Joshua Tree National Park immediately east of the Hidden Valley Campground (and 0.2 mile east of mile marker 17), turn north onto a paved road, following signs for Barker Dam. Follow this road 1.6 miles to its end at the Barker Dam parking area. You can shave off 0.4 mile by turning right onto the dirt Queen Valley Rd. immediately before reaching the parking area. Proceed 0.2 mile, then veer left on an unnamed road and follow it 0.3 mile to the parking area at the end.

Bill Keys built the Wall Street Mill in 1930 to process gold ore. The ore was carted to the top of the mill, then dumped through a crusher and smashed into sand by two great stamps. The sand was mixed with water and mercury; the gold adhered to the mercury, while the worthless gravel washed away. Keys ceased operations in 1966 and the mill was placed on the National Register of Historic Sites. It is one of the better-preserved examples of early 20th Century mining technology. A short hike through the desert brings you to inspect the structure.

Hike north from the Barker Dam Trailhead for 100 yards, and then turn right at a signed junction. Follow the trail northeast for 0.4 mile to the alternative parking location described in the driving directions above. Just beyond, pass two side trails on the left leading to old foundations and a rusted car. The main trail (an old dirt road) then passes the Desert Queen Well, where a

Wall Street Mill

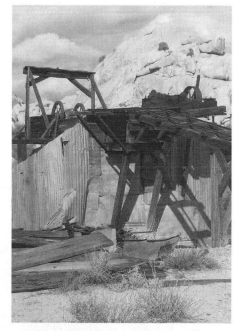

creaky old windmill once raised water from the ground for mill operations. Beyond, a stone marks the spot where Keys killed Worth Bagley in a 1943 shootout over a land dispute. After five years in jail, Keys

was found not guilty on the grounds of self-defense. The path enters a wash and soon arrives at Wall Street Mill.

Explore the site, being careful around the old structures. Return the way you came.

trip 15.10 Quail Mtn.

Distance	13 miles (out-and-back)
Hiking Time	7 hours
Elevation Gain	1800'
Difficulty	Strenuous
Trail Use	Suitable for backpacking
Best Times	October–April
Agency	Joshua Tree National Park
Required Map	Trails Illustrated *Joshua Tree* or *Keys View*, *Indian Cove* 7.5'

see maps on pp. 325 & 334

DIRECTIONS From the main Park Blvd. through Joshua Tree National Park, 0.8 mile east of mile marker 16, turn south on Keys View Rd. In 1.1 miles, park on the west side of the road at the signed Juniper Flats Trailhead.

Quail Mtn. (5813') is the highest point in Joshua Tree National Park. The mountain is at the southeast end of a long and complex ridge separating Covington Flat from the main part of Joshua Tree National Park. It is situated far from any roads and there is a lengthy approach across Lost Horse Valley.

Follow the California Riding and Hiking Trail west through healthy stands of Joshua trees. In 1.7 miles, pass a turnoff to the south for the Stubbe Spring Loop, then in another 1.9 miles, pass another turnoff

to the south for the other end of the loop. In 1 more mile, reach a dirt road (closed) crossing the trail at the aptly named Juniper Flats.

Turn right (north) on the road and follow it 0.5 mile to the end. Two peaks are visible to the northwest. The true summit is the rightmost, farther one. Take a good look so you can identify it later, before you enter more complicated terrain ahead. Also, identify landmarks at the end of the road so you can find your way back. Hike across the flats toward the peak, and climb either the

Quail Mtn. Summit Rocks

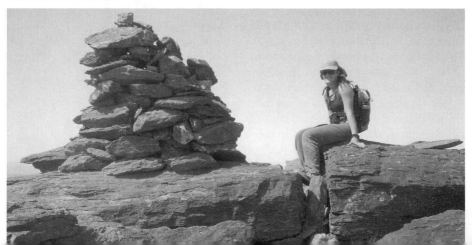

southeast ridge, or the canyon immediately south of the ridge. This is a good area to watch for wildlife.

You may notice some pieces of aircraft wreckage near the summit. In 1999, two civilian T-28's crashed into the west side of the mountain near the 5300-foot level when clouds obscured the peak.

The summit offers panoramic views on a clear day. Four other major high points in the park (Eureka Peak to the west, Inspiration Point to the southeast, Ryan Mtn. to the east, and Queen Mtn. to the northeast) are all visible. On the horizon are the highest points in three more distant ranges: San Gorgonio in the San Bernardino Mountains, San Jacinto in the San Jacinto Mountains, and Toro Peak in the Santa Rosas. After enjoying the view, return the way you came.

trip 15.11 Lost Horse Mine and Mtn.

Distance	4 miles (out-and-back) or 6 miles (loop)
Hiking Time	2 hours or 3 hours
Elevation Gain	500' or 1000'
Difficulty	Moderate
Trail Use	Good for children
Best Times	October–April
Agency	Joshua Tree National Park
Recommended Map	Trails Illustrated *Joshua Tree* or *Keys View* 7.5'

see map on p. 334

Joshua Tree National Park

DIRECTIONS From the main Park Blvd. through Joshua Tree National Park 0.8 mile east of mile marker 16, turn south on Keys View Rd. In 2.5 miles, turn left at a signed dirt road to Lost Horse Mine. The road ends in one mile at a parking area with an outhouse. This road is open for day use only.

The Lost Horse Mine was one of the few highly profitable gold mines in Southern California, yielding 10,000 ounces of gold between 1894 and 1931. The story of the mine was related by William Keys, a long-time resident of the area. Johnny Lang, a cattle rancher, explored the area when his horse vanished one night. He learned of the mine from a prospector and bought the rights to the mine for $1000, naming it Lost Horse. Five years later, J.D. Ryan joined the partnership and hauled in a massive steam-powered ten-stamp mill. The mill crushed the ore from the mine; the resulting powder was mixed with water to form a slurry. The slurry was treated with mercury to separate the gold from the debris. The amalgam was smelted to separate the gold and mercury; the mercury was reused, while the gold was shipped in 200-pound bricks to Banning. To power the steam mill, Ryan ran a pipeline 3.5 miles from the well at his ranch and up 750 feet to the mine. The hills around the mine are still sparsely vegetated because so many trees were cut to generate the steam. According to Keys, Ryan caught Lang stealing gold from the night shift and forced Lang to sell out. Lang later retrieved some of the bullion that he had secreted away near the mine, but he died of exposure along Keys View Rd. in the winter of 1925, and was buried by Keys near the Lost Horse Mine turnoff. As you hike this popular trail to the mine, imagine this Wild West drama unfolding and take care that your hiking partner doesn't double cross you.

The wide trail, formerly a wagon road, begins at the east end of the parking area. It starts up the wash, but promptly veers left at a sign. Enjoy the junipers, Mojave yuccas, and nolinas that are common throughout this area. The trail tends east beneath a hill strewn with volcanic rocks. For an interesting detour, scramble up to the top of the hill to find five and six-sided basalt columns naturally formed as the magma cooled and then split apart. One has to travel to Devil's Postpile in the Sierra Nevada to find an equally good example of basalt columns.

The trail then gradually climbs to the southeast. In a mile it crosses a low ridge and views open up to the east; soon after, the Lost Horse Mine comes into view. In another mile, reach a trail and an old road-bed forking left toward the mine.

The mill is fenced off. The shaft formerly reached a depth of 500 feet, with lateral tunnels branching every 100 feet. As the wooden frame decayed and the tunnels began to collapse, a sinkhole began to form. The Park Service has plugged the shaft and shored up the mill, but stay clear of the fence for your safety. You can also explore the foundations of the old cabins and the old cyanide settling tanks.

VARIATION

If you would like to climb Lost Horse Mtn., continue southeast up the right fork of the main trail to the saddle at the end of the valley. At the saddle, turn right and hike cross-country up to the top of the ridge. There are three small bumps of nearly equal height on the top of the ridge; the farthest one is the highest and is home to the summit register. The summit offers panoramic views, including Lost Horse Valley and San Gorgonio and San Jacinto to the west, Ryan Mtn. to the north, and the black Malapai Hill in Pleasant Valley to the east. This excursion adds a mile and 300 feet of elevation gain to your adventure.

ALTERNATIVE FINISH

For an even better trip that is only 2 miles longer, make a loop rather than retracing your steps. Continue southeast up the right fork of the main trail to a saddle in 0.2 mile, where you have a good view of Malapai Hill's basalt slopes. (This saddle is the departure point for the Lost Horse Mtn. variation described above.) Descend the steep and rugged remains of a former mining road into a beautiful system of ridges and gullies. In 0.5 mile, reach the remains of Lang Mine.

Follow the trail as it climbs onto a ridge, then turns west along the south flank of Lost Horse Mtn. In another 0.5 mile, pass a chimney at the site of the former Optimist Mine. The deep mineshaft can be found above a large pile of tailings. It is not fenced, so treat it with healthy respect.

In another 1.3 miles, the trail crosses a dry wash. The trail generally follows the wash, sometimes along the side and sometimes straight down the sandy center, through a secluded valley full of Joshua trees. In 2.2 miles, reach the dirt road at an unmarked junction, which is difficult to identify. Turn right (east) and hike up the road for 0.1 mile to the trailhead where you began.

Lost Horse Mine mill

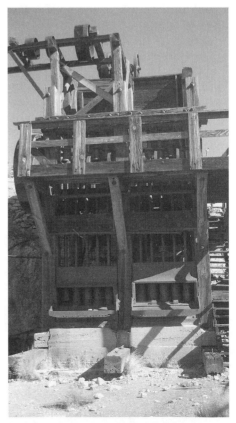

trip 15.12 Mt. Inspiration

Distance	2 miles (out-and-back)
Hiking Time	1.5 hours
Elevation Gain	700′
Difficulty	Easy
Best Times	October–April
Agency	Joshua Tree National Park
Optional Map	Trails Illustrated *Joshua Tree* or *Keys View* 7.5′

see map on p. 334

DIRECTIONS From the main Park Blvd. through Joshua Tree National Park, 0.8 mile east of mile marker 16, turn south on Keys View Rd. Proceed 5.3 miles to the parking area at the end of the road.

Keys View, atop the Little San Bernardino Mountains, is a popular automobile destination for park visitors, offering overlooks of the Coachella Valley. Hikers willing to venture up the short but steep trail to Mt. Inspiration are rewarded with even better panoramic views on a clear day. Those who are observant, quiet, and lucky might even catch sight of the elusive desert bighorn sheep. Mt. Inspiration is one of the park's major summits over 5000 feet.

Take the signed trail from the northwest side of the parking area up the steep hill to the north. The trail is rocky and sometimes poorly defined. After passing numerous junipers and yuccas, reach the top of the hill marked with a large cairn. Descend the trail northwest to a saddle, then up to a second rocky hill, Point 5559′. This is a satisfying summit with grand views, but purists will want to continue on over a third minor bump to the Inspiration benchmark, the true high point.

The views from the top on a clear day include the Coachella Valley and Salton Sea to the south, San Jacinto and San Gorgonio towering to the west, and the valleys, hills, and rock formations of Joshua Tree to the north. Sunrise and sunset are especially good times. Unfortunately, smog from the

Joshua Tree National Park

Bighorn sheep below Mt. Inspiration

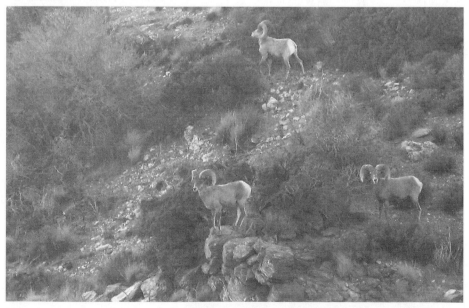

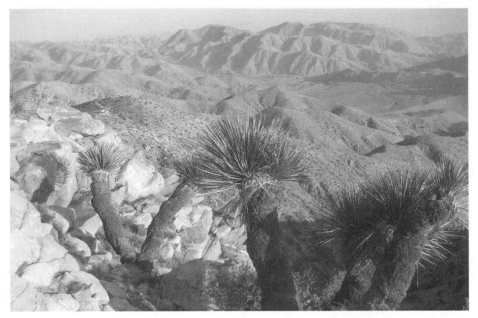

Nolina at sunset

Los Angeles Basin tends to blow eastward, obscuring the views as much as half of the time.

VARIATION

Adventurous mountaineers can reach Keys View and Mt. Inspiration from the south. The best place to start is on an aque-duct access road leading northeast from the junction of Dillon Rd. and Thousand Palms Canyon Rd. Ascend an old jeep track and a wash past Hidden Gold Mine. This route involves about 7 miles and 4200 feet of climbing one-way.

trip 15.13 Ryan Mtn.

Distance	3 miles (out-and-back)
Hiking Time	2 hours
Elevation Gain	1000′
Difficulty	Moderate
Best Times	October–April
Agency	Joshua Tree National Park
Recommended Map	Trails Illustrated *Joshua Tree* or *Indian Cove, Keys View* 7.5′

see map on p. 334

DIRECTIONS From the main Park Blvd. through Joshua Tree National Park at mile marker 13, park at the large signed Ryan Mtn. Trailhead parking lot on the south side of the road.

Jep and Thomas Ryan owned the lucrative Lost Horse Mine. They built a homestead around 1900, and the bright red adobe walls are still visible. The mountain overlooking their homestead has come to be known as Ryan Mtn. At 5461 feet, it is one of the tallest peaks in Joshua Tree National Park. Ryan Mtn. offers perhaps the best panoramic view in the park. In the distance, the tall summits of San Jacinto

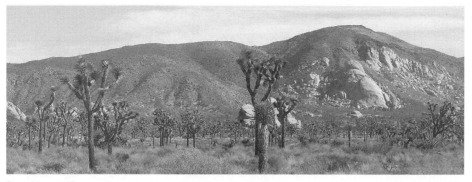

Ryan Mtn.

and San Gorgonio, capped with snow in the winter and spring, rise above the scenic features of Joshua Tree.

From the signed trailhead on the south side of the parking area, walk south past huge boulders. The wide and well-built trail soon begins climbing steadily and continues at a nearly constant grade all the way to the summit. Many rock steps are built into the mountainside. In 0.2 mile, pass a signed junction with a trail on the left com-

ing in from Sheep Pass Campground (near site #1). As the trail rounds the corner of the mountain, the enormous Saddle Rocks come into view. Look for climbers on the longest technical routes in the park. Eventually, the trail crosses a small wash and follows the east side of the mountain before it ends at a sign and huge rock pile on the summit. After enjoying the views, return the way you came.

Joshua Tree National Park

trip 15.14 Queen Mtn.

Distance	3.75 miles (out-and-back)
Hiking Time	3 hours
Elevation Gain	1200′
Difficulty	Moderate
Best Times	October–March
Agency	Joshua Tree National Park
Required Map	Trails Illustrated *Joshua Tree* or *Queen Mountain* 7.5′

see map on p. 334

DIRECTIONS From Park Blvd. through Joshua Tree National Park, near Queen Valley, 0.4 mile east of mile marker 11, turn north on the good dirt Big Horn Pass Rd. Drive north, staying right at a fork in 0.4 mile, then continue straight at a four-way junction, arriving at road's end 1.8 miles from the paved road.

Queen Mtn. (5687′) is the second tallest summit in Joshua Tree National Park and is one of the most fun scrambles in the park. This cross-country adventure features a walk along a sandy wash, followed by a scramble up a rocky gully to the summit rocks. Queen Mtn. offers grand views over Queen Valley, the Wonderland of Rocks, and out to the high ridges of San Gorgonio

and San Jacinto. Queen Mtn. is in a day-use area; no camping is allowed.

From the parking area, look north toward the mountain to identify your route. The two highest points are separated by a prominent saddle on the ridge. The true summit is the one to the left of the saddle. A rocky gully leads to the saddle; it is your route. Also, closely note where you are

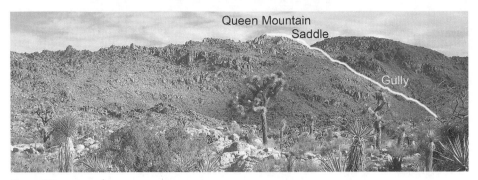

Queen Mtn. approach

leaving your vehicle. You will be returning cross-country to this spot and may not be able to see the vehicle until you are very close. A GPS can be helpful if you are not an experienced desert navigator.

Hike due east across the desert for 0.25 mile to the second wash. A trail once led in this direction, but few traces remain. Turn left at the wash and follow it northeast. Watch for old man prickly pear and cholla cacti. Climb some rock slabs as you pass between two low hills, then continue northeast up the wash. Look for another wash, strewn with light-colored rocks, coming straight down from the south face of the peak. When you come close to this wash, depart from the wash you have been follow-

ing and walk up the left (west) side toward the main gully coming down from the notch. Hike up the gully or along a dirt use trail on the left side of the gully. Pass some huge prickly pear cacti along the way.

At the saddle atop the gully is a flat sandy clearing. The true high point is a slab to the west (left), partially hidden behind a large rock outcrop. You may find a faint path marked with cairns passing around the south side of the outcrop, then leading up the huge slab to the summit.

Return the way you came, taking care to exit the wash at the right place to reach the road's end. There are some low hills to the west of the parking area.

trip 15.15 Desert Queen Mine

Distance	1 mile (loop)
Hiking Time	30 minutes
Elevation Gain	300'
Difficulty	Easy
Trail Use	Good for children
Best Times	October–April
Agency	Joshua Tree National Park
Recommended Map	Trails Illustrated *Joshua Tree* or *Queen Mountain* 7.5'

see map on p. 334

DIRECTIONS From the main Park Blvd. through Joshua Tree National Park 0.1 mile east of mile marker 10 and directly opposite the Geology Tour Rd., turn north on the good dirt Desert Queen Mine Rd. and proceed 1.3 miles to the parking area at the Pine City backcountry board.

Most gold miners in California toiled hard to extract a meager existence from marginally productive veins. The owners of the Desert Queen Mine were some of the rare few to make substantial profits. According to the United States

Bureau of Mines, 3,845 ounces of gold were extracted from the mine between 1895 and 1961. Nevertheless, owning the mine was no stroke of luck. Frank James discovered gold here in 1894 but his time to enjoy it was short. Jim McHaney took over the mine after his henchman shot James "in self defense" under suspicious circumstances. But Jim's mining career was terminated in 1900 when he was arrested in San Bernardino for counterfeiting. In subsequent years, the mine changed hands under other unfortunate circumstances. In 1976, the mine was placed on the National Register of Historic Places. This short hike tours the site and invites you to imagine the heady heyday of the gold rush. The National Park Service has covered most of the shafts for safety. Nevertheless, keep a close eye on children so that they do not wander into trouble.

The mine can be reached by an old dirt road or by a steep trail with a good view. This trip describes a loop going out on the trail and back on the road. Hikers with inadequate footwear or who are unsure of their balance may prefer to take the road in both directions.

In either case, begin hiking east from the parking area on a dirt road. Reach a junction in 0.1 mile. For the easiest walking, turn left (south) and follow the dirt road into a wash. But for a better view, continue straight 0.2 mile past the ruins of an old stone cabin to a point overlooking Desert Queen Canyon. This point offers a view of the entire mining camp. Beyond, a loose dirt trail switchbacks down into the canyon bottom, then up to join a dirt mining road on the far side above some covered mineshafts. Take some time to explore the area. More shafts are located farther up the hill.

To return, follow the dirt road south into the canyon bottom, then west up a wash past creosotes, yuccas, junipers, and pinyon pines. When you arrive back at the junction, turn left and hike 0.1 mile back to the trailhead.

Desert Queen Mine

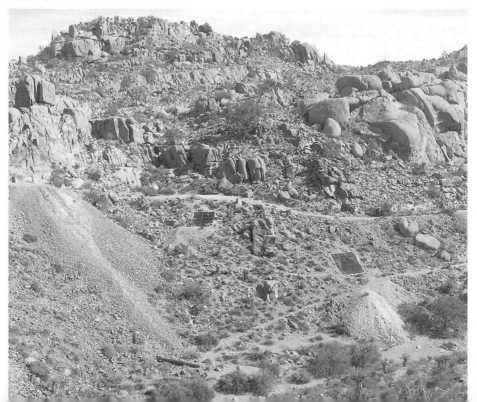

trip 15.16 Malapai Hill

Distance	1.5 miles
Hiking Time	1.5 hours
Elevation Gain	500'
Difficulty	Moderate
Trail Use	Good for children
Best Times	October–March
Agency	Joshua Tree National Park
Recommended Map	Trails Illustrated *Joshua Tree* or *Malapai Hill* 7.5'

see map on p. 334

DIRECTIONS From Park Blvd. through Joshua Tree National Park, 0.1 mile east of mile marker 10, turn south on the dirt Geology Tour Rd. This road is listed as a 4WD route, but is usually passable to Malapai Hill in an ordinary passenger car. At the start of the road, look for a small box containing a pamphlet about the sights along the Geology Tour Rd.; these are sold on the honor system for 25 cents and are well worth the investment. Drive south for 4.4 miles to marker #7 and park off the road.

Malapai Hill is a black double-humped basalt mound, the remnant of a recent intrusion of magma into the monzogranite. The hike to the summit of the hill from the Geology Tour Rd. is shorter than it looks, and is a fun excuse to get out of the car and put your hands on some geology.

The right (northern) hump of Malapai Hill is the high point. From the parking area, head straight across the desert toward the summit. A large monzogranite rock pile blocks your way and it is slightly easier to bypass on the left (south). Watch out for the plentiful cactus. Ascend the hill any way you like, either on the steep dirt or up the piles of basalt talus. From the top, enjoy the panoramic views over Queen Valley. Lost Horse and Ryan Mountains are to the west. The Hexie Mountains are to the east, and the Little San Bernardino Mountains are to the south.

On the west side, you can find a few five- and six-sided basalt columns. Test your compass on the black rocks. Some are magnetite and will deflect the needle.

Malapai Hill

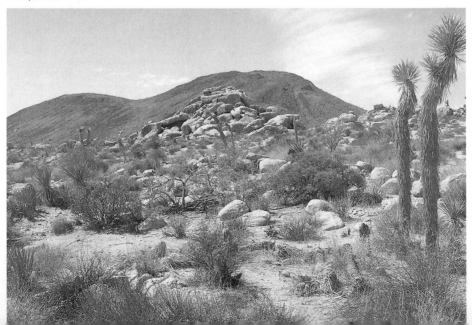

trip 15.17 Arch Rock Nature Trail

Distance	0.3 mile (loop)
Hiking Time	15 minutes
Elevation Gain	50'
Difficulty	Easy
Trail Use	Good for children
Best Times	October–April
Agency	Joshua Tree National Park
Optional Map	*Malapai Hill 7.5'*

DIRECTIONS From Highway 62 in the town of Twentynine Palms, turn south on Utah Trail. Drive through the north entrance station of Joshua Tree National Park and continue to the junction with Pinto Basin Rd. Turn left and proceed 2.7 miles to the White Tank Campground. Turn left again onto a dirt road and park near site #9 at the signed Arch Rock Trailhead.

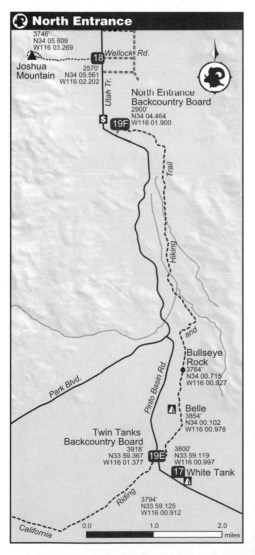

Arches and natural bridges are formed when more rapid erosion takes place on the lower parts on a rock. These formations are common in sandstone but rare in granite. Arch Rock is one of these unusual granite arches. A short nature trail explains the arch and many of the park's other prominent geological features. Arch Rock is located halfway along the loop trail.

A century ago, Joshua Tree had a climate wet enough to support limited ranching. Ranchers built small dams called tanks

Arch Rock

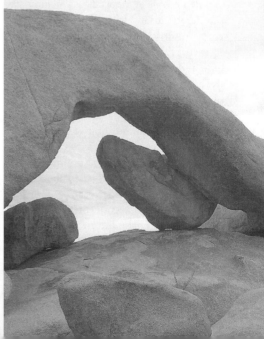

Joshua Tree National Park

across washes to retain rainwater for their cattle. The White Tank Campground and the entire White Tank monzogranite rock formation are named for one of these tanks, which is located just beyond Arch Rock. For a visit to White Tank, follow an alley south past the arch and along the base of a vertical-walled boulder. Then turn left and descend through a tunnel under a large boulder to the wash, where you can see the White Tank. This tank, like most, has filled with sand over the decades.

trip 15.18 Joshua Mtn.

Distance	3 miles (out-and-back)
Hiking Time	3 hours
Elevation Gain	1200′
Difficulty	Moderate
Best Times	October–April
Agency	Joshua Tree National Park
Recommended Map	Trails Illustrated *Joshua Tree* or *Queen Mountain* 7.5′

see map on p. 345

DIRECTIONS From Highway 62 east of downtown Twentynine Palms, turn south on Utah Trail. Pass the visitor center in 0.5 mile and continue another 2.5 miles to an intersection with Wellock Rd. Park on the shoulder of the road. Alternatively, if you are coming from the south, exit the North Entrance Station and continue 1.0 mile to the aforementioned intersection.

Joshua Mtn. would be an insignificant hill on the flank of Queen Mtn. were it not for the enormous granite block with a gigantic overhanging corner on its summit. The mountain is also known as Indian Head because imaginative travelers driving south from Twentynine Palms can make out the chiseled profile of a stern face watching over the desert. Joshua Mtn. is a short and fun cross-country hike that passes a great variety of cacti, climbs a wash, and then circles the base of the summit to an easier scramble up the backside. Children who like rock scrambling will enjoy the route, but it is not recommended for those who are unsteady on their feet or uncomfortable with heights.

From the parking area, look west to identify the prominent stone summit and the gully that leads straight up to the summit cliffs. Hike across the desert toward the base of the gully. This section of the Mojave is rich with desert plant life. Along the way you will see Mojave yuccas, silver chollas, pencil chollas, beavertail, hedgehog, barrel and pincushion cacti. Shortly before reaching the base of the gully, cross a wide deep wash.

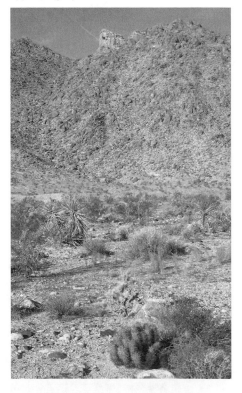

Granite peak of Joshua Mtn. above the approach gully

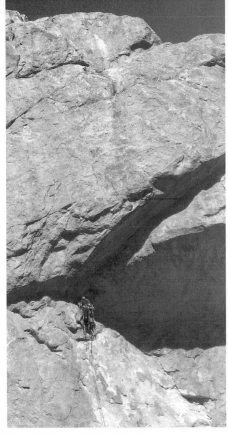

Ascend the gully. For the first part, it is easiest to stay on the slopes to the left, avoiding the larger boulders choking the center. A faint climber's trail may be seen for part of the way. Later, the bottom of the gully becomes easier, though there is plenty of easy boulder-hopping. The gully levels out beneath the summit cliffs, 1 mile from the start.

The cliffs ahead are only climbable by expert rock climbers. You may see intrepid climbers testing their skills on the huge overhanging chin of Indian Head. The gully forks beneath the cliffs; the right fork passes around the east side of the mountain, while the left fork climbs and loops around the west side. Take either fork and work your way around to the north side of the mountain, where more gradual slopes lead up a huge granite slab to the summit. Consider ascending one way and descending the other. There is a bit of rock scrambling shortly before reaching the top of Joshua Mtn. Take care with children because of the sheer drop off the edge of the summit.

Rock climbers on Joshua Mtn.

trip 15.19 California Riding and Hiking Trail

Distance	37 miles (one-way)
Hiking Time	2–5 days
Elevation Gain	2500'
Difficulty	Moderate–strenuous backpack
Trail Use	Equestrians, suitable for backpacking
Best Times	October–April
Agency	Joshua Tree National Park
Required Map	Trails Illustrated *Joshua Tree* or *Yucca Valley South, Joshua Tree South, East Deception Canyon, Keys View, Malapai Hill, Queen Mountain* 7.5'

see
map on
p. 320

DIRECTIONS This lengthy hike is divided into five segments. The driving directions for each trailhead are given below:

(A) Black Rock Campground: From Highway 62 in Yucca Valley 0.4 mile east of mile marker 062 SBD 12.00, turn south on Joshua Lane (directly opposite Highway 247). Joshua Lane veers east and then back south. At a T-junction in 4.4 miles, turn right, then immediately left onto Black Rock Canyon Rd. and drive into the campground. Shortly after entering the campground, look for the Black Rock backcountry board on the east side of the road. The road is divided here and the sign can be difficult to see. If you reach the ranger station, you have gone too far.

(B) Upper Covington Flat: From Highway 62, 0.2 mile east of mile marker 062 SBD 15.00, turn south at the traffic light onto La Contenta. In 1 mile, the road turns to good dirt. In another 2.9 miles, veer left at a sign indicating Covington Flat. The park service recommends 4WD, for this the road, but it is usually passable by low-clearance vehicles. In 6 miles the road forks, stay right; the left fork goes to the desolate Lower Covington Flat picnic area. In another 1.8 miles, turn left at a junction; the right fork goes to Eureka Peak. Finally, in another 1.9 miles, reach the Upper Covington Flat parking area at the end of the road.

(C) Keys View Rd.: From the main Park Blvd. through Joshua Tree National Park, 0.8 mile east of mile marker 16, turn south on Keys View Rd. In 1.1 miles, park on the west side of the road at the signed Juniper Flats Trailhead.

(D) Geology Tour Rd.: From the main Park Blvd. through Joshua Tree National Park, 0.1 mile east of mile marker 10, turn south on the dirt Geology Tour Rd. The first part of this road is normally passable by low-clearance vehicles. In 1.5 miles park at the backcountry board.

(E) Twin Tanks: At the Pinto Wye, 4.6 miles south of the North Entrance Station, turn onto Pinto Basin Rd. Go 2.2 miles to the Twin Tanks parking area on the west side of the road.

(F) North Entrance: From Highway 62 in Twentynine Palms, turn south on Utah Trail. Drive 4 miles to the North Entrance Station of Joshua Tree National Park. Then continue 0.4 mile. Turn east on an unmarked dirt road and go 0.2 mile to the parking area at the North Entrance backcountry board. Alternatively, from Park Blvd. 0.6 mile north of mile marker 1, turn east on the aforementioned dirt road.

The California Riding and Hiking Trails Act was passed in 1945 to establish a trail system spanning the entire state. The ambitious project was never completed, and much of it fell into disuse. However, several segments of the California Riding and Hiking Trail (CRHT) still exist, and the 37-mile part through Joshua Tree National Park offers a grand tour of the main park. There is nothing like crossing the park on foot to gain an intimate appreciation of the topography and desert life of this region.

This trip can be done as a long backpacking trip or as some combination of five shorter sections. There is no water along the way, so it is helpful to cache water ahead of time near some of the road crossings. The trail is not always clearly marked and is most suitable for experienced backcountry hikers. If you only have time for a shorter trip, the first two segments are recommended because they traverse the wildest country and the most diverse scenery.

trip 15.19 *Segment A:*
Black Rock Campground to Upper Covington Flat

see
map on
p. 322

Distance	7.5 miles (one-way)
Hiking Time	4 hours
Elevation Gain	800'
Recommended Map	Trails Illustrated *Joshua Tree* or *Yucca Valley South, Joshua Tree South* 7.5'

The first part of this trail has especially diverse and interesting desert plant life. It passes a complex warren of trails that are shown on the Trails Illustrated map but not on the USGS topos, so route-finding requires care. From the backcountry board, the sandy trail leads east and then south through a forest of Joshua trees for 0.2 mile to a signed junction. Follow the CRHT east

Covington fire burn area

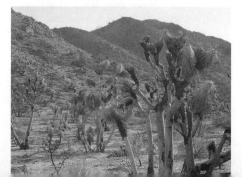

out of the wash. Look for Mojave yuccas, silver chollas, and junipers. The yuccas bloom impressively in the spring. In 1.1 miles, reach a second signed junction with the Fault Trail, which veers off to the right. In another 0.3 mile, reach a wash and look for another junction with the Short Loop going south up the wash. Beyond, reach an area that burnt in the 2006 Covington Fire. Charred Joshua trees litter the melancholy hillside.

The trail enters a sandy wash and passes two more signed junctions leading south to the Cliff Trail. In another 1.3 miles, the wash forks. Stay on the left fork. (You may see footprints from people who accidentally took the right fork; this leads to the Bigfoot Trail, which is shown on the Trails Illustrated map, but which has nearly vanished into the desert.) Then, 1.4 miles later, the wash begins to emerge from the canyon you have been following. In 0.4 mile, the Eureka Peak Trail cuts off to the right. In another 0.2 mile, reach a dirt road leading west to Eureka Peak. Stay on the CRHT paralleling the road east toward Upper Covington Flat. Soon, reach a road junction. The northeast fork descends to Lower Covington Flat and Yucca Valley, while the CRHT follows alongside the southeast fork toward the Upper Covington Flat Trailhead. The trail gradually descends through the valley full of healthy Joshua trees, heading toward a low pass between the hills to the east. Look to the right for the Upper Covington Flat parking area. If the trail becomes faint and you start following a wash down to the north, you are going the wrong way.

trip 15.19 *Segment B:* Upper Covington Flat to Keys View Rd.

Distance	11 miles (one-way)
Hiking Time	6 hours
Elevation Gain	1100'
Recommended Map	Trails Illustrated *Joshua Tree* or *Joshua Tree South, East Deception Canyon, Keys View* 7.5'

see map on p. 325

This is the most remote section of the trail, passing through seldom-visited country behind Quail Mtn. It features some of the largest Joshua trees and prickly pear cacti in the park. It also offers an opportunity for a side trip up Quail Mtn., the highest point in the park. The trail can be hard to follow in places and is not suitable for inexperienced hikers.

Two trails depart from the parking area in Upper Covington Flat: the signed Covington Crest Trail leads south (see Trip 15.3), while you should take the unmarked CRHT leading east. Note that the 1994 revision of the *Joshua Tree South* 7.5' map shows the trails diverging east of the road end; this is no longer accurate. In less than 0.1 mile, look on the right side of the trail

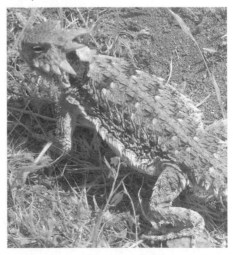

Horned Lizard (commonly known as a "horny toad")

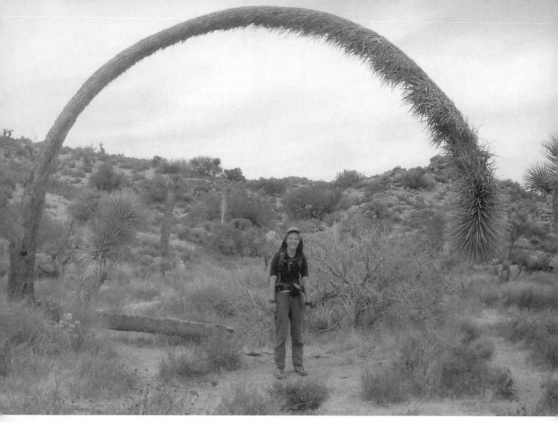

Rainbow Joshua tree along the CRHT

for the decomposing hulk of what was once the largest Joshua tree in the park. On the left side, another enormous tree still stands.

In 0.6 mile, cross a low saddle and descend into a lonely valley. Cross two washes and come to a signed junction in another 1.1 miles. The trail to the left returns to Lower Covington Flat, while the trail to the right climbs southeast up the valley for a mile. This valley is littered with the carcasses of burned Joshua trees and chollas. The complex mass of Quail Mtn. looms to the east.

Continue to the right and after reaching another broad saddle, the trail descends into the next valley to the south. Enormous tree-like pancake prickly pear cacti grow alongside the trail, along with fine groves of Joshua trees and Mojave yuccas. After rounding the south end of Quail Mtn., 2 miles down the valley, the trail turns east and begins climbing again. It crosses a saddle and in 2 miles comes to a dirt road (now closed) in Juniper Flats.

From this point, it is possible to make a 3-mile round trip north to climb Quail Mtn. (see Trip 15.10). However, the CRHT continues east. In one mile, it passes the Stubbe Spring Loop Trail leading south, and then in 1.9 more miles passes a second junction to the south with the other end of the loop. There is no reliable source of water at the spring, and to protect wildlife the Park Service does not allow camping near water sources. Beyond, Ryan Mtn. is visible to the east and Lost Horse Mine comes into view as a black speck on a hill south of Ryan Mtn. (see Trip 15.11). As you finish the last 1.7 miles through Lost Horse Valley to Keys View Rd., you pass through yet another healthy Joshua tree forest and enjoy views of landmarks including Cap Rock and the Headstone.

If you complete this trip in the early evening, consider a short drive up to Keys View to catch the sunset over the park.

trip 15.19 *Segment C:*
Keys View Rd. to Geology Tour Rd.

Distance	6.5 miles (one-way)
Hiking Time	3 hours
Elevation Gain	400'
Recommended Map	Trails Illustrated *Joshua Tree* or *Keys View, Malapai Hill* 7.5'

see map on p. 334

This stretch of trail leads past Ryan Campground and through a low pass hidden between Ryan and Lost Horse Mountains, then descends across the broad Queen Valley. It is well marked throughout.

The eastbound trail begins 0.1 mile north of the Juniper Flats parking area, on Keys View Rd., and leads through the vast Joshua tree forest of Lost Horse Valley. In 0.8 mile, it reaches the south end of Ryan Campground. Watch for rock climbers on Headstone Rock, which is crookedly balanced atop an *inselberg* at the far end of the campground. Dayhikers can start from the campground to shorten the trip, but backpackers must start at the backcountry board at Juniper Flats.

The trail then turns right and leads east toward the low point to just south of Ryan Mtn. As you climb, junipers begin to appear. In places, the path follows an old pipe used to carry water during the mining days. Beyond Ryan Campground 1.9 miles cross the broad saddle and descend into Queen Valley. In 0.4 mile, watch for the foundation of an old miner's cabin on the left (north) side of the trail. It is easy to miss, but stone markers along the edge of an old pathway provide a clue that you are close. The mature pancake prickly pear growing inside hints at the age of the ruins.

The remainder of the hike leads mostly downhill through another great forest of Joshua trees in Queen Valley, crossing the occasional dry wash en route.

Joshua Tree National Park

Ryan Mtn. from the California Riding and Hiking Trail

trip 15.19 *Segment D:*
Geology Tour Rd. to Twin Tanks

Distance	4.3 miles (one-way)
Hiking Time	2 hours
Elevation Gain	100'
Recommended Map	Trails Illustrated *Joshua Tree* or *Malapai Hill* 7.5'

see maps on pp. 334 & 345

This is the shortest and easiest section of the trail. The obvious trail leads mostly downhill across the valley between Jumbo Rocks Campground and the Hexie Mountains. The hills in this part of the park are mostly ancient gneiss, accentuated with the occasional granite outcrop. Thin dikes of light-colored aplite criss-cross the desert and in several places they cross the trail.

In about a mile, the trail leads past the south face of Crown Prince Lookout, a granite formation where a World War II airplane warning station was once perched.

The rocks near here offer some of the only sheltered camping in the sandy desert. There are views from the trail back to Ryan and Queen Mountains. San Jacinto can be seen over the shoulder of Lost Horse Mtn., and at times Toro Peak can be seen behind the Little San Bernardino Mountains. Soon views open up into the enormous Pinto Basin to the east. When the trail reaches the paved Pinto Basin Rd., the Twin Tanks parking lot can be seen 0.2 mile north along a spur trail.

Mojave yucca in bloom

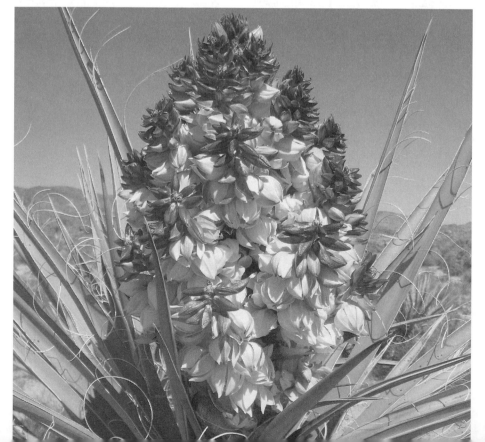

trip 15.19 *Segment E:* **Twin Tanks to North Entrance**

Distance	7.1 miles (one-way)
Hiking Time	3.5 hours
Elevation Gain	100'
Recommended Map	Trails Illustrated *Joshua Tree* or *Malapai Hill, Queen Mountain* 7.5'

see map on p. 345

This section of the trail parallels the paved road and is almost entirely downhill. The trail is set just far enough back from the road so that vehicles are occasionally seen and seldom heard. The first part passes beside a field of house-sized granite boulders. The northern stretch becomes harder to follow in places as it descends along a series of washes.

The trail crosses the paved Pinto Basin Rd. 0.2 mile south of the Twin Tanks backcountry board. In 1.1 miles, it passes along the east edge of Belle Campground. In 0.7 mile, look for Bullseye Rock, the northernmost boulder along the route. The rock is visible to the east immediately after passing a pile of boulders close to the trail.

In another 0.6 mile, the trail crosses a paved mining road near Pinto Wye. It becomes fainter as it crosses a wash and climbs the rise around the east side of a hill. Beyond, the trail drops into a maze of washes. The vegetation here includes Mojave yuccas, silver and pencil chollas, and bladderpods. The elevation here is lower than most of the park, so it is a good place to see early wildflowers in March. If the trail has been obliterated by winter storms, just hike north between the road and hills, watching for wooden posts marking the route. In 4 miles, just beyond where the paved road turns left, the trail also turns left, leading generally toward the stone summit of Joshua Mtn. In another 0.7 mile, reach the North Entrance backcountry board marking the end of the trail.

Bullseye Rock

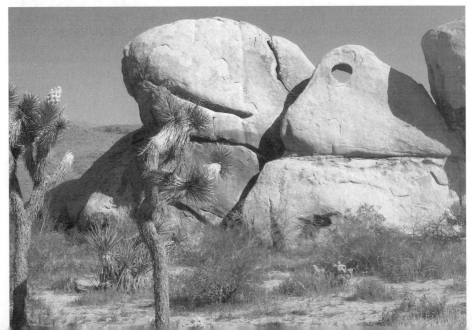

Joshua Tree
National Park

trip 15.20 Indian Cove Nature Trail

Distance	0.6 mile
Hiking Time	30 minutes
Elevation Gain	100'
Difficulty	Easy
Trail Use	Good for children
Best Times	September–April
Agency	Joshua Tree National Park
Optional Map	none

see map on p. 327

DIRECTIONS From Highway 62, 0.4 mile east of mile marker 062 SBD 27.00, turn south on Indian Cove Rd. Drive past the entrance station and past a dirt road leading west to the group campsites. At the main campground, turn right and drive all the way west through the maze of campsites to the end of the road, just beyond campsite #90. Park near the signed start of the Indian Cove Nature Trail. Alternatively, the trail can be accessed from the west end of the group campsites.

This short nature trail at the west end of the Indian Cove Campground is a good place to take a stroll and learn about the plant and animal life of this unusual corner of the Mojave Desert. The trail circles through the desert and along a sandy wash. In the creek, it threads past desert willows. Above, look for pencil and silver cholla cacti, Mojave yuccas, desert almonds, creosote and jojoba bushes.

Mojave yucca at Indian Cove

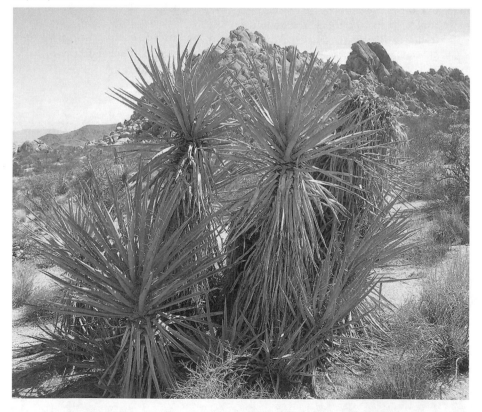

trip 15.21 Gunsight Loop

Distance	3 miles
Hiking Time	2.5 hours
Elevation Gain	800'
Difficulty	Moderate, with extensive boulder scrambling
Best Times	October–March
Agency	Joshua Tree National Park
Recommended Map	Trails Illustrated *Joshua Tree* or *Indian Cove* 7.5'

see map on p. 327

DIRECTIONS From Highway 62, 0.4 mile east of mile marker 062 SBD 27.00, turn south on Indian Cove Rd. Drive past the entrance station and past a dirt road leading west to the group campsites. At the main campground, turn right and drive all the way west through the maze of campsites to the end of the road, just beyond campsite #90. Park near the signed start of the Indian Cove Nature Trail.

The Wonderland of Rocks casts a siren's spell to curious explorers. The otherworldly boulders, buttresses, and towers of monzogranite are a marvel to discover, but are a challenge to both movement and navigation. More than one hiker has become lost overnight, and the body of a stray hiker took years to discover. Gunsight Loop samples the pleasures of the Wonderland. This relatively short hike requires challenging boulder scrambling that is not suitable for young children or those with less than excellent balance. Rock climbers would rate the route third class, meaning there is hands-on climbing but no rope is required. Nobody should stray into the Wonderland without good cross-country navigation skills, and a compass or GPS receiver. The Wonderland of Rocks is a day-use area; no camping is allowed.

The Wonderland of Rocks forms a forbidding ridge south of Indian Cove separating the cove from the rest of Joshua Tree National Park. From the parking area, look southwest to the obvious low point in the ridge. This is Gunsight Notch. This cross-country route climbs up the boulder-filled canyon through the notch into a small valley on the other side, then curves right and descends through the next canyon to the west via dry waterfalls before returning through a wash.

Walk south past the Nature Trail a few yards and look for traces of an old dirt road. Follow it for a short distance as it heads toward Gunsight Notch; soon the road veers left and you make a beeline for the canyon. Watch for the silver and pencil chollas and the cat's claw acacias that threaten unwary hikers.

The canyon is full of huge boulders. Pick your favorite route; if one path is blocked with overhanging rocks, you can usually find another more moderate way nearby. After the most difficult lower stretch, the canyon momentarily opens into a small wash before closing in again. Continue up the main canyon and cross over Gunsight Notch into a sandy wash, 0.6 mile from the start.

The walking is now much easier. Go 0.3 mile and round a bend into a valley. The wash forks. The main branch continues southwest and eventually emerges from the Wonderland near the Boy Scout Trail. This loop, however, takes the right (west) fork, which soon becomes partially choked with rocks and bushes. Follow the wash as it climbs and curves right before it gains a crest and enters another small flat valley in another 0.3 mile.

Hike across the valley and through another wash, veering right around the rocks to aim for the lowest point to the north. You may find some cairns along the way, but the walking is mostly cross-country. In 0.3 mile, come to the top of a canyon descending to the northeast. Look for the

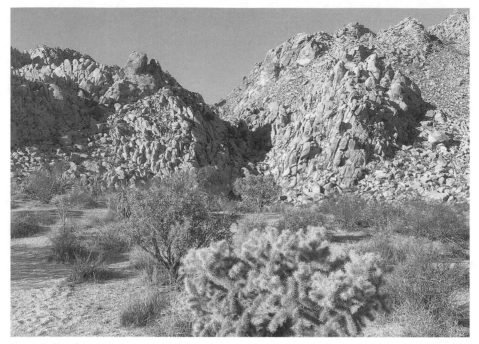

Gunsight Notch

wash at the bottom among the rocky buttresses. The first part of the descent to a small flat area is moderate, but the canyon soon plunges steeply into the desert below. The climbing is generally easier than Gunsight Notch, but the two cruxes involve descending dry waterfalls.

In 0.5 mile, emerge from the canyon at the sandy wash. Follow the wash, avoiding copious cat's claws. In 0.6 mile, come to a junction with the Indian Cove Nature Trail wash. Turn right and walk upstream for 100 feet to rocky steps exiting on the left that lead 0.2 mile back to the trailhead.

trip 15.22 Rattlesnake Canyon

Distance	2.5 miles (out-and-back)
Hiking Time	2 hours
Elevation Gain	400′
Difficulty	Moderate
Best Times	October–April
Agency	Joshua Tree National Park
Recommended Map	Trails Illustrated *Joshua Tree* or *Indian Cove* 7.5′

see map on p. 327

DIRECTIONS From Highway 62, 0.4 mile east of mile marker 062 SBD 27.00, turn south on Indian Cove Rd. Pass the entrance station in 1.1 miles, and then continue 1.9 miles to the campground. Turn left (east) and pass through the campsites and in 1.3 miles reach the picnic area at Rattlesnake Canyon.

The Wonderland of Rocks is a fascinating but formidable barrier to travel in Joshua Tree National Park. Rattlesnake Canyon climbs into the Wonderland from the picnic area east of Indian Cove Campground. It treats the hiker to a number of remarkable geological formations, including a rare slot canyon carved through the monzogranite. Although this hike is short, it involves plenty of boulder hopping and easy rock scrambling, so it is not suited for those who are unsure of foot. However, it is a fun romp for carefully supervised children. The Wonderland of Rocks is a day-use area; no camping is allowed.

From the picnic area, hike down into the wash and turn right to follow it upstream into the mouth of a canyon. You will soon encounter easy boulder hopping. Look for the granite boulders sprinkled with enormous pinkish feldspar crystals. In 0.3 mile, the main canyon turns abruptly left. Look for a steep rise, where the creek has carved an unusual slot canyon. It is interesting to explore potholes at the canyon bottom, which hold life-sustaining water for desert wildlife; you may encounter frogs or killer bees in the pools.

Bypass the slot canyon by moving right (west) past the cliffs and scrambling up past several oak trees to a notch. Beyond the notch, descend back to the sandy floor of Rattlesnake Canyon. If there is no water running, it is interesting to walk back to the top of the slot and peer down the impressive drop-off.

The canyon continues south. The ancient brownish Pinto gneiss forming the slopes of Queen Mtn. to the east stands in vivid contrast to the much younger White Tank monzogranite rock that forms most of the Wonderland.

Soon, the canyon turns sharply to the right. You can follow it for a half mile or more before turning around and retracing your steps. Beware of snakes in the aptly named Rattlesnake Canyon, especially when passing near brush.

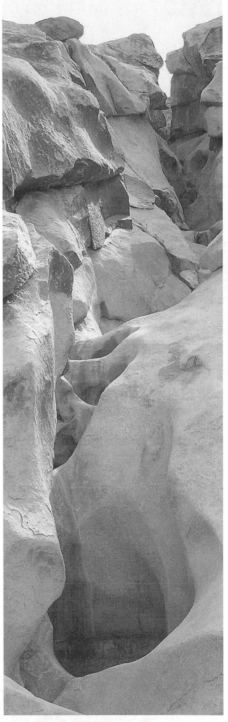

The slot in Rattlesnake Canyon

trip 15.23 Fortynine Palms Oasis

Distance	3 miles (out-and-back)
Hiking Time	2 hours
Elevation Gain	600'
Difficulty	Easy
Trail Use	Good for children
Best Times	October–April
Agency	Joshua Tree National Park
Recommended Map	Trails Illustrated *Joshua Tree* or *Queen Mountain* 7.5'

DIRECTIONS From Highway 62, 0.2 mile east of mile marker 062 SBD 29.00, turn south on Canyon Rd. Follow it south and then west 1.6 miles to the trailhead at the end.

The Fortynine Palms Oasis is one of five palm oases scattered about Joshua Tree National Park. The attractive location, nestled in a steep-walled canyon, and its relatively easy access make this a very popular hike. If you come on a pleasant weekend, expect to have plenty of company. If you have time for a longer hike, the Lost Palms Oasis (see Trip 15.25) is even more spectacular and has more interesting cacti and rock formations along the route.

The well-built trail climbs a series of steps to reach a ridge. Just before reaching the ridge, look for a vista point on the left with great views over the town of Twenty-nine Palms. There are several other minor

◉ Fortynine Palms Oasis

To Hwy. 62
Canyon Rd.

0.0   0.25   0.5
miles

23

2736'
N34 07.153
W116 06.728

Overlook

3100'

Fortynine Palms Canyon

2804'
N34 06.374
W116 06.327

Fortynine
Palms Oasis

Fortynine Palms Oasis

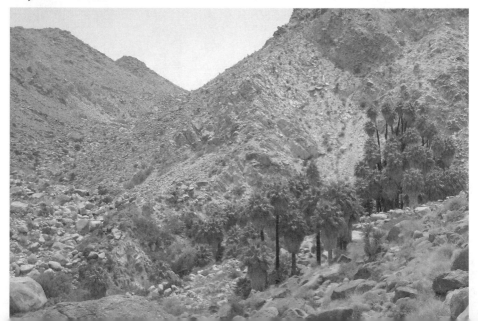

paths branching off the main trail, but they tend to lead to difficult boulder hopping; stay on the main trail.

The top of the ridge marks the halfway point. From here, you can glimpse part of the oasis in Fortynine Palms Canyon to the south. The trail descends past creosote and brittle bushes and barrel cacti into the canyon. Arrive at the oasis, where a flat rock shaded by palms makes a perfect lunch stop. Notice how many of the California

fan palms are missing their lower fronds. A series of fires over the years have burnt the trunks clean without killing the trees.

It is possible to follow the trail into the heart of the oasis, although the footing becomes more difficult. Adventurous souls can try rock-hopping south along Fortynine Palms Canyon for another mile and a half to its head, but the route is challenging because of large boulders and small cliffs barring the way.

trip 15.24 Mastodon Peak Loop

Distance	2.6 miles (loop)
Hiking Time	1.5 hours
Elevation Gain	400'
Difficulty	Easy, but some scrambling on the summit rocks
Trail Use	Good for children
Best Times	October–March
Agency	Joshua Tree National Park
Recommended Map	Trails Illustrated *Joshua Tree* or *Cottonwood Spring* 7.5'

DIRECTIONS Drive east on Interstate 10, 32 miles past Indio, then exit north on Cottonwood Springs Rd. to Joshua Tree National Park. Drive 7.2 miles to the Cottonwood Visitor Center, where you pay your park admission fee. Turn right (east) and proceed 1.1 miles to the Cottonwood Spring Trailhead parking at the end of the road.

This short loop hike in the southeastern part of Joshua Tree National Park treats you to an oasis, traces of an ancient Cahuilla Indian village, fun scrambling up the rocky summit of Mastodon Peak, ruins of two old mines, and a signed nature trail, all in less than a league of walking.

From the trailhead, descend southeast into the Cottonwood Spring Oasis. The Cahuilla Indians once inhabited this lush and shady site; in the late 1800s it became popular among miners seeking precious water. The California fan palms that now occupy the oasis were introduced after 1920.

Continue southeast to a signed junction at 0.6 mile. Turn left (north) and follow the trail 0.3 mile to another signed junction at the base of the rocky Mastodon Peak. Can you find the vantage point from

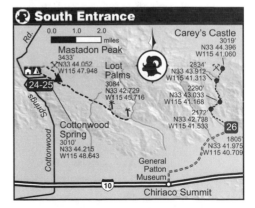

which prospectors imagined the mountain to be an enormous elephant head? Turn right and circle around the peak 0.1 mile until you find a faint trail scrambling up the east side of the mountain. The climb to the summit is steep and exposed, but not

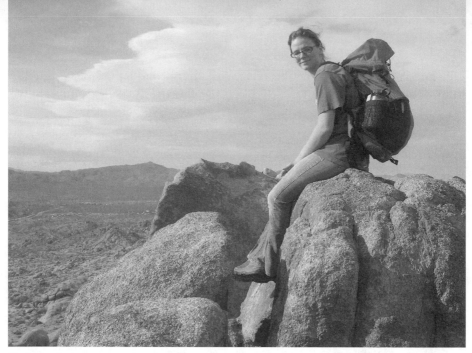

Mastodon Peak

difficult. Enjoy the far-reaching views from the summit extending over the Salton Sea to the Santa Rosa Mountains and San Jacinto.

Return to the junction at the base of the peak and continue north. Pass ruins of the Mastodon Mine, which was worked by the Hulsey family from 1934 to 1971. Be careful around old mines; the shafts and timbers are notoriously unstable.

After passing the mine, the trail wanders in and out of a wash for a mile until arriving at another trail junction near the foundations of the old Winona Mill, a gold mill worked by George Husley in the 1920s. The Cottonwood Campgrounds are to the right, but your path continues straight, following a signed nature trail for another 0.4 mile until it returns to the parking area.

trip 15.25 Lost Palms Oasis

Distance	7.5 miles
Hiking Time	4 hours
Elevation Gain	700'
Difficulty	Moderate
Best Times	October–March
Agency	Joshua Tree National Park
Recommended Map	Trails Illustrated *Joshua Tree* or *Cottonwood Spring* 7.5'

see map on p. 359

DIRECTIONS Drive east on Interstate 10, 32 miles past Indio, then exit north on Cottonwood Springs Rd. to Joshua Tree National Park. Drive 7.2 miles to the Cottonwood Visitor Center, where you pay your park admission fee. Turn right (east) and proceed 1.1 miles to the Cottonwood Spring Trailhead parking at the end of the road.

The Lost Palms Oasis hike showcases Joshua Tree National Park at its best. You will hike across cactus-covered hills on a clearly marked and well-kept trail. The oasis, hidden in a deep canyon studded with trademark Joshua Tree quartz monzonite, is home to the largest stand of California fan palms in the park. Lost Palms is in a day-use area; no camping is allowed.

From the trailhead, descend southeast into the Cottonwood Spring Oasis. This oasis was once home to the Cahuilla Indians. The bean pods from the thorny mesquite tree were a major food source for the Indians. Look for deep mortars in the granite boulders where the women ground the beans into flour.

Continue southeast to a signed junction at 0.6 mile. The left fork leads to Mastodon Peak (see Trip 15.24), but you should take the right fork, following the arrow for Lost Palms Oasis. The hike will take you across the flat desert past countless cholla cacti, yuccas, and ocotillos, then in and out of dry washes in the badlands before reaching another signed trail junction at the canyon rim, 3.5 miles from the start.

You can take a short detour to the right for an overlook of Lost Palms Oasis. Look for a smaller collection of palms in an upper side canyon. The main trail to the left makes a steep and rocky descent into the oasis on the canyon floor. Your efforts are rewarded at the bottom of the canyon when you stand among the largest collection of fan palm trees in Joshua Tree National Park. Once you are finished basking at the oasis, you can return via the same trail. Alternatively, if you are feeling adventurous, you can choose to take a short detour to Mastodon Peak (see Trip 15.24). This adds 2 miles to your day, but offers fun rock scrambling, spectacular views, and a taste of mining history.

Joshua Tree
National Park

Lost Palm Oasis

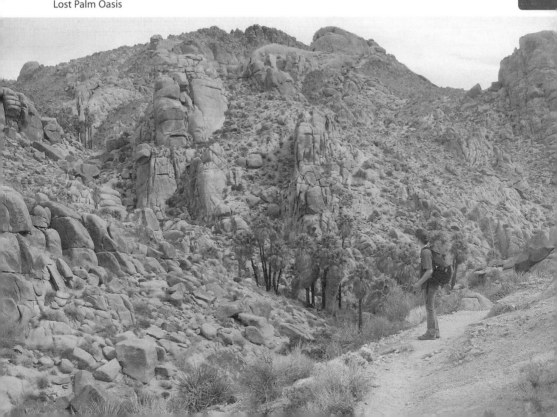

trip 15.26 Carey's Castle

Distance	8 miles (out-and-back)
Hiking Time	6 hours
Elevation Gain	1200'
Difficulty	Moderate
Best Times	October–April
Agency	Joshua Tree National Park
Recommended Map	Trails Illustrated *Joshua Tree* or *Hayfield* 7.5'

see map on p. 359

DIRECTIONS From Interstate 10 east of Indio, exit at Chiriaco Summit (Exit 173). The General Patton Museum is located northeast of the interchange. Look for a dirt road leading north along the east edge of the museum property. Follow it north 0.5 mile, then turn right (east) on another dirt road along a buried aqueduct. If you reach the fenced boundary of Joshua Tree National Park, you went north 0.1 mile too far. Drive for 3.4 miles to a dirt turnout on the left side of the road. If the road bends sharply right at the base of the mountain, you went 0.1 mile too far.

A prospector named Carey worked a mine in the remote Eagle Mountains in the 1940s. Near his mine, he built his "castle," a one-room dwelling under an overhanging boulder. Now within the border of Joshua Tree National Park at the head of Red Butte Wash, Carey's Castle has become a legendary destination for adventurous hikers. Getting to the castle involves 4 miles of spectacular cross-country travel up the twisty wash. The mountains are full of outlandish rock formations and exotic desert vegetation; they are especially attractive when the desert bursts into bloom after the winter storms. Solid navigational skills are necessary to locate the hidden site; a GPS receiver is handy but good old-fashioned route-finding is perfectly sufficient.

From the parking area, a trace trail leads over a small hump into a wash. This is one of the braids of Red Butte Wash, which gently slopes up northwest into the Eagle

Carey's Castle

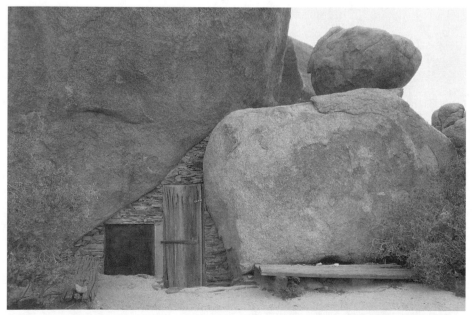

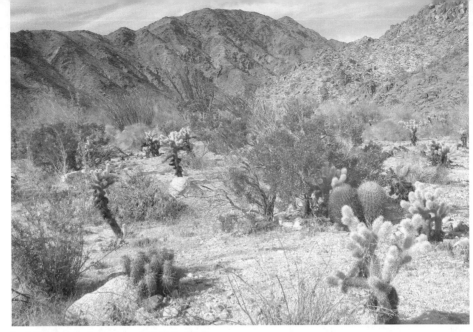
Lush desert vegetation near Red Butte Wash

Mountains. The main part of the wash is about 0.2 mile farther west. The vegetation is most impressive here, and features ocotillos, palo verdes, smoke bushes, and many species of cacti. Identify the mouth of the biggest canyon to the northwest and pick a path up the wash toward it. Eventually, the wash you are in will merge into the wider sandy bottom of Red Butte Wash, where you are likely to see footprints or cairns left by prior explorers.

Another large canyon opens up from the left (west), but stay in Red Butte Wash as it turns north. In 1.3 miles, the wash forks. The left fork goes up what appears to be the largest canyon, while the right fork turns a corner and heads toward huge cliffs of light tan granite that stand in contrast to the reddish-brown rock you have been passing. Turn right. In 0.5 mile, at the first break in the canyon's north wall, veer left and continue up the sandy wash. Soon, find yourself occasionally hopping over the polished granite boulders on the canyon floor. In 0.3 mile, stay left again at another fork. As you gain elevation, the canyon walls become shorter. Watch for brittle bushes, desert lavenders, and Mojave yuccas. In 1.1 miles, the wash forks again. The main branch leads left, but this hike veers right. Soon, the wash

is choked with boulders. Pick a path up the rocks to the sand beyond. In 0.7 mile, the wash opens into a small valley strewn with huge boulders. At the top of the valley, look for a faint trace of trail that was once an old mining road.

Carey's Castle is to the right, hidden on the north side of an enormous boulder. You can open the wooden door and inspect the premises, which includes windows, shelves, a table, and bed springs. Walls of stones and mortar fill the gaps between the boulders. Be careful to leave the place exactly as you found it so that others can enjoy the same adventure. Dates on magazines found in a cave nearby suggest that Carey lived here in the 1940s.

The mineshaft is located 0.1 mile from the castle. Follow the faint trail/road, as it leads west, then veers south. Look for a metal grate sealing the top of the shaft. Pieces of a rotting wooden ladder can still be seen leading down into the deep hole.

Return the way you came. Navigation is easy – just hike down the wash. If you stay in the main part of the wash, you may emerge at the dirt road a few hundred yards west of your vehicle; if so, turn left and make the short jaunt back.

trip 15.27 Spectre Point

Distance	14 miles (semi-loop)
Hiking Time	9–12 hours
Elevation Gain	3200'–4000' (depending on the number of peaks)
Difficulty	Strenuous
Best Times	October–April
Agency	Joshua Tree National Park
Required Map	Trails Illustrated *Joshua Tree* or *Cadiz Valley* SW 7.5'

see map on p. 365

DIRECTIONS From Highway 62 about 40 miles east of Twentynine Palms, park at a turnout on the south side of the road 0.8 mile east of mile marker 72.

While driving on lonely desert highways, mountain climbers sometimes pass imposing jagged desert peaks and wonder what they would be like to climb. The Coxcomb Mountains, located in the remote northeast corner of Joshua Tree National Park, are emblematic of these kinds of mysterious summits. The crest of the Coxcombs is a triple-peaked massif. The highest peak is called Spectre Point. The northern peak is called Aqua (or Tensor), and has a USGS benchmark. And the most difficult summit to climb is called Dyadic. These challenging cross-country climbs belong on the must-do list of any serious desert mountaineer. The northern Coxcomb Mountains are in a day-use area; no camping is allowed.

This hike can be done as a semi-loop. It begins with a long but easy walk across the desert along an old road to the base of

the northern Coxcombs Mountains. Then the route makes a beeline up a steep and boulder-filled series of canyons to the summit plateau. Spectre and Aqua are both rated class two, Dyadic involves fourth-class climbing on crumbling weathered granite, so a 100-foot rope and some slings are recommended if you choose to climb that summit. Bag as many of the peaks as you desire, then explore an alternate descent that is longer but arguably easier before returning via the old road.

From the parking area, a sandy jeep road (now closed to vehicles) leads south through the creosote-studded desert. After passing some rock mounds, it veers left (southeast) toward the distinctive low saddle between the high parts of the dramatic Coxcomb Mountains. In 3.6 miles, the jeep road drops into the broad wash leading

The Coxcomb Mountains

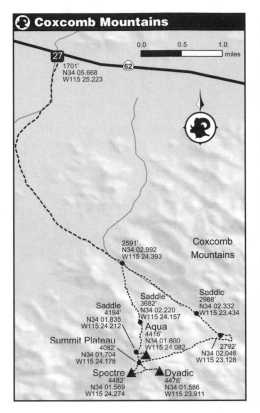

Coxcomb Mountains

it looks. Climb to the top, and then follow a wash that continues up the valley beyond. At the top of the valley, it is easiest to stay left as you climb to another saddle. You have now traveled 1.0 difficult mile since leaving the main wash.

Descend into the canyon beyond and turn right. Hike up the canyon, staying left at several forks, to a point just below the pinyon-clad Aqua Peak; continue up the canyon to a saddle on the right (west) side of Aqua 0.6 mile from the last saddle. There are great views from here into the Pinto Basin.

South of this saddle, and slightly obscured from view, is the summit plateau. If you plan to climb Aqua Peak, turn left (east) and follow the easy ridge to the 4416-foot summit. Climbing Aqua is also worthwhile because it offers good views to help you plan your path to the other summits. Otherwise, go south to the plateau. From the plateau, Aqua is located to the north, Spectre to the southwest, and Dyadic to the east, all within a quarter mile but hard to distinctly identify until you start to climb out of the hole. The easiest climb to Spectre is via the north face or northeast ridge. Dyadic has a challenging summit fin that is best accessed by any of several options from the south side. Descending the north face is not recommended; it involves very loose

toward the saddle. Continue up for 0.2 mile. Look for a prominent gully to the south leading to a broad gap immediately left of the highest rocks. Leave the main wash and head south up an easy side wash to the base of the gully, which is rocky but easier than

Joshua Tree
National Park

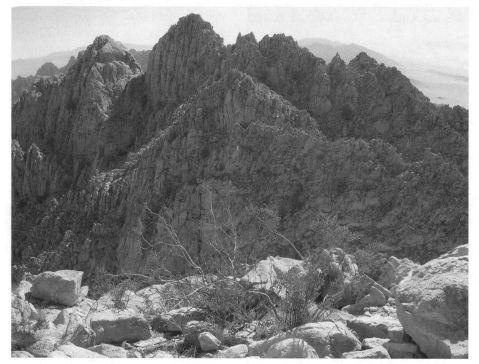

Dyadic Peak from Aqua

downclimbing and some bad rappels. All of the summits have awesome views of the rugged Coxcomb Mountains and desolate Pinto Basin.

You can return the way you came, but an enjoyable loop option is to follow the drainage east from the summit plateau. The wash drops down a step, then becomes wide and sandy, then descends a dry waterfall in the narrows, then becomes easy again. After 1.0 mile of boulder hopping, the wash dumps into a main northwest/southeast trending wash. You may find signs of a shortcut use

trail that leads north 100 yards over a low ridge, into the wash leading northwest. If you miss the shortcut, continue into this main wash, turn left, and follow its serpentine path northwest to where you may see a cairn marking the other end of the shortcut. In any event, continue 0.4 mile northwest to the distinctive saddle that you approached early in the trip, then 1.4 miles down rejoin the jeep road where it exits the left side of the wash. Finally, follow this road 3.6 easy downhill miles back to the highway.

chapter 16

Mojave National Preserve

The vast Mojave National Preserve was established by Congress in 1994 to protect 1.6 million acres of pristine desert in eastern California. Located between Joshua Tree and Death Valley National Parks, this area receives scant attention compared to its better-known neighbors, yet the scenery is no less varied and remarkable. The preserve includes sand dunes, limestone caverns, volcanic craters, granite peaks, Joshua tree forests, petroglyphs, and even a river that emerges from underground before sinking back into the desert sands. Four-wheeling enthusiasts trace the historic Mojave Road, where pioneers once hauled their wagons across the harsh desert. Settlements here are few and far between, and you must be prepared to handle any unforeseen difficulties yourself.

Mojave Preserve features a rich and complex geological history. The area was once submerged under a warm sea. The seabed accumulated expansive deposits of carbonate sediment, the skeletal remains of invertebrate shellfish. About 140 million years ago, during the Cretaceous period, collisions along the San Andreas Fault forced California upward out of the sea. The Mojave Desert was thrust upward to form a huge plateau and the gradual process of erosion carried away much of the now exposed seabed sediment. More recent

Sunbeam through a skylight at the lava tube (Trip 16.6)

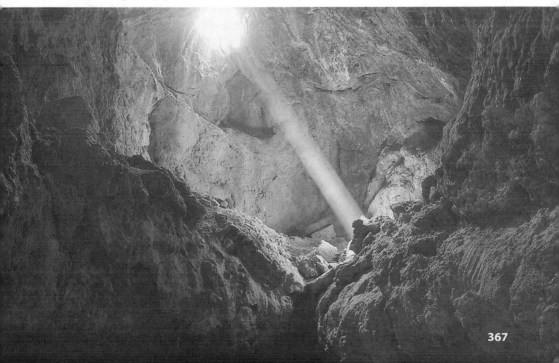

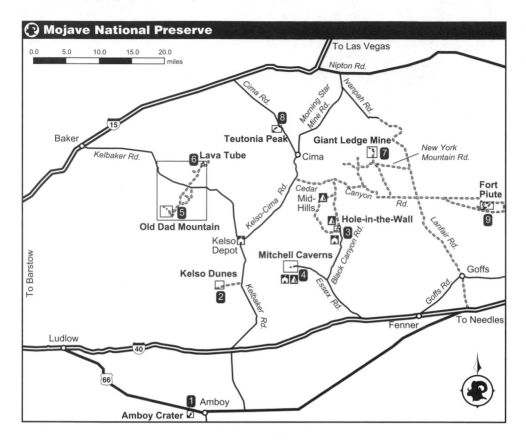

Mojave National Preserve

0.0   5.0   10.0   15.0   20.0
miles

To Las Vegas

Nipton Rd.

Cima Rd.

Morning Star Mine Rd.

Ivanpah Rd.

8

Baker

Teutonia Peak

15

Kelbaker Rd.

6 Lava Tube

Giant Ledge Mine

New York Mountain Rd.

7

Cima

Fort Piute

9

Cedar Canyon Rd.

Mid-Hills

Old Dad Mountain

5

Kelso-Cima Rd.

Hole-in-the-Wall

3

Kelso Depot

Mitchell Caverns

Lanfair Rd.

To Barstow

Kelso Dunes

2

4

Goffs

Kelbaker Rd.

Essex Rd.

Black Canyon Rd.

Goffs Rd.

Fenner

To Needles

Ludlow

40

66

1 Amboy

Amboy Crater

tectonic activity pushed up many of the chains of mountains that border the Mojave Desert. Until relatively recently, the area received far more rainfall and resembled Africa's verdant savannahs; herds of mastodons, rhinoceros, and camels roamed the great plains and their fossils can still be seen. At the end of the last Ice Age, about 10,000 years ago, rainfall patterns changed and the desert as we now know it came into existence. The great rivers and lakes dried up, but their traces can still be found in the landscape. Meanwhile, recent volcanic activity has left a chain of cinder cones and lava flows across the desert.

Native Americans carried on a precarious existence in this difficult environment. The Chemehuevi were the predominant tribe in the area, but their numbers were estimated at only about 1000 spread over the enormous desert. The Spanish were the first Europeans to visit the area. In 1776, Francisco Garces, a Franciscan priest, was dispatched to find a route from Santa Fe to Monterey. From the Colorado River, he crossed what is now the Mojave National Preserve, following Piute Creek, then passing the New York and Providence Mountains and the Kelso Dunes before reaching the Mojave River near Barstow. The American trapper, Jedediah Smith, took a similar route 50 years later, but had such a bad experience with hostile Indians and hunger that few others dared follow. Finally, in 1857, the War Department commissioned Edward Beale to build a wagon road along the 35th parallel. In a marginally successful experiment, Beale imported camels as pack animals. Forts were established a day's journey apart, but the Mojave Road's heyday was short lived. The construction of the transcontinental railroad farther south in the 1880s and 1890s put an end to the wagon traffic. By the turn of the century, miners and ranchers came to the area, but farming proved unprofitable in all but the wettest years. In the late 20th Century, the region began drawing recreational users. Unfortunately, off-road vehicle use, vandalism, and poaching led to the destruction of archeological sites and the loss of the desert tortoise and other threatened desert life. The establishment of the Mojave National Preserve promises to protect the region for future generations to enjoy.

Tourism in the area took off in the 1930s when Jack Mitchell began guiding visitors by lantern light through a spectacular pair of limestone caverns. He sold the area to the state of California in 1954. Now ranger-led tours of the Mitchell Caverns are offered in the Providence Mountains State Recreation Area, a state park within the National Preserve.

The Mitchell Caverns and the famous Kelso Dunes are not to be missed, but much of the charm of the Mojave National Preserve comes from exploring the back roads and lesser-visited trails. Distances are great and services are few in the eastern Mojave. Fill up with gas in Baker, Barstow, or Needles before you visit. (In a pinch, some of the most expensive gas in California can also be found at Fenner on Interstate 40.) Cell phone coverage is spotty, so bring a reliable vehicle and come prepared to take care of yourself if you stray from the beaten path. Let somebody know where you are going and when you expect to return. A high-clearance 4WD vehicle is helpful for exploring the back roads, though most of the hikes in this chapter can be reached in an ordinary passenger vehicle. Carry a good map, extra food, and plenty of water. Temperatures are also widely variable, and fluctuations between day and night can be extreme. The summers are almost unbearably hot in the desert, while the winters bring snow to the taller peaks.

One of the best ways to enjoy the Mojave National Preserve is to make a several-day visit during the cooler months. Although there are established campgrounds at Hole-in-the-Wall, Mid-Hills, and Mitchell Caverns, there is also a long tradition of free camping in the open desert. Camping by your vehicle is allowed alongside dirt roads in any site that has traditionally been used for the purpose (look for beaten ground with a fire ring; many such areas are indicated on the Tom Harrison map).

Visitor information is available at the Kelso Depot, a magnificent Union Pacific railroad station that has recently been renovated by the Park Service. Another visitor center is located near the Hole-in-the-Wall Campground. Information is also available at the Preserve Headquarters in Barstow and at the Needles Desert Information Center. At the time of this writing, there are no entrance fees and no permits required except for large groups and special events such as weddings.

Mojave
National Preserve

trip 16.1 Amboy Crater

Distance	3 miles (out-and-back)
Hiking Time	2 hours
Elevation Gain	400'
Difficulty	Easy
Trail Use	Dogs, good for children
Best Times	October–April
Agency	BLM (Needles Field Office)
Optional Map	*Amboy Crater* 7.5'

DIRECTIONS From Interstate 40, 28 miles east of Ludlow, take Exit 78, Kelbaker Rd. Drive south 11 miles to a T-junction with National Trails Highway (historic Route 66). Turn right (west) and continue 6 miles into Amboy, then 1 more mile west to a signed turnoff for Amboy Crater National Natural Landmark. Follow the good dirt Crater Rd. south 0.5 mile to the trailhead parking area. Amboy can also be reached from the south via a scenic drive from Twentynine Palms.

Amboy Crater is a volcanic cone of ash and cinders rising out of a lava flow. It has erupted at least four times; the most recent eruption happened 10,000 years ago. This short hike leads through the basalt flows and up a breach in the crater wall to the center of the cone. After the winter rains, the fields of purple sand verbena and desert lily along this route are especially photogenic. This trip has enough attractions to keep a child captivated, and the steady stream of freight trains on the Atchison, Topeka & Santa Fe line blowing their whistles at Amboy lend a certain atmosphere that some may find appealing. The crater is located on BLM land outside the boundaries of Mojave National Preserve.

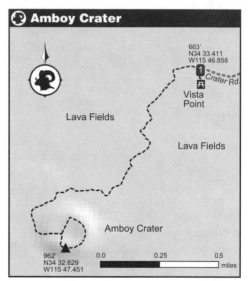

Amboy Crater

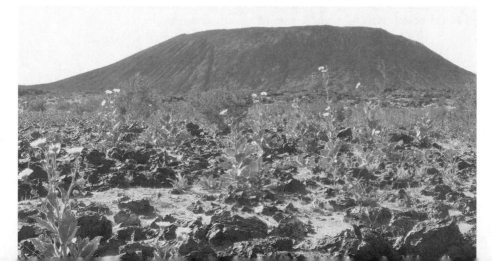

WARNING: The Twentynine Palms Marine Corps Air Ground Combat Center is located immediately west of Amboy Crater. This is a live bombing range and is still active. DO NOT enter the bombing range, and do not handle unexploded stray ammunition.

There are two trails from the parking area. At the southeast end, a wheelchair-accessible path leads 100 yards to a shaded viewing platform. The main trail departs from the west end near the outhouses. It snakes through the lava flows along an old jeep track toward the crater, passing some shaded benches en route. Sometimes the path can be faint, but look for footprints and occasional trail markers if you are in doubt.

Do not climb the main wall of the crater directly; this contributes to unsightly erosion. Instead, follow the trail as it curves around to the right (west) side and enters the crater via a hidden break. From the center of the crater, consider taking one of the paths up to the rim and circumnavigating the lip of the volcano. There are good views of the lava flow and the Bristol dry lake to the south. Return the way you came.

trip 16.2 Kelso Dunes

Distance	3 miles (out-and-back)
Hiking Time	3 hours
Elevation Gain	500'
Difficulty	Moderate
Trail Use	Dogs, good for children
Best Times	October–April
Agency	Mojave National Preserve
Optional Map	Trails Illustrated *Mojave National Preserve* or *Kelso Dunes* 7.5'

DIRECTIONS From Interstate 40, 28 miles east of Ludlow and 65 miles west of Needles, take Exit 78, Kelbaker Rd. Go 16 miles north to the signed Kelso Dunes turnoff. Alternatively, from Kelso Depot, go 7 miles south to the same turnoff. Follow the excellent dirt road west 2.8 miles to the signed trailhead and outhouse.

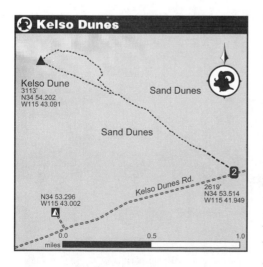

The Kelso Dunes are the third highest sand dunes in the United States, and are the highlight of many visits to Mojave National Preserve. Winds pick up the fine sands from the Mojave River Sink and carry them across the Devil's Playground. Eddies formed by the Granite and Providence Mountains cause the winds to drop their loads, creating the ever-shifting Kelso Dunes. Although this trip to the top of the highest dune is relatively short, the climb up loose sand can be exhausting. It is easy for groups to split up before the final climb because the route is in view all the way and because there are plenty of smaller hills to enjoy along the way. Primitive camping is also available another mile west by a lonely

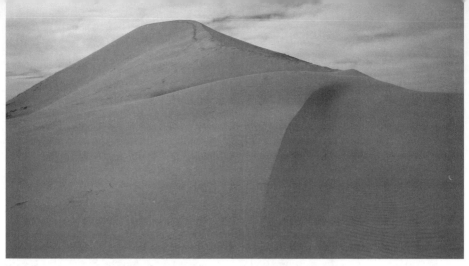

Kelso Dune Summit

wind-swept tree; there is no camping at the trailhead.

The Kelso Dunes are also known as "booming dunes" because under the right conditions they emit a sound like low thunder. The phenomenon is found only in relatively few dunes in the world and is an active subject of scientific investigation. The best way for you to investigate it yourself is to slide down the steep face of the biggest dune!

From the signed trailhead, follow the well-defined trail northwest through the creosote bushes. Soon, the sands begin. Unless a recent sandstorm has obliterated the tracks, footprints clearly lead toward the highest dune. In 1 mile, veer right and head for a point just left of the saddle between the two biggest dunes. This route avoids climbing the steepest sections of sand. Once you reach the ridge, turn left and climb a spectacular razorback ridge of sand to the summit. There are fine views of the Granite Mountains to the south, the rugged limestone-cliffed Providence Mountains to the east, and the Devil's Playground to the north.

Return by descending straight down the face of the dune and walking directly back to the trailhead, rejoining the main trail in about 0.4 mile.

Kelso Dunes trailhead

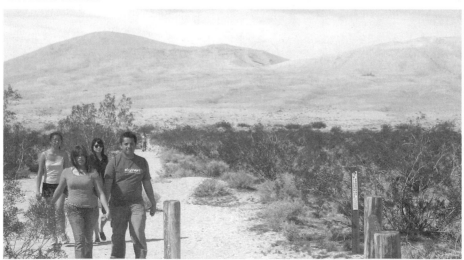

trip 16.3 Hole-in-the-Wall

Distance	1.5 miles (loop)
Hiking Time	1 hour
Elevation Gain	200′
Difficulty	Easy
Trail Use	Dogs, good for children
Best Times	September–May
Agency	Mojave National Preserve
Optional Map	Trails Illustrated *Mojave National Preserve* or *Columbia Mountain 7.5′*

DIRECTIONS From Interstate 40, 50 miles east of Ludlow and 43 miles west of Needles, take Exit 100, Essex Rd. Drive north 10 miles to a junction, then stay right on Black Canyon Rd. and continue another 10 miles. Turn left on a good dirt road at a signed junction for the Hole-in-the-Wall Ranger Station, and park at the ranger station.

A volcanic eruption 18 million years ago in the Mojave Desert emitted dense blasts of super-heated ash. The ash, dust, and volcanic gas from the eruption compacted and cemented together as it cooled, forming what is known as volcanic tuff. This popular loop hike explores the narrow Banshee Canyon that snakes through the fascinating and colorful rock formation. Gas trapped in the ash created pockets in the tuff resembling eternally moaning mouths, and the wind howls as it blows through the canyon. The hike descends a short vertical section in the narrow slot canyon; metal rings have been set in the rock to provide holds. A person of ordinary physical ability

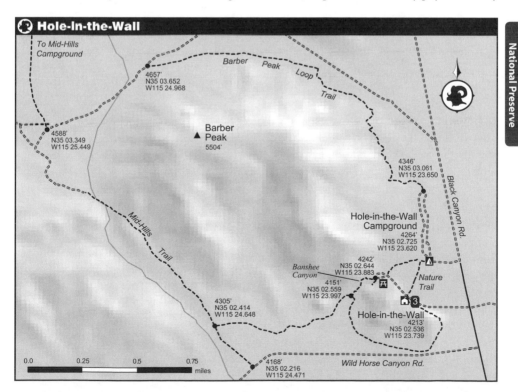

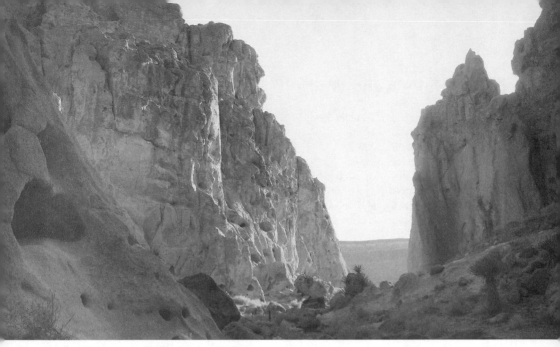

Banshee Canyon

can negotiate the rings, but young children may need a boost and some hikers may find the slot claustrophobic. Dogs must be lifted or pushed up the two narrow chutes where the rings are located.

VARIATION

Hole-in-the-Wall is located next to a popular campground. A quarter mile nature trail leads from the south end of the campground to the ranger station. This is a worthwhile walk for those staying at the campground and it is a good way to learn to identify the cacti, yuccas, and bushes common to the eastern Mojave Desert.

From the trail marker at the ranger station parking area, curve east and then south around the base of the volcanic formation, passing close by Wild Horse Canyon Rd. As the trail passes some upthrust rocks, look carefully for several small petroglyphs. Skin oils can stain the rock art, so do not touch or damage the petroglyphs. The trail continues through a lush desert landscape of Mojave yuccas, buckhorn chollas, and barrel cacti. It curves to the right and comes to a junction.

VARIATION

The left fork leads 8 miles across the desert to Mid-Hills Campground. This is a good one-way hike or round-trip backpack for those who love solitude. The trail is marked with brown posts and cairns. It gains 800 feet of elevation. Because this is one of the higher parts of Mojave National Preserve, it tends to be cooler (and can be downright cold in the winter). The trail passes through a pinyon-juniper woodland that burned in the catastrophic 2005 Hackberry Fire, and reaches the road opposite the entrance of Mid-Hills Campground (at GPS coordinates N35 07.388 W115 25.967 5485′).

This trip follows the right fork into the spectacular Banshee Canyon. Take a few minutes to explore the many holes in the wall. A trail marker indicates the narrowing of the canyon and the approach to the vertical slots. Climb the rocks leading to the two chutes, and use the metal rings for hand and foot holds. Continue up the rocks to reach a picnic area. A short side trail to the right leads to an overlook into Banshee Canyon. When you are done, follow the dirt road 0.2 mile back to the ranger station.

VARIATION —————————————

The Barber Peak Loop Trail was constructed in this area in spring 2008, too late to be included in this edition. The 6-mile trail circles Barber Peak, the dramatic volcanic formation immediately west of the campground. This trail starts at the northeast end of the picnic area above Banshee Canyon and leads to the nature trail at the south end of Hole-in-the-Wall Campground. Follow the campground road to the extreme north end of the campground, where the trail resumes adjacent to the tent camping sites. The trail climbs to a rise with good views, drops down a stone staircase, and circles around the rhyolite cliffs of Barber Peak until it can follow the Mid-Hills to Hole-in-the-Wall Trail back to Banshee Canyon and up the slot. The loop traverses spectacular country and is a worthwhile longer hiking alternative. The total elevation gain is about 1000′.

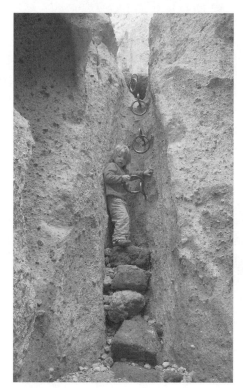

Rings Trail

trip 16.4 Mitchell Caverns

Distance	1 mile (out-and-back)
Hiking Time	1.5 hours
Elevation Gain	100′
Difficulty	Easy
Best Times	September–May
Agency	Providence Mountains State Recreation Area
Optional Map	Trails Illustrated *Mojave National Preserve* or *Fountain Peak* 7.5′

see map on p. 376

DIRECTIONS From Interstate 40, 50 miles east of Ludlow and 43 miles west of Needles, take Exit 100, Essex Rd. Drive north 10 miles to a junction. Stay left and continue another 6 miles to park at the Providence Mountains State Park Ranger Station.

Mitchell Caverns is a spectacular system of limestone caves in the Providence Mountains. Visitors to the caverns will see stalactites, stalagmites, shields, draperies, soda straws, and other rare and beautiful formations. Cavern tours run at 1:30 P.M. daily and last 1.5 hours. Additional tours are offered at 10:00 A.M. and 3:00 P.M. on weekends and holidays between Memorial Day and Labor Day. School and special groups must make reservations one month in advance by calling (760) 928-2586. Reservations for the general public are not required, but are recommended on busy weekends and holidays because there is a limit of 25 visitors per tour. The cost is $5 for adults. The caves are 65°F year round, but the half-mile trail to them can be sizzling in the summer or icy in the winter. A six-site campground with no facilities for RVs or large groups is located across from the ranger station.

The Providence Mountains were once part of an ancient seabed. Around 250 million years ago, vast layers of shells accumulated on the sea floor and were compressed to form limestone. More recently, the limestone was thrust upward and partially covered with volcanic rhyolite; the mountains now consist of an upper core of rhyolite and a lower layer of limestone. Some 12 million years ago, when there was significantly more rainfall in the area, mildly acidic rainwater percolated down and dissolved the limestone forming chambers which the Chemehuevi Indians call "Eyes of the Mountains." Businessman and prospector Jack Mitchell purchased the area in 1932 and developed the caverns as a tourist attraction, offering full-day tours by lantern. He had a flair for drama and his tours involved crawling through narrow tunnels and visiting features that he called "The Queen's Chamber" and "The Bottomless Pit." The state of California acquired the caverns in 1954 and further "improved" the caverns for easier travel; young children will have no difficulty with the walk. Now the Providence Mountains State Recreation Area is a state park within the boundaries of the Mojave National Preserve. The ranger-led tours are less romantic than Mitchell's, but far more factually accurate.

If you have additional time before or after a tour, several short and enjoyable trails start at Mitchell Caverns parking area.

Mary Beal Nature Study Trail: 0.5 mile. Starting at the north end of the parking lot this trail loops through a wonderful variety of cacti and other desert plants. Obtain a booklet at the trailhead or ranger station describing the numbered attractions. The

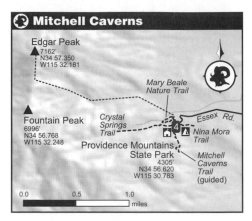

Entrance to Mitchell Caverns

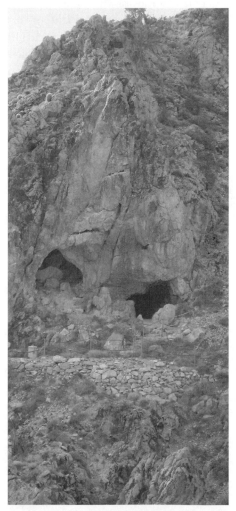

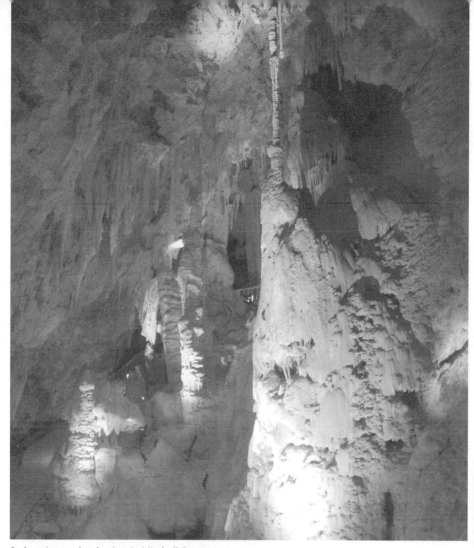
Stalagmites and stalactites in Mitchell Caverns

trail is named for an amateur naturalist who spent half a century exploring the area and collecting botanical specimens.

Nina Mora Trail: 0.5 mile. Starting at the east end of the campground this trail follows a ridge covered with cacti and yuccas past the grave of Nina Mora, the infant daughter of a Mexican miner who worked the mines here a century ago. The trail leads to a viewpoint above the Clipper Valley.

Crystal Springs Trail: 1.2 miles, 600′ elevation gain. The trail starts adjacent to the Mitchell Caverns Trail near the ranger station, steeply climbs through areas of cacti, junipers, and pinyon pines into the volcanic rhyolite formations of the upper Providence Mountains, and reaches a spring in the dramatic Crystal Canyon.

Edgar Peak: 5 miles (out-and-back), 2900′ elevation gain. It is also possible to climb a strenuous cross-country route up to Edgar Peak (7162′), the high point of the Providence Mountains. Check in at the ranger station for more information. Climb cross-country from the Mary Beal Trail up the main canyon (not the Crystal Canyon) to a fork at 5900 feet, then stay right and climb to the top of the ridge. Turn right (north) and continue 0.3 mile to the true summit, avoiding some more difficult false summits along the ridge.

trip 16.5 Old Dad Mtn.

Distance	3.5 miles (out-and-back)
Hiking Time	4 hours
Elevation Gain	1800'
Difficulty	Strenuous
Best Times	October–April
Agency	Mojave National Preserve
Required Map	Trails Illustrated *Mojave National Preserve* or *Old Dad Mountain* 7.5'

DIRECTIONS A 4WD vehicle is recommended because this approach follows sandy washes. Be prepared to dig yourself out if you get stuck, and carry plenty of water and supplies. The drive is confusing because there are many minor access road forks; do it in daylight if possible. From Interstate 15 at Baker, take Exit 246, Kelbaker Rd. and follow it east, then south, for 19 miles to the unmarked Aiken Mine Rd., a dirt road that crosses Kelbaker Rd. just south of a line of cinder cones. The turnout on the east side of the road at the intersection is the only large parking area along this part of Kelbaker Rd. Alternatively, from Kelso Depot, follow Kelbaker Rd. 15 miles north to Aiken Mine Rd. Turn southwest and follow the dirt road 1.6 miles to a T-junction. Turn right and follow the road, which curves around to the south. In 2.5 miles, stay right at a fork and follow a sandy wash near three rows of transmission lines. Follow the wash for 1.0 mile to a fork. Stay left and go 1.2 miles, passing under one set of transmission lines, to a four-way junction in a wash. Turn right (north) and drive under the other two transmission lines. Park in 0.5 mile where the road turns right and begins to climb out of the wash. NOTE: It is possible to take a shortcut back following this road to the right, but it involves climbing a steep 4WD hill.

Old Dad Mtn. was humorously named in response to the nearby Old Woman Mountains. It is a short but steep and fun climb to the 4252-foot volcanic summit. The mountain hike appears difficult at first, but with careful route-finding, it is possible to stay on class two scrambling. Bighorn sheep frequent this area, and lucky visitors may see them.

From the parking area, hike northwest for 1.0 mile up the wash. Look for a prominent canyon on the east face of Old Dad Mtn. Climb the ridge just north of this canyon to 4000 feet. This involves fun scrambling up

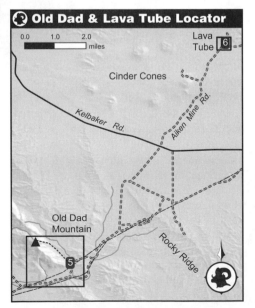

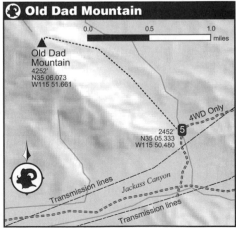

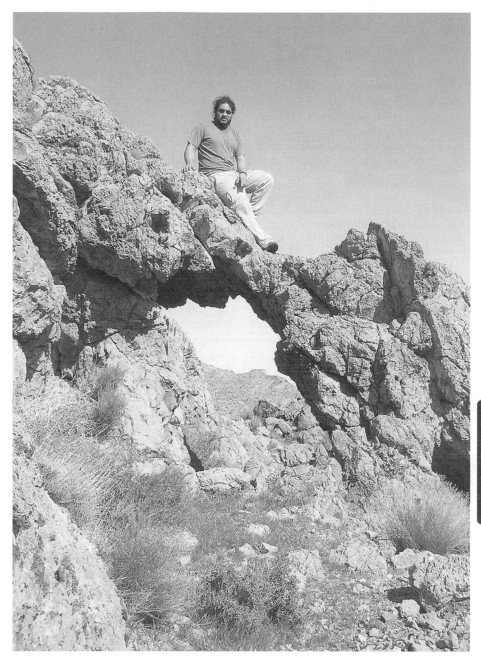

Scrambling up Old Dad Mtn.

interesting rock, but should not be too difficult if you are on route. Then turn left and hike up gentler slopes to the summit.

From the top, enjoy views of the Devil's Playground, Soda Dry Lake, the lava beds, and the Kelso Sand Dunes. On a clear winter day, the snow-capped summits of San Jacinto, San Gorgonio, Mt. Charleston, and Telescope Peak are all visible. Return the way you came.

trip 16.6 Lava Tube

Distance	0.5 mile (out-and-back)
Hiking Time	30 minutes
Elevation Gain	100'
Difficulty	Easy
Trail Use	Good for children
Best Times	October–April
Agency	Mojave National Preserve
Optional Map	Trails Illustrated *Mojave National Preserve* or *Indian Spring* 7.5'

see maps on pp. 381 & 378

DIRECTIONS From Interstate 15 at Baker, take Exit 246, Kelbaker Rd. and follow it east, then south, for 19 miles to the unmarked Aiken Mine Rd., a dirt road that crosses Kelbaker Rd. just south of a line of cinder cones. The turnout on the east side of the road at the intersection is the only large parking area along Kelbaker Rd. Alternatively, from Kelso Depot, follow Kelbaker Rd. 15 miles north to Aiken Mine Rd. Follow the excellent dirt road 4.6 miles northeast to an unmarked fork. Turn left onto a narrow and sandy dirt road, which leads north past a corral and ends at a parking area in 0.3 mile. Be careful of the sand; it is usually not a problem, but passenger cars have become mired here.

Among the many notable geological features of Mojave National Preserve are a chain of cinder cones and lava flows located between Baker and Kelso Depot. In one of the lava beds is a lava tube, which formed when the surface of the lava flow cooled and hardened into a crust while the molten center flowed on. This short trip leads into the tube. Make sure to bring a flashlight.

From the parking area, hike up a closed road north onto the lava flow. In 0.2 mile near the crest of the flow, look for a clearing

Lava Tube

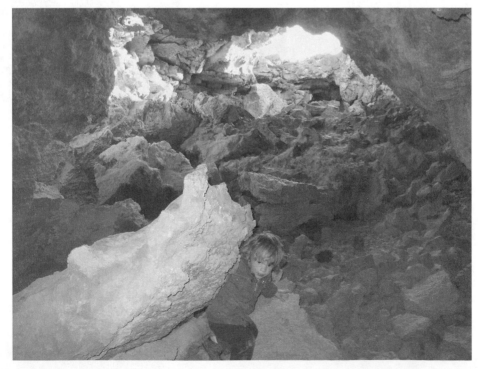

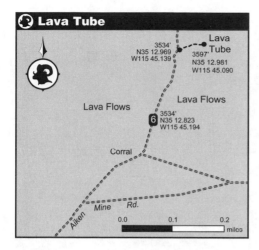

Lava Tube

3534'
N35 12.969
W115 45.139

Lava Tube
3597'
N35 12.981
W115 45.090

Lava Flows

Lava Flows

6 3534'
N35 12.823
W115 45.194

Corral

Aiken Mine Rd.

0.0   0.1   0.2
miles

and trail on the right (east); it may be marked by a metal stake. Follow the trail east for 100 yards as it gently climbs through the black lava flow. Pass a pair of sinister-looking "eyes" marking the bottom end of the lava tube, and then reach the gaping main entrance. A sturdy metal staircase was installed in 2008, providing an easy descent to the floor of the lava tube.

Follow a tunnel that leads back toward the eyes and opens up into a large chamber, then return the way you came.

trip 16.7 Giant Ledge Mine

Distance	2.5 miles (out-and-back)
Hiking Time	1.5 hours
Elevation Gain	400'
Difficulty	Easy
Trail Use	Dogs, good for children
Best Times	September–May
Agency	Mojave National Preserve
Recommended Map	Trails Illustrated *Mojave National Preserve* or *Pinto Valley, Ivanpah* 7.5'

see maps on pp. 368 & 382

DIRECTIONS A 4WD vehicle is recommended to reach this trailhead. From Interstate 40 at Fenner, 57 miles east of Ludlow and 36 miles west of Needles, take Exit 107, Goffs Rd. Drive north 10 miles to the old Goffs Schoolhouse, and then turn left on Lanfair Rd. Drive north for 21 miles to the OX Ranch. The first 10 miles are paved and the remainder is graded dirt, eventually changing name to Ivanpah Rd. Then turn left (west) onto the signed occasionally graded dirt New York Mountain Rd. Proceed 5.4 miles, then turn right (north) at an unsigned junction onto a fair dirt road. Go 1.8 miles toward the mountains, passing an old windmill and water tank along the way. Stay on the main road, tending right at forks. Shortly after crossing a sandy wash, look for a large turnout on the right that makes a good parking spot. 2WD vehicles may park before the wash to avoid getting stuck in the sand.

The New York Mountains, named for their dramatic skyline, are over 7000 feet tall and offer refreshingly cool camping and hiking in the remote heart of the Mojave National Preserve. Caruthers Canyon penetrates the range from the south and leads to the abandoned Giant Ledge copper mine. This short but scenic hike leads along a creek bed to the mine site. Botanists are especially interested in this canyon because it is home to a unique mutant of the single-leaf pinyon pine (*Pinus monophylla*) with

Giant Ledge Mine

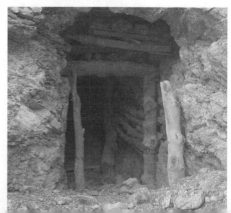

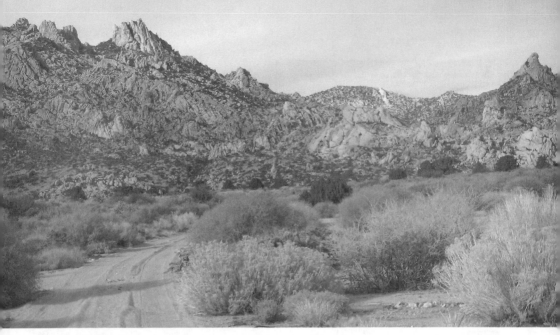

New York Mountains

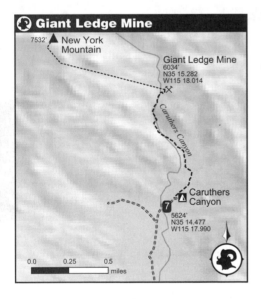

Giant Ledge Mine

7532' ▲ New York Mountain

Giant Ledge Mine
6034'
N35 15.282
W115 18.014

Caruthers Canyon

Caruthers Canyon

7

5624'
N35 14.477
W115 17.990

0.0   0.25   0.5
miles

beneath the granite spires of the New York Mountains. In 0.6 mile, cross the creek bed. Soon reach the top of a small rise, where you can enjoy fine views back to the south.

Shortly thereafter, arrive at Giant Ledge Mine nestled among the trees in a valley. You may first see the remains of a broken-down wooden chute. A side trail leads to the top of the chute, where several tunnels are supported by timbers. You may find bits of bright blue ore scattered along the trail. Leave the rocks for future hikers to enjoy and do not enter the shafts; old mines are extremely dangerous. Return the way you came.

VARIATION

Motivated mountaineers may choose to continue on to the 7532-foot summit of New York Mountain. It is less than a mile to the west, but 1500 feet higher than the mine. Ascend a gully to the left of the prominent pinnacle to the west. The true high point is 0.2 mile west of the pinnacle and is most easily climbed by passing around on the south to the west side, then climbing a third-class crack near the top.

bundled pairs of needles rather than the normal single needle.

Hike north on the dirt road, which rapidly deteriorates to 4WD only and soon becomes impassable to all vehicles. There are numerous fine primitive camping sites along the road; a fork to the right (east) leads to one with a picnic table and fire pit. Follow the main road up the canyon

trip 16.8 Teutonia Peak

Distance	3.2 miles (out-and-back)
Hiking Time	2 hours
Elevation Gain	700'
Difficulty	Moderate
Trail Use	Dogs
Best Times	October–April
Agency	Mojave National Preserve
Recommended Map	Trails Illustrated *Mojave National Preserve* or *Cima Dome* 7.5'

DIRECTIONS From Interstate 15, 25 miles east of Baker, take Exit 272, Cima Rd. Proceed south 11 miles to a small turnout on the right (west) with a trail maker. Alternatively, the trailhead can be reached by driving 6 miles north on the Cima Rd. from Cima.

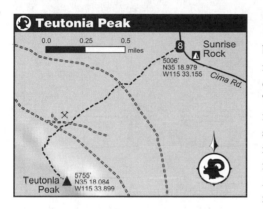

Cima Dome appears unremarkable at first, but careful inspection reveals it to be an unusual formation: a nearly symmetrical hump of monzonite nearly 10 miles in diameter protruding from the desert floor. The igneous dome formed underground from an ancient upwelling of magma. The softer overlying rock eroded away, leaving the dome. Its size is best appreciated from a distance; there is a good view from Interstate 15 near the Cima Rd. exit. On its northeast flank, the rocky Teutonia Peak

Teutonia Peak Trail

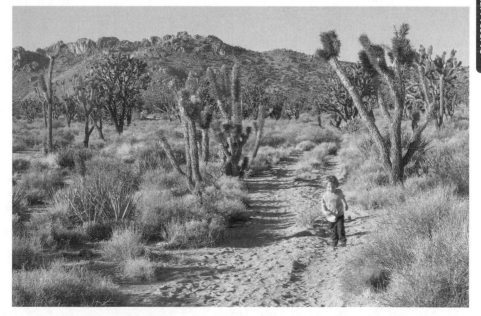

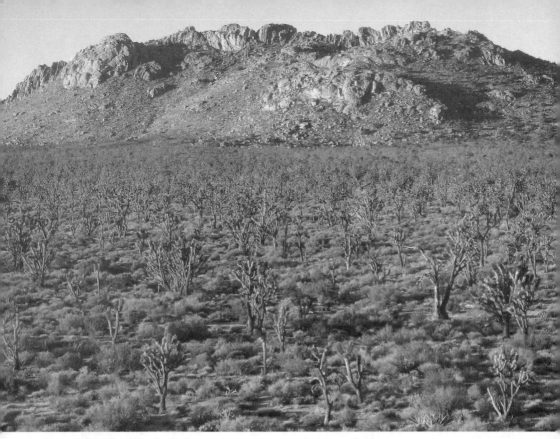

Teutonia Peak from Sunrise Rock

(5755´) breaks the symmetry, and is slightly taller than the center of the dome itself. This hike leads to the peak through one of the world's largest Joshua tree forests.

There is an excellent primitive camping site at Sunrise Rock, 0.1 mile south of the Cima Dome Trailhead. Turn east on a dirt road along the north side of the rock and pick a site among the junipers and Joshua trees.

The beginning of the trail is marked with a picture of a hiker and an interpretive panel about the Joshua tree forest in the desert woodland, but there is no mention of Teutonia Peak itself. The trail leads southwest directly toward Teutonia Peak. This is a lush region of desert full of Joshua trees, blue yuccas, and buckhorn cacti. Occasional exposed granite slabs remind you of the geologic origin of Cima Dome. In 0.5 mile, cross a dirt road. In another 0.5 mile, cross a second network of dirt roads near an old mine. The proper path is marked with trail

signs. If you are feeling adventurous, take a 100-yard detour right (west) toward a deep mine shaft that is now fenced off. The trail soon begins to climb, making a few switchbacks before reaching the ridge. As you gain elevation, the Joshua tree forest gives way to junipers and pancake prickly pear cacti. The trail turns left (south-southeast) and follows the ridge just west of its crest. There are good views of the gently sloping Cima Dome to the west. At 0.6 mile from the mine, the trail reaches the ridge again at a notch between some of the huge toothlike summit boulders. Here, you can enjoy views to the east of the Ivanpah Mountains and of the jagged New York Mountains to the southeast.

Return the way you came. A fainter trail leads on part way around the boulders to the south, but soon ends. The summit rocks are tricky and a rope and climbing skills are recommended if you choose to scale them.

trip 16.9 **Fort Piute**

Distance	5 miles (out-and-back), or 6 miles (loop)
Hiking Time	3–4 hours
Elevation Gain	1000'
Difficulty	Moderate
Trail Use	Dogs
Best Times	October–April
Agency	Mojave National Preserve
Recommended Map	Trails Illustrated *Mojave National Preserve* or *Signal Hill, Homer Mountain* 7.5'

DIRECTIONS A 4WD vehicle is recommended to reach this trailhead. Always check on road conditions after heavy rains. From Interstate 40 at Fenner, 57 miles east of Ludlow and 36 miles west of Needles, take Exit 107, Goffs Rd. Drive north 10 miles to the old Goffs Schoolhouse, and then turn left on Lanfair Rd. Drive north for 10 miles until the road turns to dirt, then another 5.7 miles to the signed junction with the Cedar Canyon Rd. Immediately north of the junction, turn right (east) onto a utility road (you may see an arrow labeled PT&T). Proceed 3.6 miles to an unmarked V-junction. Stay right and continue 5.8 miles across the Lanfair Valley, crossing some sandy washes. Just before reaching the Piute Mountains, turn left on a dirt road and proceed north 0.5 mile to a wide clearing marked with cairns.

The Mojave Road was once a trade route for Native Americans crossing the desert between the Colorado River and the Pacific Ocean. Before the Civil War, it became a wagon road, and after the war, forts were established a day's travel apart to protect travelers from hostile Indians displaced by white settlers. The forts were rendered obsolete in 1883 when the Southern Pacific Railroad was completed farther south of the Mojave Road. Fort Piute is one of these derelict garrisons, located at the base of the Piute Mountains. The area is also noteworthy because of Piute Spring, which flows year-round to support lush vegetation, its waters then sinking back into the desert sands. This hike follows the Mojave Road past some petroglyphs to the fort overlooking the creek, and then offers the option of returning via the spectacular Piute Gorge.

Mojave
National Preserve

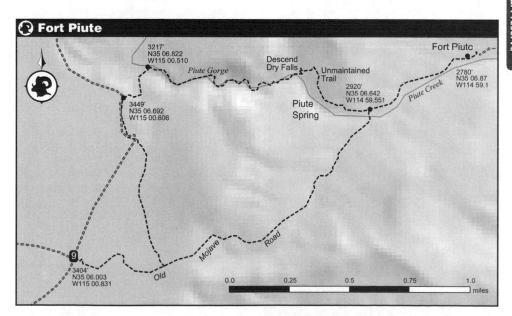

Entering the gorge involves some third-class rock scrambling down dry waterfalls.

From the parking area, walk due east past some posts marking the wilderness boundary; vehicles are not permitted beyond the posts. The path is initially faint, but soon becomes the well-defined old Mojave Road, which switchbacks up the slope. As you climb, the creosote bushes yield to Mojave yuccas and buckhorn, barrel, and hedgehog cacti. In 0.6 mile, reach the crest of the ridge and begin descending the exceedingly rocky road.

After rounding a corner to the left, the canyon bottom comes into view. The Mojave Road descends to the bottom of a dry wash and follows it for some distance, then exits at a clearly marked point on the left side where the wash turns right, 1.1 miles down from the ridge. Immediately after leaving the wash, look for petroglyphs on a boulder beside the trail. Sharp-eyed hikers may notice several more petroglyphs along the route. The Mojave Road descends a band of red rock. Wheel tracks can still be seen gouged into the rock where the wagon teams struggled up the steep hill. In 0.2 mile, arrive at the perennial Piute Creek. Such a reliable source of water is rare in the Mojave Desert and has attracted animals and humans through the ages.

The trail jogs left upstream, then promptly crosses and climbs up the north bank to a junction. Turn right (east) and follow the trail through rich fields of yuccas and cacti overlooking Piute Creek. This area was once a lush riparian zone of cottonwood, willow, and mesquite, which provided vital nourishment to birds, toads, and much desert wildlife. In September 2004, careless visitors triggered a wildfire that burned twelve acres along the creek; the trees are gradually beginning to recover. In 0.6 mile, arrive at the low stone walls, which

Cactus near Fort Piute Trail

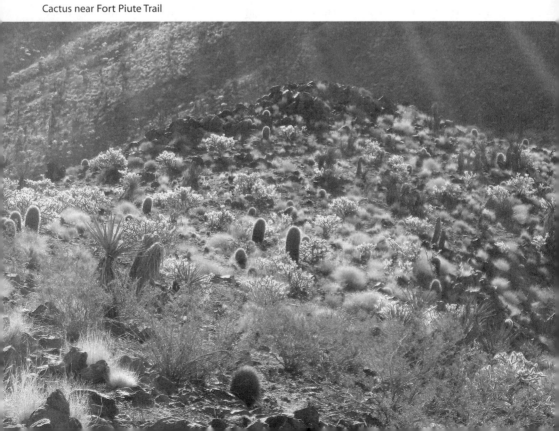

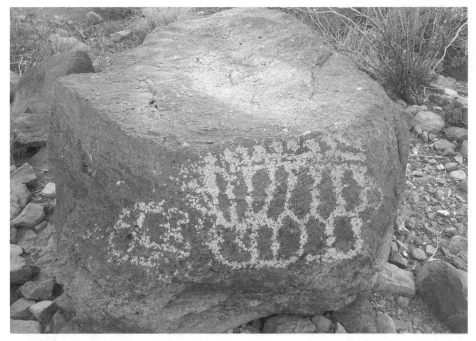

Petroglyph

are all that remains of Fort Piute. Enjoy the exhibits and imagine what a solider's life might have been like at such a remote outpost. Please do not climb, sit on, or disturb the fragile historic fort walls. After exploring, you may return the way you came.

ALTERNATIVE FINISH

Alternatively, at the trail junction immediately north of the Piute Creek crossing, an unmaintained trail leads west above the creek. In 0.3 mile, reach a vista atop steep loose cliffs where you can see Piute Spring, clearly identifiable by the lush vegetation below and the barren sandy wash above. (The path stays above the cliff to avoid bushwhacking through the vegetation in the canyon.) The route becomes somewhat difficult to identify here, but is marked with cairns as it switchbacks up and leads 0.2 mile north toward a side canyon entering from the north. The trail descends into this gully, which cuts through red, purple, and brown volcanic rocks. The gully drops into Piute Gorge. This is the crux of the hike, involving climbing down dry water-

falls (third class on unstable rock). Look for paths bypassing some of the falls.

The route turns right (west) and enters the spectacular narrows of Piute Gorge, passing through many-hued volcanic rock formations and threading past house-sized boulders that plummeted off the canyon walls into the creek bed. The route follows the meandering canyon for 0.9 mile upstream until the steep walls abruptly end as the creek enters a zone of tan sedimentary rock. A good trail exits on the left side and climbs steeply 0.2 mile up to the road at a parking area.

The other trailhead is 0.9 mile south across the flat desert. You can follow the road or a trail that parallels it for 0.3 mile to a jog in the road overlooking the next ravine. From here, the road and trail diverge. The road leads straight back to your vehicle, while the trail veers up the hill, climbing to meet the old Mojave Road just below the ridge crest.

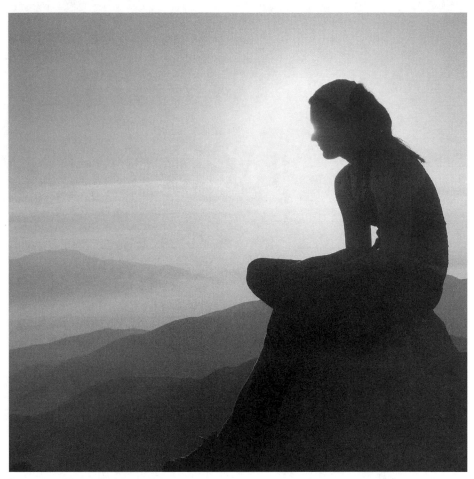

Sunset near Mt. Inspiration

Best Hikes

Big Three Mountain Climbs

Mt. Baldy *(Trip 1.1)* — 10,064′ monarch of the San Gabriel Mountains.

San Gorgonio Mtn. *(Trip 5.1 or 5.12)* — 11,499′ crown of the San Bernardino Mountains.

San Jacinto Peak *(Trip 9.21 or 9.16)* — 10,804′ pinnacle of the San Jacinto Mountains.

More Great Peaks

Cucamonga Peak *(Trip 1.10)* — Wilderness experience with magnificent views over the Inland Empire.

Iron Mtn. *(Trip 1.13)* — Challenging climb up Big Bad Iron. Don't get stuckka by yucca.

Cornell Peak *(Trip 9.20)* — Beautiful forest approach to a classic pyramid with an airy summit block.

Antsell Rock *(Trip 10.1)* — Stimulating summit rocks on the rugged Desert Divide.

Murray Hill *(Trip 12.2)* — Surprisingly vigorous for a low summit, with cactus and panoramic views.

Best Oases

Lower Palm Canyon *(Trip 11.10)* — World's largest California fan palm oasis.

McCallum Grove *(Trip 14.1)* — Short hike to two oases and a reflecting pond.

Lost Palms Oasis *(Trip 15.25)* — Cross the fiery Joshua Tree badlands to a hidden oasis.

Best Spring Wildflowers

Los Santos Loop *(Trip 8.4)* — Some of the Inland Empire's best wildflowers in March and April of a wet year.

Black Rock Canyon Panorama Loop *(Trip 15.1)* — Blooming Joshua trees, Mojave yuccas, cacti, and wildflowers, along with terrific views.

Best Fall Colors

Aspen Grove *(Trip 5.15)*   A rare grove of quaking aspens along a creek on San Gorgonio's northeast flank. Visit in October.

Best Bird Watching

Sylvan Meadows *(Trip 8.2)*   Diverse birds and gorgeous Engelmann oaks at the Santa Rosa Ecological Preserve.

Big Morongo Preserve *(Trip 14.3)*   Birds and birdwatchers flock to this rare wetland between the San Bernardino Mountains and Joshua Tree.

Best Sunsets

Sunset Peak *(Trip 2.8)*   A steep scramble up a firebreak, then enjoy a picnic and the golden light on Mt. Baldy before descending the fire road.

Mt. Inspiration *(Trip 15.12)*   Brilliant sunsets over San Jacinto on a partly cloudy evening.

Best Mines

Lost Horse Mine *(Trip 15.11)*   Treachery in the desert. A well-preserved ten-stamp mill at a highly profitable gold mine.

Desert Queen Mine *(Trip 15.15)*   Cursed gold brought the owners more grief than fortune.

Best Full Moon Hikes

Museum Trail *(Trip 11.3)*   The desert becomes mysterious by moonlight.

Boy Scout Trail *(Trip 15.5)*   Eerie rock formations in the Wonderland of Rocks.

Best Geology Tours

Owl Canyon *(Trip 6.3)*   Wild colors, dry falls, and even a natural tunnel near the Barstow syncline.

Ladder and Painted Canyons *(Trip 13.1)*   Scale a slot canyon using a system of ladders, then descend the brilliant Painted Canyon.

Mitchell Caverns *(Trip 16.4)*   Rare and spectacular formations in the limestone caverns.

Best Hot Springs

Deep Creek Hot Springs *(Trip 3.1)* — Trek across the desert to the Inland Empire's favorite skinny dipping pool.

Best Hikes with Kids

Heart Rock *(Trip 3.3)* — Easy walking through the woods to a waterfall and pool with a remarkable rock formation.

Cougar Crest *(Trip 4.3)* — A perennial favorite walk in the woods above Big Bear Lake.

Big Falls *(Trip 5.4)* — Play along Mill Creek en route to the falls.

Vernal Pool *(Trip 8.5)* — Young naturalists can explore the pool from a boardwalk in March of a good rain year.

Kelso Dunes *(Trip 16.2)* — An unforgettable slide down the tallest of the booming dunes.

Hole-in-the-Rock *(Trip 16.3)* — A thrilling climb down a slot into Banshee Canyon, then loop back through areas of yuccas and cacti.

Best Strenuous Hikes

The Three T's *(Trip 1.11)* — A classic hike near Mt. Baldy over Timber, Telegraph, and Thunder.

Pines-to-Palms *(Trip 11.12)* — Follow Palm Canyon all the way from Highway 74 to the oasis near Palm Springs. Full spectrum of desert flora arranged by elevation.

Art Smith Trail *(Trip 12.6)* — A gem of the Santa Rosa Mountains, with cacti, oases, and outlandish rocks. Descend the Hahn Buena Vista Trail for fantastic views of San Jacinto.

Boo Hoff Loop *(Trip 12.10)* — Follow an ancient Indian footpath on the slopes of Martinez Mtn. with views of the Salton Sea, and descend a huge dry waterfall in Lost Canyon.

Wonderland Traverse *(Trip 15.7)* — Can you find your way through the maze-like Wonderland of Rocks? Rock-hopping on huge boulders, and a visit to a hidden "fortress."

Best Monster Hikes

Nine Baldy Peaks *(Trip 1.12)* — All the major summits around Baldy. The toughest adventure in this book.

San Antonio Ridge *(Trip 1.14)*   Cross-country romp from Iron Mtn. to Baldy along a truly gnarly ridge.

San Gorgonio Nine Peaks Challenge *(Trip 5.18)*   Grand traverse of the San Bernardino Ridge.

Nine Peaks of the Desert Divide *(Trip 10.7)*   Awesome scenery along the Pacific Crest Trail's most rugged stretch south of the Sierra Nevada.

Cactus-to-Clouds *(Trip 11.4)*   Palm Springs to San Jacinto. A Southern California classic, and North America's biggest continuous ascent by trail.

Rabbit Peak *(Trip 12.16)*   Only 6640', but the most strenuous mountain in Southern California. Amazing cacti and agaves.

Three Saints *(Trips 1.1, 5.1, and 9.21)*   San Jacinto, San Gorgonio, and San Antonio (Mt. Baldy), in 24 hours or bust!

Agency Contact Information

Forest Service

Arrowhead Ranger Station   (909) 382-2782
www.fs.fed.us/r5/sanbernardino/contact/skyforest.shtml
28104 Highway 18
P.O. Box 350
Skyforest, CA 92385
Mon–Sat 8–5

Big Bear Discovery Center   (909) 382-2790
www.fs.fed.us/r5/sanbernardino/contact/fawnskin.shtml
41397 North Shore Dr. (Highway 38)
P.O. Box 290
Fawnskin, CA 92333
Daily 8:30–4:30

Big Pines Information Center   (760) 249-3504
Angeles Crest Highway (Highway 2)
Wrightwood CA 92397
Fri–Sun 8:30–4:00

Cajon/Lytle Creek Ranger Station   (909) 382-2850
www.fs.fed.us/r5/sanbernardino/contact/lytlecreek.shtml
1209 Lytle Creek Rd.
Lytle Creek, CA 92358
Daily 8–4:30

Mill Creek/San Gorgonio Ranger Station   (909) 382-2881
www.fs.fed.us/r5/sanbernardino/contact/millcreek.shtml
34701 Mill Creek Rd. (corner of Highway 38 and Bryant)
Mentone, CA 92359
Thu–Mon 8–4:30 (closed Tue–Wed)
Wilderness & Camping Permits: www.sgwa.org/permit.htm

Mt. Baldy Visitor Center   (909) 982-2829
Mt. Baldy Road
Mt. Baldy, CA 91759
Daily 8–4:30

San Gabriel River Ranger District   (626) 335-1251
110 N. Wabash Ave.
Glendora, CA 91741
Mon–Fri 8–4:30

Idyllwild Ranger Station   (909) 382-2921

                                                            FAX: (951) 659-2107

www.fs.fed.us/r5/sanbernardino/contact/sanjacinto.shtml

54270 Pine Crest (corner of Highway 243 and Pine Crest)

P.O. Box 518

Idyllwild, CA 92549

Mon–Fri 8–12, 1–3:30; Sat–Sun 8–4:30

Wilderness & Camping Permits: www.fsva.org/pdf/Wilderness Permit App MSJW.pdf

Santa Rosa and San Jacinto Mountains National Monument

Visitor Center   (760) 862-9984

(Jointly administered by the Bureau of Land Management and the Forest Service)

www.fs.fed.us/r5/sanbernardino/contact/sanrosa.shtml

51500 Highway 74

Palm Springs, CA 92260

Daily 9–4

National Park Service

Joshua Tree National Park   (760) 367-5500

www.nps.gov/jotr

74485 National Park Dr.

Twentynine Palms, CA 92277

Oasis Visitor Center

Utah Trail & National Park Drive in Twentynine Palms

Daily 8–5

Joshua Tree Visitor Center

Park Blvd. one block south of Highway 62 in Joshua Tree

Daily 8–5

Cottonwood Visitor Center

Eight miles north of Interstate 10 at Cottonwood Spring

Daily 9–3

Mojave National Preserve

www.nps.gov/moja

Barstow Headquarters   (760) 252-6100

2701 Barstow Rd. (south of Interstate 15)

Mon–Fri 8–4:30

Kelso Depot Visitor Center   (760) 252-6108

Kelso (on Kelbaker Road between Interstates 15 and 40)

Daily 9–5

BLM

Barstow Field Office (760) 252-6000
2601 Barstow Rd.
Barstow, CA 92311

Palm Springs South Coast Field Office (760) 251-4800
690 W. Garnet Ave.
P.O. Box 581260
North Palm Springs, CA 92258-1260

County Parks

Los Angeles Department of Parks and Recreation
Frank G. Bonelli Regional Park (909) 599-8411
Marshall Canyon Regional Park (909) 593-3036

Riverside County Regional Park and Open-Space District (800) 234-7275

San Bernardino County Regional Parks District (909) 387-2757

San Bernardino Special Districts (909) 387-6076

California State Parks

California Citrus State Historic Park (951) 780-6222

Lake Perris State Recreation Area (951) 940-5600

Mt. San Jacinto State Park (951) 659-2607
P.O Box 308
25905 Highway 243
Idyllwild, CA 92549
Wilderness & Camping Permits: www.parks.ca.gov/pages/636/files/dpr409.pdf

Providence Mountains State Recreation Area (760) 928-2586

Other

Big Morongo Canyon Preserve (760) 363-7190

City of Claremont Human Services Department (909) 399-5490

City of Riverside Parks & Recreation Department (951) 826-2000

Coachella Valley Preserve (760) 343-1234

Crafton Hills Open Space Conservancy
P.O. Box 1475
Yucaipa, CA 92399

Appendixes

Herman Garner Biological Preserve
Pomona College Biology Department   (909) 607-2993

Indian Canyons Trading Post   (760) 323-6018
www.theindiancanyons.com
South end of Palm Canyon Dr. near Palm Springs

The Living Desert   (760) 346-5694
www.livingdesert.org

Rim of the World Interpretive Association
www.heapspeakarboretum.com
P.O. Box 1958
Lake Arrowhead, CA 92352

Santa Rosa Plateau Ecological Reserve   (951) 677-6951

The Wildlands Conservancy

    Oak Glen Headquarters   (909) 797-8507
    Whitewater Preserve   (760) 325-7222
    Desert Field Office (Mission Creek & Pipes Canyon)   (760) 369-7105

Activity Groups

Hiking with an organized group is a great way to visit new places, learn new skills, and make new friends. Southern California has a variety of local and regional hiking groups. Some of the groups include:

Sierra Club

The Angeles Chapter of the Sierra Club organizes over 4000 outings of all sorts each year in Southern California. Most are open to non-members. For more information, visit angeles.sierraclub.org or join the club to receive the Schedule of Activities published three times a year.

Coachella Valley Hiking Club

The CVHC is the largest hiking group in the California desert, offering over 150 hikes a year in the desert and surrounding mountains. Non-members are invited. For more information, visit www.cvhikingclub.net.

Desert Trails Hiking Club

Desert Trails organizes hikes from October–June around the Coachella Valley and nearby mountains. Non-members are welcome but are charged a $5 guest fee. www.deserttrailshiking.com

Outdoors Club

A web-based club organized by volunteers leading outdoor activities of many types. First three activities are free for non-members. www.outdoorsclub.org

The Forest Service and Bureau of Land Management are chronically underfunded and have few staff to patrol or maintain the trails. Much of the trail work is done by volunteer groups, such as the ones listed below. Joining one of these groups is a good way to spend time outside and meet other hikers as well as to enjoy the satisfaction of caring for the trails.

San Gabriel Mountains Trailbuilders	www.sgmtrailbuilders.org
San Gorgonio Wilderness Association	www.sgwa.org
Forest Service Volunteer Association (San Jacinto District)	www.fsva.org
Friends of the Desert Mountains	www.desertmountains.org

There are also hikes organized from time to time by many managing agencies such as the Forest Service. Many of these trips include expert commentary by naturalists. Check with the ranger stations or visitor centers for more information.

References

Hiking

Ferranti, Philip, with Hank Koenig. *140 Great Hikes In and Near Palm Springs*. Westcliffe Publishers, 2007.

Furbush, Patty. *On Foot in Joshua Tree National Park*. 5th Edition. Moose: M.I. Adventure Publishers, 2005.

McKinney, John. *California's Desert Parks: A Day Hiker's Guide*. 1st Edition. Berkeley: Wilderness Press, 2006.

Robinson, John, with David Money Harris. *San Bernardino Mountain Trails: 100 Hikes in Southern California*. 6th Edition. Berkeley: Wilderness Press, 2006.

Schad, Jerry. *Afoot and Afield in Los Angeles County*. 2nd Edition. Berkeley: Wilderness Press, 2000.

Backcountry Roads

Massey, Peter. *Backcountry Adventures Southern California: The Ultimate Guide to the Backcountry for Anyone With a Sport Utility Vehicle*. Castle Rock: Adler Publishing Company, 2006.

Nature

Croissant, Ann, and Gerald Croissant, with Shirly Debraal. *Wildflowers of the San Gabriel Mountains*. Las Vegas: Stephens Press, 2007.

Hickman, James C. *The Jepson Manual: Higher Plants of California*. Berkeley: University of California Press, 1993.

Ingram, Stephen. *Cacti, Agaves, and Yuccas of California and Nevada*. Los Olivos: Cachuma Press, 2008.

Knute, Adrienne. *Plants of the East Mojave*. Rev. Edition. Barstow: Mojave River Valley Museum, 2003.

Lanner, Ronald M. *Conifers of California*. Los Olivos: Cachuma Press, 1999.

Munz, Philip A. *Introduction to California Desert Wildflowers*. Berkeley: University of California Press, 2004.

Pavlik, Bruce M., Pamela Muick, and Sharon Johnson. *Oaks of California*. Los Olivos: Cachuma Press, 1993.

Quinn, Ronald D., and Sterling C. Keeley, with Marianne D. Wallace. *Introduction to California Chaparral*. Berkeley: University of California Press, 2006.

Trent, D.D., and Richard W. Hazlett. *Joshua Tree National Park Geology*. Joshua Tree: Joshua Tree National Park Association, 2002.

Historical

Olander, Ann, and Farley Olander. *Call Of The Mountains: The Beauty and Legacy of Southern California's San Jacinto, San Bernardino and San Gabriel Mountains.* Las Vegas: Stephens Press, 2005.

Robinson, John. *The San Bernardinos: The Mountain Country From Cajon Pass to Oak Glen, Two Centuries of Changing Use.* Arcadia: Big Santa Anita Historical Society, 2001.

Robinson, John. *San Gabriels: Southern California Mountain Country.* San Marino: Golden West Books, 1977.

Robinson, John. *San Gorgonio: A Wilderness Preserved.* San Gorgonio: San Gorgonio Volunteer Association, 1991.

Robinson, John. *The San Jacintos.* Arcadia: Big Santa Anita Historical Society, 1993.

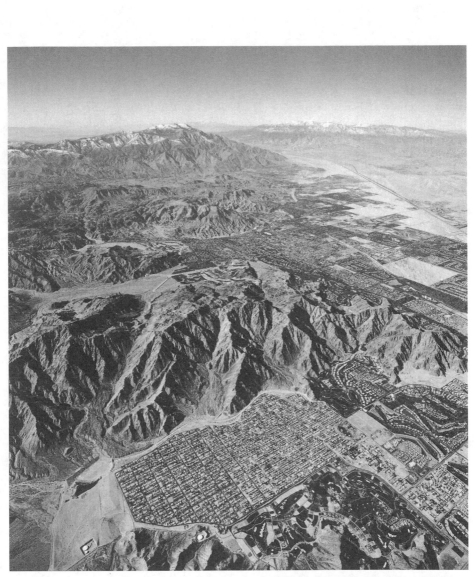

Aerial view of the Coachella Valley, with San Jacinto, San Antonio, and San Gorgonio on the skyline

Index

About the Authors

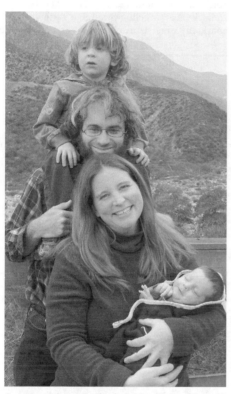

From top to bottom: Abraham, David, Jennifer and Samuel Money Harris

photo by Daniel Harris

David grew up rambling about the Desolation Wilderness as a toddler in his father's pack and later roamed the High Sierra as a Boy Scout. As a Sierra Club trip leader, he organized mountaineering trips throughout the Sierra Nevada. For the past decade, he has explored the mountains and deserts of Southern California. David teaches Engineering at Harvey Mudd College. He is the co-author of the 6th edition of *San Bernardino Mountain Trails.*

Jennifer teaches English composition and studies Early Modern English Literature. She is also interested in preserving the oral histories and languages of indigenous South American peoples.

David and Jennifer Money Harris live in Upland, CA with their two sons. Since the birth of their first son, David and Jennifer have discovered the joy of dayhiking with children.

Other Southern California Books from Wilderness Press

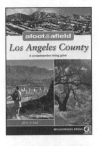

Afoot & Afield Los Angeles County

Covering all the best L.A. adventures, from strolling along at Malibu Lagoon State Beach to trekking up a mountain on Catalina Island. The 200 trips explore the City of Angels' own backyard, traveling through a variety of climate zones and revealing a remarkably diverse array of plant and animal life.

ISBN 978-0-89997-499-6

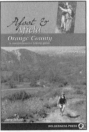

Afoot & Afield Orange County

In 87 hikes in the parks, preserves, designated open spaces, and public lands surrounding Orange County's densely populated coastal plain, this book provides fresh inspiration for trips along the coast from Huntington Beach to San Clemente, in the rugged Santa Ana Mountains, and through the foothills from Anaheim to the Santa Rosa Plateau Ecological Reserve.

ISBN 978-0-89997-397-5

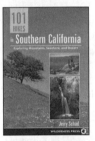

101 Hikes in Southern California

The book that proves there's more to SoCal than theme parks and strip malls. From the San Gabriel Mountains to the Anza-Borrego Desert and everywhere in between, this guide offers an incredible selection of exciting trips covering scores of hidden places just beyond the urban horizon.

ISBN 978-0-89997-351-7

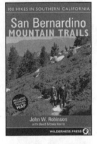

San Bernardino Mountain Trails

The classic guide to three mountain ranges in Southern California: the San Bernardinos, the San Jacintos, and the Santa Rosas. Covers 100 of the best hikes in these mountains; includes a separate foldout sheet map.

ISBN 978-0-89997-409-5

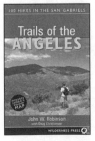

Trails of the Angeles

The authoritative volume to hiking in the San Gabriel Mountains includes 100 classic trips in the Angeles National Forest. The hikes range from one-hour strolls to challenging two-day backcountry trips. Comes with a separate foldout sheet map.

ISBN 978-0-89997-377-7

For ordering information, contact your local bookseller or Wilderness Press, www.wildernesspress.com